Breast Cancer

SOURCEBOOK

SIXTH EDITION

Breast Cancer
SOURCEBOOK

SIXTH EDITION

Basic Consumer Health Information about the Prevalence, Risk Factors, and Symptoms of Breast Cancer, Including Ductal and Lobular Carcinoma *in Situ*, Invasive Carcinoma, Paget Disease, Triple-Negative Breast Cancer, and Breast Cancer in Men and Pregnant Women

Along with Facts about Benign Breast Changes, Breast-Cancer Screening and Diagnostic Tests, Treatments Such as Surgery, Radiation Therapy, Chemotherapy, and Hormonal and Biologic Therapies, Tips on Managing Treatment Side Effects and Complications, a Glossary of Terms, and a Directory of Resources for Additional Help and Information

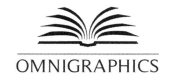

OMNIGRAPHICS

615 Griswold, Ste. 901, Detroit, MI 48226

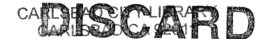

Bibliographic Note
Because this page cannot legibly accommodate all the copyright notices, the Bibliographic Note portion of the Preface constitutes an extension of the copyright notice.

* * *

OMNIGRAPHICS
Angela L. Williams, *Managing Editor*

* * *

Copyright © 2019 Omnigraphics
ISBN 978-0-7808-1687-9
E-ISBN 978-0-7808-1688-6

Library of Congress Cataloging-in-Publication Data

Names: Omnigraphics, Inc., issuing body.

Title: Breast cancer sourcebook: basic consumer health information about the prevalence, risk factors, and symptoms of breast cancer, including ductal and lobular carcinoma in situ, invasive carcinoma, inflammatory breast cancer, and breast cancer in men and pregnant women; along with facts about benign breast changes, breast cancer screening and diagnostic tests, treatments such as surgery, radiation therapy, chemotherapy, and hormonal and biologic therapies, tips on managing treatment side effects and complications, a glossary of terms, and a directory of resources for additional help and information / Angela Williams, managing editor.

Description: Sixth edition. | Detroit, MI: Omnigraphics, [2019] | Series: Health reference series | Includes bibliographical references and index.

Identifiers: LCCN 2018057792 (print) | LCCN 2018058663 (ebook) | ISBN 9780780816886 (ebook) | ISBN 9780780816879 (print)

Subjects: LCSH: Breast--Cancer--Popular works.

Classification: LCC RC280.B8 (ebook) | LCC RC280.B8 B6887 2019 (print) | DDC 616.99/449--dc23

LC record available at https://lccn.loc.gov/2018057792

JUN 2 7 2019

Table of Contents

Part II: Types of Breast Cancer

Part III: Risk Factors, Symptoms, and Prevention of Breast Cancer

Part IV: Screening, Diagnosis, and Stages of Breast Cancer

ix

Part VI: Managing Side Effects and Complications of Breast-Cancer Treatment

Part VII: Living with Breast Cancer

Part VIII: Clinical Trials and Breast-Cancer Research

Part IX: Additional Help and Information

Preface

About This Book

Breast cancer is one of the most commonly diagnosed cancers in women, and it is estimated that approximately 12.4 percent of women in the United States will be diagnosed with breast cancer at some point during their lifetime. Although breast cancer still claims the lives of nearly 41,000 women annually, there has been progress in the battle against it. Thanks to treatment advances, earlier detection, screening techniques, and increased awareness of symptoms, the number of deaths attributable to breast cancer each year has declined since 1990. Furthermore, according to a recent National Cancer Institute (NCI) report, in 2015, there were more than 3.4 million breast-cancer survivors living in the United States.

Breast Cancer Sourcebook, Sixth Edition provides updated information about breast cancer and its causes, risk factors, diagnosis, and treatment. Readers will learn about the types of breast cancer, including ductal carcinoma *in situ*, lobular carcinoma *in situ*, invasive carcinoma, and inflammatory breast cancer, as well as common breast-cancer treatment complications such as pain, fatigue, lymphedema, hair loss, and sexuality and fertility issues. Information on preventive therapies, nutrition and exercise recommendations, and tips on living with breast cancer are also included, along with a glossary of related terms and a directory of organizations that offer additional information to breast-cancer patients and their families.

How to Use This Book

This book is divided into parts and chapters. Parts focus on broad areas of interest. Chapters are devoted to single topics within a part.

Part I: Introduction to Breast Cancer identifies the parts of the breasts and lymphatic system, discusses common changes in the breast that pose no threat to health, and offers general information about breast cancer in women and men. It also offers statistical information on the prevalence of breast cancer in the United States.

Part II: Types of Breast Cancer identifies the most common types of breast cancer, including ductal carcinoma *in situ* (DCIS), lobular carcinoma *in situ* (LCIS), invasive carcinoma of the breast, inflammatory breast cancer, Paget disease of the nipple, triple-negative breast cancer, and other rare types of breast cancers.

Part III: Risk Factors, Symptoms, and Prevention of Breast Cancer provides information about hereditary and nonhereditary factors that increase the risk of developing breast cancer, including age, family health history, exposure to radiation, alcohol consumption, use of hormone replacement therapy, reproductive risk factors, and obesity. Genetic counseling for breast-cancer risk is discussed, along with information about preventing breast cancer in people who are susceptible.

Part IV: Screening, Diagnosis, and Stages of Breast Cancer identifies tests and procedures used to screen, diagnose, and stage breast cancer, including breast examinations, mammograms, and breast biopsies. It also provides information on how to understand laboratory tests and breast pathology reports.

Part V: Breast-Cancer Treatments discusses how to find a treatment facility or doctor and offers information about considerations to make before undergoing breast-cancer treatment. Surgical treatments for breast cancer, such as mastectomy, lumpectomy, and breast reconstruction, are discussed, and facts about radiation therapy, chemotherapy, hormone therapy, biologic therapies, and complementary and alternative medicine treatments for breast cancer are provided. The part also includes a discussion of the treatment of breast cancer in pregnant women, men, and patients with recurrent breast cancer.

Part VI: Managing Side Effects and Complications of Breast-Cancer Treatment Disorders describes anemia, delirium, fatigue, hot flashes and night sweats, infection, lymphedema, pain, sexual and fertility issues, and hair loss associated with breast-cancer treatment. Information about complementary and alternative therapies that may relieve physical discomfort or emotional anxiety is also provided.

Part VII: Living with Breast Cancer discusses strategies for coping with the difficult emotions produced by a breast-cancer diagnosis and offers information about talking to family members and friends about cancer. In addition, the part identifies nutrition and exercise recommendations after cancer treatment, tips for dealing with cancer in the workplace, information and suggestions for caregivers of breast-cancer patients.

Part VIII: Clinical Trials and Breast-Cancer Research provides information on current clinical trials related to breast cancer and latest breast-cancer researches.

Part IX: Additional Help and Information provides a glossary of important terms related to breast cancer and directory of organizations that offer financial assistance to people with breast cancer and a directory that offers other information about breast cancer.

Bibliographic Note

This volume contains documents and excerpts from publications issued by the following U.S. government agencies: Centers for Disease Control and Prevention (CDC); Centers for Medicare & Medicaid Services (CMS); Genetic and Rare Diseases Information Center (GARD); National Cancer Institute (NCI); National Center for Biotechnology Information (NCBI); National Center for Complementary and Integrative Health (NCCIH); National Human Genome Research Institute (NHGRI); National Institute of Environmental Health Sciences (NIEHS); National Institutes of Health (NIH); NIH Osteoporosis and Related Bone Diseases—National Resource Center (NIH ORBD—NRC); Office on Women's Health (OWH); U.S. Department of Labor (DOL); U.S. Department of Veterans Affairs (VA); and U.S. Food and Drug Administration (FDA).

It may also contain original material produced by Omnigraphics and reviewed by medical consultants.

About the Health Reference Series

The *Health Reference Series* is designed to provide basic medical information for patients, families, caregivers, and the general public.

Each volume takes a particular topic and provides comprehensive coverage. This is especially important for people who may be dealing with a newly diagnosed disease or a chronic disorder in themselves or in a family member. People looking for preventive guidance, information about disease warning signs, medical statistics, and risk factors for health problems will also find answers to their questions in the *Health Reference Series*. The *Series*, however, is not intended to serve as a tool for diagnosing illness, in prescribing treatments, or as a substitute for the physician/patient relationship. All people concerned about medical symptoms or the possibility of disease are encouraged to seek professional care from an appropriate healthcare provider.

A Note about Spelling and Style

Health Reference Series editors use *Stedman's Medical Dictionary* as an authority for questions related to the spelling of medical terms and the *Chicago Manual of Style* for questions related to grammatical structures, punctuation, and other editorial concerns. Consistent adherence is not always possible, however, because the individual volumes within the *Series* include many documents from a wide variety of different producers, and the editor's primary goal is to present material from each source as accurately as is possible. This sometimes means that information in different chapters or sections may follow other guidelines and alternate spelling authorities. For example, occasionally a copyright holder may require that eponymous terms be shown in possessive forms (Crohn's disease vs. Crohn disease) or that British spelling norms be retained (leukaemia vs. leukemia).

Medical Review

Omnigraphics contracts with a team of qualified, senior medical professionals who serve as medical consultants for the *Health Reference Series*. As necessary, medical consultants review reprinted and originally written material for currency and accuracy. Citations including the phrase "Reviewed (month, year)" indicate material reviewed by this team. Medical consultation services are provided to the *Health Reference Series* editors by:

Dr. Vijayalakshmi, MBBS, DGO, MD
Dr. Senthil Selvan, MBBS, DCH, MD
Dr. K. Sivanandham, MBBS, DCH, MS (Research), PhD

Our Advisory Board

We would like to thank the following board members for providing initial guidance on the development of this series:

- Dr. Lynda Baker, Associate Professor of Library and Information Science, Wayne State University, Detroit, MI

- Nancy Bulgarelli, William Beaumont Hospital Library, Royal Oak, MI

- Karen Imarisio, Bloomfield Township Public Library, Bloomfield Township, MI

- Karen Morgan, Mardigian Library, University of Michigan-Dearborn, Dearborn, MI

- Rosemary Orlando, St. Clair Shores Public Library, St. Clair Shores, MI

Health Reference Series *Update Policy*

The inaugural book in the *Health Reference Series* was the first edition of *Cancer Sourcebook* published in 1989. Since then, the *Series* has been enthusiastically received by librarians and in the medical community. In order to maintain the standard of providing high-quality health information for the layperson the editorial staff at Omnigraphics felt it was necessary to implement a policy of updating volumes when warranted.

Medical researchers have been making tremendous strides, and it is the purpose of the *Health Reference Series* to stay current with the most recent advances. Each decision to update a volume is made on an individual basis. Some of the considerations include how much new information is available and the feedback we receive from people who use the books. If there is a topic you would like to see added to the update list, or an area of medical concern you feel has not been adequately addressed, please write to:

Managing Editor
Health Reference Series
Omnigraphics
615 Griswold, Ste. 901
Detroit, MI 48226

Part One

Introduction to Breast Cancer

Chapter 1

Breast and Lymphatic System Basics

Breast Anatomy

The breasts of an adult woman are milk-producing, tear-shaped glands. They are supported by and attached to the front of the chest wall on either side of the breast bone or sternum by ligaments. They rest on the major chest muscle, the pectoralis major.

The breast has no muscle tissue. A layer of fat surrounds the glands and extends throughout the breast.

The breast is responsive to a complex interplay of hormones that cause the tissue to develop, enlarge and produce milk. The three major hormones affecting the breast are estrogen, progesterone, and prolactin, which cause glandular tissue in the breast and the uterus to change during the menstrual cycle.

Each breast contains 15 to 20 lobes arranged in a circular fashion. The fat (subcutaneous adipose tissue) that covers the lobes gives the breast its size and shape. Each lobe is comprised of many lobules, at the end of which are tiny bulb-like glands, or sacs, where milk is produced in response to hormonal signals.

This chapter includes text excerpted from "Breast Anatomy," Surveillance, Epidemiology and End Results Program (SEER), National Cancer Institute (NCI), March 1, 2003. Reviewed February 2019.

Ducts connect the lobes, lobules, and glands in nursing mothers. These ducts deliver milk to openings in the nipple. The areola is the darker-pigmented area around the nipple.

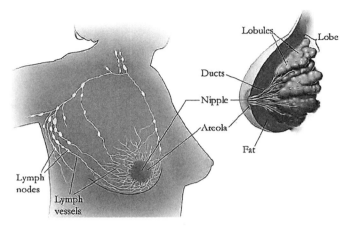

Figure 1.1. *Anatomy of Breast*

*Mammary Glands**

Functionally, the mammary glands produce milk; structurally, they are modified-sweat glands. Mammary glands, which are located in the breast overlying the pectoralis major muscles, are present in both sexes, but usually are functional only in the female.

Externally, each breast has a raised nipple, which is surrounded by a circular pigmented area called the "areola." The nipples are sensitive to touch, due to the fact that they contain smooth muscle that contracts and causes them to become erect in response to stimulation.

Internally, the adult-female breast contains 15 to 20 lobes of glandular tissue that radiate around the nipple. The lobes are separated by connective tissue and adipose. The connective tissue helps support the breast. Some bands of connective tissue, called "suspensory (Cooper's) ligaments," extend through the breast from the skin to the underlying muscles. The amount and distribution of the adipose tissue determine the size and shape of the breast. Each lobe consists of lobules that contain the glandular units. A lactiferous duct collects the milk from the lobules within each lobe and carries it to the nipple. Just before

* Excerpted from "Mammary Glands," Surveillance, Epidemiology and End Results Program (SEER), National Cancer Institute (NCI), July 1, 2002. Reviewed February 2019.

the nipple, the lactiferous duct enlarges to form a lactiferous sinus (ampulla), which serves as a reservoir for milk. After the sinus, the duct again narrows and each duct opens independently on the surface of the nipple.

Mammary-gland function is regulated by hormones. At puberty, increasing levels of estrogen stimulate the development of glandular tissue in the female breast. Estrogen also causes the breast to increase in size through the accumulation of adipose tissue. Progesterone stimulates the development of the duct system. During pregnancy, these hormones enhance the further development of the mammary glands. Prolactin from the anterior pituitary stimulates the production of milk within the glandular tissue, and oxytocin causes the ejection of milk from the glands.

Regional Lymph Nodes

Blood and lymph vessels form a network throughout each breast. Breast tissue is drained by lymphatic vessels that lead to axillary nodes (which lie in the axilla) and internal mammary nodes (which lie along each side of the breast bone). When breast cancer spreads, it is frequently to these nodes.

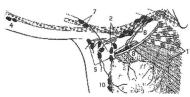

2. Axillary lymphatic plexus
4. Cubital lymph nodes *
5. Superficial axillary (low axillary)
6. Deep axillary lymph nodes
7. Brachial axillary lymph nodes
8. Interpectoral axillary lymph nodes (Rotter nodes)
10. Paramammary or intramammary lymph nodes
11. Parasternal lymph nodes (internal mammary nodes)

Figure 1.2. *Regional Lymph Nodes*

Chapter 2

Understanding Breast Changes

Chapter Contents

Section 2.1

Noncancerous Breast Changes

This section contains text excerpted from the following sources: Text in this section begins with excerpts from "Breast Changes and Conditions," National Cancer Institute (NCI), October 23, 2018; Text under the heading "Details That You Should Share with Your Healthcare Provider" is excerpted from "Understanding Breast Changes," National Cancer Institute (NCI), February 2014. Reviewed February 2019.

Some breast changes can be felt by a woman or her healthcare provider, but most can be detected only during an imaging procedure such as a mammogram, magnetic resonance imaging (MRI), or ultrasound. Whether a breast change was found by your doctor or you noticed a change, it's important to follow up with your doctor to have the change checked and properly diagnosed.

Breast Changes of Concern

Check with your healthcare provider if your breast looks or feels different, or if you notice one of these symptoms:

- **Lump or firm feeling in your breast or under your arm**. Lumps come in different shapes and sizes. Normal breast tissue can sometimes feel lumpy. Doing breast self-exams can help you learn how your breasts normally feel and make it easier to notice and find any changes, but they are not a substitute for mammograms.

- **Nipple changes or discharge**. Nipple discharge may be different colors or textures. It can be caused by birth control pills, some medicines, and infections. But because it can also be a sign of cancer, it should always be checked.

- **Skin that is itchy, red, scaled, dimpled, or puckered**

Breast Changes during Your Lifetime That Are Not Cancer

Most women have changes in the breasts at different times during their lifetime.

- **Before or during your menstrual periods**, your breasts may feel swollen, tender, or painful. You may also feel one or more lumps during this time because of extra fluid in your breasts. Your healthcare provider may have you come back for a return visit at a different time in your menstrual cycle to see if the lump has changed.

- **During pregnancy**, your breasts may feel lumpy. This is usually because the glands that produce milk are increasing in number and getting larger. While breastfeeding, you may get a condition called "mastitis." This happens when a milk duct becomes blocked. Mastitis causes the breast to look red and feel lumpy, warm, and tender. It may be caused by an infection and it is often treated with antibiotics. Sometimes the duct may need to be drained.

- **As you approach menopause**, your hormone levels change. This can make your breasts feel tender, even when you are not having your menstrual period. Your breasts may also feel lumpier than they did before.

- **If you are taking hormones** (such as menopausal hormone therapy (MHT), birth control pills, or injections) your breasts may become denser. This can make a mammogram harder to interpret. Be sure to let your healthcare provider know if you are taking hormones.

- **After menopause**, your hormone levels drop. You may stop having any lumps, pain, or nipple discharge that you used to have.

Details That You Should Share with Your Healthcare Provider

It can help to prepare before you meet with your healthcare provider. Use the list below. Write down the breast changes you notice, as well as your personal medical history and your family medical history before your visit.

Tell your healthcare provider about breast changes or problems:

- The breast changes or problems that you have noticed.

- What the breast change looks or feels like? For example: Is the lump hard or soft? Does your breast feel tender or swollen? How big is the lump? What color is the nipple discharge? and so on.

- The place of breast change. For example: What part of the breast feels different? Do both breasts feel different or only one breast?

- When did you first notice the breast change?

- Since then, this is the change you have noticed. For example: Has it stayed the same or gotten worse?

Share your personal medical history:

- The breast problems you had in the past

- The breast exams and tests that you have had

- The date of your last mammogram

- The date on which your last menstrual period began

- The list of medicines or herbs that you take

- Your present status such as whether you have breast implants, or in case you are pregnant or breastfeeding, or if you have had this type of cancer before

Share your family medical history:

- Details of breast problems or diseases that your family members had

- Details of the family members who had breast cancer and the age when they were diagnosed with breast cancer

Section 2.2

Breast Changes That May Become Cancer

This section includes text excerpted from "Understanding Breast Changes," National Cancer Institute (NCI), February 2014. Reviewed February 2019.

Ductal carcinoma *in situ* (DCIS): DCIS is a condition in which abnormal cells are found in the lining of a breast duct. These cells have not spread outside the duct to the breast tissue. This is why it is called "*in situ*," which is a Latin term that means "in place." You may also hear DCIS called Stage 0 breast carcinoma *in situ* or noninvasive cancer.

Since it's not possible to determine which cases of DCIS will become invasive breast cancer, it's important to get treatment for DCIS. Talk with a doctor who specializes in breast health to learn more. Treatment for DCIS is based on how much of the breast is affected, where DCIS is in the breast, and its grade. Most women with DCIS are cured with proper treatment.

Treatment choices for DCIS include:

- **Lumpectomy**. This is a type of **breast-conserving surgery** or **breast-sparing surgery**. It is usually followed by **radiation therapy.**

- **Mastectomy**. This type of surgery is used to remove the breast or as much of the breast tissue as possible.

- **Tamoxifen**. This drug may also be taken to lower the chance that DCIS will come back, or to prevent invasive breast cancer.

- **Clinical trials**. Talk with your healthcare provider about whether a clinical trial is a good choice for you.

Breast Cancer

Breast cancer is a disease in which cancer cells form in the tissues of the breast. Breast-cancer cells:

- Grow and divide without control

- Invade nearby breast tissue

- May form a mass called a **tumor**

- May **metastasize**, or spread, to the lymph nodes or other parts of the body

- After breast cancer has been **diagnosed**, tests are done to find out the extent, or **stage**, of cancer. The stage is based on the size of the tumor and whether cancer has spread. Treatment depends on the stage of cancer.

Getting the Support You Need

It can be upsetting to notice a breast change, to get an abnormal test result, or to learn about a new condition or disease. But knowledge is power and we hope that this sourcebook answers some of your questions and calms some of your fears as you talk with your healthcare provider and get the follow-up care you need.

Many women choose to get extra help and support for themselves. It may help to think about people who have been there for you during challenging times in the past.

- Ask friends or loved ones for support. Take someone with you while you are learning about your testing and treatment choices.
- Ask your healthcare provider to:
  - Explain medical terms that are new or confusing
  - Share with you how other people have handled the types of feelings that you are having
  - Tell you about specialists that you can talk to learn more

Table 2.1. Breast Conditions and Follow-Up Care

Condition	Features	What Your Doctor May Recommend
Adenosis	• Small round lumps, lumpiness, or you may not feel anything at all • Enlarged breast lobules • If there is scar-like fibrous tissue, the condition is called sclerosing adenosis. It may be painful. • Some studies have found that women with sclerosing adenosis may have a slightly increased risk of breast cancer.	• A core biopsy or a surgical biopsy may be needed to make a diagnosis.
Atypical lobular hyperplasia (ALH)	• Abnormal cells in the breast lobules • ALH increases your risk of breast cancer.	Regular follow-up, such as: • Mammograms • Clinical breast exams Treatment, such as: • Tamoxifen (for all women) or raloxifene (for postmenopausal women)
Atypical ductal hyperplasia (ADH)	• Abnormal cells in the breast ducts • ADH increases your risk of breast cancer.	Regular follow-up, such as: • Mammograms • Clinical breast exams Treatment, such as: • Tamoxifen (for all women) or raloxifene (for postmenopausal women)

Table 2.1. Continued

Condition	Features	What Your Doctor May Recommend
Breast cancer	• Cancer cells found in the breast, with a biopsy • A lump in or near your breast or under your arm • Thick or firm tissue in or near your breast or under your arm • A change in the size or shape of your breast • A nipple that's turned inward (inverted) into the breast • Skin on your breast that is itchy, red, scaly, dimpled, or puckered • Nipple discharge that is not breast milk	Treatment depends on the extent or stage of cancer. Tests are done to find out if cancer has spread to other parts of your body. Treatment may include: • Surgery • Chemotherapy • Radiation therapy • Hormonal therapy • Biological therapy Clinical trials may be an option for you. Talk with your doctor to learn more.
Cysts	• Lumps filled with fluid • Often in both breasts • Maybe painful just before your menstrual period begins • Some cysts may be felt. Others are too small to be felt. • Most common in women 35–50 years old	• Cysts may be watched by your doctor over time, since they may go away on their own. • Ultrasound can show if the lump is solid or filled with fluid. • Fine needle aspiration may be used to remove fluid from the cyst.

Table 2.1. Continued

Condition	Features	What Your Doctor May Recommend
Ductal carcinoma *in situ* **(DCIS)**	• Abnormal cells in the lining of a breast duct • Unlike cancer cells that can spread, these abnormal cells have not spread outside the breast duct. • Maybe called noninvasive cancer or Stage 0 breast carcinoma *in situ*.	Treatment is needed because doctors don't know which cases of DCIS may become invasive breast cancer. Treatment choices include: • **Lumpectomy.** This is a type of breast-conserving surgery or breast-sparing surgery. It is usually followed by radiation therapy. • **Mastectomy.** Surgery to remove the breast. • **Tamoxifen.** This drug may be taken to lower the chance that DCIS will come back after treatment or prevent invasive breast cancer. • **Clinical trials.** Talk with your doctor about whether a clinical trial is a good choice for you.
Fat necrosis	• Round, firm lumps that usually don't hurt • May appear after an injury to the breast, surgery, or radiation therapy • Formed by damaged fatty tissue • Skin around the lump may look red, bruised, or dimpled • A benign (not cancer) breast condition	• A biopsy may be needed to diagnose and remove fat necrosis since it often looks like cancer. • Fat necrosis does not usually need treatment.

Table 2.1. Continued

Condition	Features	What Your Doctor May Recommend
Fibroadenoma	• Hard, round lumps that move around easily and usually don't hurt • Often found by the woman • Appear on a mammogram as smooth, round lumps with clearly defined edges • The most common benign breast tumors • Common in women under 30 years old • Most fibroadenomas do not increase your risk of breast cancer. However, complex fibroadenomas do slightly increase your risk.	• A biopsy may be needed to diagnose fibroadenoma. • A minimally invasive technique such as ultrasound-guided cryoablation or an excisional biopsy may be used to remove the lumps. • These growths may be watched by your doctor over time, since they may go away on their own.
Intraductal papilloma	• A wart-like growth inside the milk duct, usually close to the nipple • May cause pain and a lump • May cause clear, sticky, or bloody discharge • Most common in women 35–55 years old • Unlike single papillomas, multiple papillomas increase your risk of breast cancer.	• A biopsy may be needed to diagnose the growth and remove it.

Table 2.1. Continued

Condition	Features	What Your Doctor May Recommend

Lobular carcinoma *in situ* (LCIS)	• A condition in which abnormal cells are found in the breast lobules
	• LCIS increases your risk of breast cancer.
		Regular follow-up, such as:
		• Mammograms
		• Clinical breast exams
		• Treatment choices:
		  • Tamoxifen (for all women) or raloxifene (for postmenopausal women) may be taken.
		  • A small number of women with LCIS and high-risk factors for breast cancer may choose to have surgery.
		  • Clinical trials may be an option for you. Talk with your doctor to learn more.

Microcalcifications	• Calcium deposits in the breast that look like small white dots on a mammogram • Often caused by aging • Cannot be felt • Usually benign (not cancer) • Common in women over 50 years old	• Another mammogram may be needed to have a closer look at the area. • Treatment is usually not needed.
Microcalcifications	• Calcium deposits in the breast that look like tiny white specks on a mammogram • Not usually a sign of cancer. However, if found in an area of rapidly dividing cells or grouped together in a certain way, they may be a sign of DCIS or invasive breast cancer.	• Another mammogram or a biopsy may be needed to make a diagnosis.

Chapter 3

What You Need to Know about Breast Cancer

Cancer is a disease in which cells in the body grow out of control. Except for skin cancer, breast cancer is the most common cancer in women in the United States. Deaths from breast cancer have declined over time, but remains the second leading cause of cancer death among women overall and the leading cause of cancer death among Hispanic women.

Each year in the United States, about 237,000 cases of breast cancer are diagnosed in women and about 2,100 in men. About 41,000 women and 450 men in the United States die each year from breast cancer. Over the last decade, the risk of getting breast cancer has not changed for women overall, but the risk has increased for black women and Asian and Pacific Islander women. Black women have a higher risk of death from breast cancer than white women.

The risk of getting breast cancer goes up with age. In the United States, the average age when women are diagnosed with breast cancer is 61. Men who get breast cancer are diagnosed usually between 60- and 70-years old.

This chapter includes text excerpted from "Basic Information about Breast Cancer," Centers for Disease Control and Prevention (CDC), July 25, 2017.

What Is Breast Cancer?

Breast cancer is a disease in which cells in the breast grow out of control. There are different kinds of breast cancer. The kind of breast cancer depends on which cells in the breast turn into cancer.

Breast cancer can begin in different parts of the breast. A breast is made up of three main parts: lobules, ducts, and connective tissue. The lobules are the glands that produce milk. The ducts are tubes that carry milk to the nipple. The connective tissue (which consists of fibrous and fatty tissue) surrounds and holds everything together. Most breast cancers begin in the ducts or lobules.

Breast cancer can spread outside the breast through blood vessels and lymph vessels. When breast cancer spreads to other parts of the body, it is said to have metastasized.

Kinds of Breast Cancer

The most common kinds of breast cancer are:

- **Invasive ductal carcinoma (IDC).** The cancer cells grow outside the ducts into other parts of the breast tissue. Invasive-cancer cells can also spread, or metastasize, to other parts of the body.

- **Invasive lobular carcinoma (ILC).** Cancer cells spread from the lobules to the breast tissues that are close by. These invasive-cancer cells can also spread to other parts of the body.

There are several other less common kinds of breast cancer, such as Paget disease, external medullary, mucinous, and inflammatory breast cancer (IBC).

Ductal carcinoma *in situ* (DCIS) is a breast disease that may lead to breast cancer. The cancer cells are only in the lining of the ducts and have not spread to other tissues in the breast.

What Are the Symptoms of Breast Cancer?

Different people have different symptoms of breast cancer. Some people do not have any signs or symptoms at all.

Some warning signs of breast cancer include:

- New lump in the breast or underarm (armpit)

- Thickening or swelling of part of the breast

- Irritation or dimpling of breast skin

- Redness or flaky skin in the nipple area or the breast
- Pulling in of the nipple or pain in the nipple area
- Nipple discharge other than breast milk, including blood
- Any change in the size or the shape of the breast
- Pain in any area of the breast

Keep in mind that these symptoms can happen with other conditions that are not cancer.

If you have any signs or symptoms that worry you, be sure to see your doctor right away.

What Is a Normal Breast?

No breast is typical. What is normal for you may not be normal for another woman. Most women say their breasts feel lumpy or uneven. The way your breasts look and feel can be affected by getting your period, having children, losing or gaining weight, and taking certain medications. Breasts also tend to change as you age.

What Do Lumps in Your Breast Mean?

Many conditions can cause lumps in the breast, including cancer. But most breast lumps are caused by other medical conditions. The two most common causes of breast lumps are fibrocystic breast condition and cysts.

- **Fibrocystic condition** causes noncancerous changes in the breast that can make them lumpy, tender, and sore.
- **Cysts** are small fluid-filled sacs that can develop in the breast.

What Are the Risk Factors for Breast Cancer?

Studies have shown that your risk for breast cancer is due to a combination of factors. The main factors that influence your risk include being a woman and getting older. Most breast cancers are found in women who are 50 years old or older.

Some women will get breast cancer even without any other risk factors that they know of. Having a risk factor does not mean you will get the disease, and not all risk factors have the same effect. Most women have some risk factors, but most women do not get breast cancer. If you have breast-cancer risk factors, talk with your doctor about ways you can lower your risk and about screening for breast cancer.

21

Risk Factors You Cannot Change

Some of the risk factors you can change. Such as:

- **Getting older.** The risk of breast cancer increases with age; most breast cancers are diagnosed after age 50.

- **Genetic mutations.** Inherited changes (mutations) to certain genes, such as *BRCA1* and *BRCA2*. Women who have inherited these genetic changes are at higher risk of breast and ovarian cancer.

- **Reproductive history.** Early menstrual periods before age 12 and starting menopause after age 55 expose women to hormones longer, raising their risk of getting breast cancer.

- **Having dense breasts.** Dense breasts have more connective tissue than fatty tissue, which can sometimes make it hard to see tumors on a mammogram. Women with dense breasts are more likely to get breast cancer.

- **Personal history of breast cancer or certain noncancerous breast diseases.** Women who have had breast cancer are more likely to get breast cancer a second time. Some noncancerous breast diseases such as atypical hyperplasia or lobular carcinoma *in situ* are associated with a higher risk of getting breast cancer.

- **Family history of breast cancer.** A woman's risk for breast cancer is higher if she has a mother, sister, or daughter (first-degree relative) or multiple family members on either her mother's or father's side of the family who has had breast cancer. Having a first-degree male relative with breast cancer also raises a woman's risk.

- **Previous treatment using radiation therapy.** Women who had radiation therapy to the chest or breasts (such as for treatment of Hodgkin's lymphoma) before age 30 have a higher risk of getting breast cancer later in life.

- **Women who took the drug diethylstilbestrol (DES),** which was given to some pregnant women in the United States between 1940 and 1971 to prevent miscarriage, have a higher risk. Women whose mothers took DES while pregnant with them are also at risk.

Risk Factors You Can Change

The risk factors that you can change include:

- **Not being physically active.** Women who are not physically active have a higher risk of getting breast cancer.

- **Being overweight or obese after menopause.** Older women who are overweight or obese have a higher risk of getting breast cancer than those at a normal weight.

- **Taking hormones.** Some forms of hormone replacement therapy (HRT) (those that include both estrogen and progesterone) taken during menopause can raise risk for breast cancer when taken for more than five years. Certain oral contraceptives (OC) (birth control pills) also have been found to raise breast-cancer risk.

- **Reproductive history.** Having the first pregnancy after age 30, not breastfeeding, and never having a full-term pregnancy can raise breast-cancer risk.

- **Drinking alcohol.** Studies show that a woman's risk for breast cancer increases with the more alcohol she drinks.

Research suggests that other factors such as smoking, being exposed to chemicals that can cause cancer, and changes in other hormones due to night shift working also may increase breast-cancer risk.

Who Is at High Risk for Breast Cancer?

If you have a strong family history of breast cancer or inherited changes in your *BRCA1* and *BRCA2* genes, you may have a high risk of getting breast cancer. You may also have a high risk of ovarian cancer. Talk to your doctor about ways of reducing your risk, including any physical and emotional side effects:

- Medicines that block or decrease estrogen in your body

- Surgery to reduce your risk of breast cancer

- Mastectomy (removal of breast tissue)

- Salpingo-oophorectomy (removal of the ovaries and fallopian tubes)

It is important that you know your family history and talks to your doctor about how you can lower your risk.

23

What Can I Do to Reduce My Risk of Breast Cancer?

Many factors can influence your breast-cancer risk, and most women who develop breast cancer do not have any known risk factors or a history of the disease in their families. However, you can help lower your risk of breast cancer in the following ways—

- Keep a healthy weight.

- Exercise regularly (at least four hours a week).

- Get enough sleep.

- Don't drink alcohol, or limit alcoholic drinks to no more than one per day.

- Avoid exposure to chemicals that can cause cancer (carcinogens).

- Try to reduce your exposure to radiation during medical tests like mammograms, X-rays, CT scans, and PET scans.

- If you are taking, or have been told to take, hormone replacement therapy or oral contraceptives (birth control pills), ask your doctor about the risks and find out if it is right for you.

- Breastfeed your babies, if possible.

Although breast-cancer screening cannot prevent breast cancer, it can help find breast cancer early, when it is easier to treat. Talk to your doctor about which breast-cancer screening tests are right for you, and when you should have them.

If you have a family history of breast cancer or inherited changes in your *BRCA1* and *BRCA2* genes, you may have a higher breast-cancer risk. Talk to your doctor about these ways of reducing your risk—

- Antiestrogens or other medicines that block or decrease estrogen in your body.

- Surgery to reduce your risk of breast cancer—

- Prophylactic (preventive) mastectomy (removal of breast tissue).

- Prophylactic (preventive) salpingo-oophorectomy (removal of the ovaries and fallopian tubes).

It is important that you know your family history and talk to your doctor about screening and other ways you can lower your risk.

What Screening Tests Are There?

Breast-cancer screening means checking a woman's breasts for cancer before there are signs or symptoms of the disease. Three main tests are used to screen the breasts for cancer. Talk to your doctor about which tests are right for you, and when you should have them.

Mammogram

A mammogram is an X-ray of the breast. Mammograms are the best way to find breast cancer early when it is easier to treat and before it is big enough to feel or cause symptoms. Having regular mammograms can lower the risk of dying from breast cancer. The United States Preventive Services Task Force recommends that if you are 50 to 74 years old, be sure to have a screening mammogram every two years. If you are 40 to 49 years old, talk to your doctor about when to start and how often to get a screening mammogram.

Clinical Breast Exam

A *clinical breast exam* is an examination by a doctor or nurse, who uses his or her hands to feel for lumps or other changes.

Breast Self-Exam

A *breast self-exam* is when you check your own breasts for lumps, changes in size or shape of the breast, or any other changes in the breasts or underarm (armpit).

Which Tests to Choose

Having a clinical breast exam or a breast self-exam have not been found to decrease the risk of dying from breast cancer. At this time, the best way to find breast cancer is with a mammogram. If you choose to have clinical breast exams and to perform breast self-exams, be sure you also get mammograms regularly.

Where Can I Go to Get Screened?

Most likely, you can get screened for breast cancer at a clinic, hospital, or doctor's office. If you want to be screened for breast cancer, call your doctor's office. They can help you schedule an appointment. Most health insurance companies pay for the cost of breast-cancer screening tests.

What Is a Mammogram and When Should I Get One?

A *mammogram* is an X-ray picture of the breast. Doctors use a mammogram to look for early signs of breast cancer.

Regular mammograms are the best tests doctors have to find breast cancer early, sometimes up to three years before it can be felt. When their breast cancer is found early, many women go on to live long and healthy lives.

When Should I Get a Mammogram?

The United States Preventive Services Task Force recommends that women should have mammograms every two years from age 50 to 74 years. Talk to your health professional if you have any symptoms or changes in your breast, or if breast cancer runs in your family. He or she may recommend that you have mammograms before age 50 or more often than usual.

How Is a Mammogram Done?

You will stand in front of a special X-ray machine. A technologist will place your breast on a clear plastic plate. Another plate will firmly press your breast from above. The plates will flatten the breast, holding it still while the X-ray is being taken. You will feel some pressure. The other breast will be X-rayed in the same way. The steps are then repeated to make a side view of each breast. You will then wait while the technologist checks the four X-rays to make sure the pictures do not need to be re-done. Keep in mind that the technologist cannot tell you the results of your mammogram.

What Does Having a Mammogram Feel Like?

Having a mammogram is uncomfortable for most women. Some women find it painful. A mammogram takes only a few moments, though, and the discomfort is over soon. What you feel depends on the skill of the technologist, the size of your breasts, and how much they need to be pressed. Your breasts may be more sensitive if you are about to get or have your period. A doctor with special training, called a radiologist, will read the mammogram. He or she will look at the X-ray for early signs of breast cancer or other problems.

When Will I Get the Results of My Mammogram?

You will usually get the results within a few weeks, although it depends on the facility. A radiologist reads your mammogram and then reports the results to you or your doctor. If there is a concern, you will hear from the mammography facility earlier. Contact your health professional or the mammography facility if you do not receive a report of your results within 30 days.

What Happens If My Mammogram Is Normal?

Continue to get regular mammograms. Mammograms work best when they can be compared with previous ones. This allows your doctor to compare them to look for changes in your breasts.

What Happens If My Mammogram Is Abnormal?

If it is abnormal, do not panic. An abnormal mammogram does not always mean that there is cancer. But you will need to have additional mammograms, tests, or exams before the doctor can tell for sure. You may also be referred to a breast specialist or a surgeon. It does not necessarily mean you have cancer or need surgery. These doctors are experts in diagnosing breast problems.

Tips for Getting a Mammogram

- Try not to have your mammogram the week before you get your period or during your period. Your breasts may be tender or swollen then.

- On the day of your mammogram, don't wear deodorant, perfume, or powder. These products can show up as white spots on the X-ray.

- Some women prefer to wear a top with a skirt or pants, instead of a dress. You will need to undress from your waist up for the mammogram.

How Is Breast Cancer Diagnosed?

Doctors often use additional tests to find or diagnose breast cancer.

- **Breast ultrasound.** A machine uses sound waves to make detailed pictures, called sonograms, of areas inside the breast.

- **Diagnostic mammogram.** If you have a problem in your breast, such as lumps, or if an area of the breast looks abnormal on a screening mammogram, doctors may have you get a diagnostic mammogram. This is a more detailed X-ray of the breast.

- **Magnetic resonance imaging (MRI).** A kind of body scan that uses a magnet linked to a computer. The MRI scan will make detailed pictures of areas inside the breast.

- **Biopsy.** This is a test that removes tissue or fluid from the breast to be looked at under a microscope and do more testing. There are different kinds of biopsies (for example, fine-needle aspiration, core biopsy, or open biopsy).

Staging

If breast cancer is diagnosed, other tests are done to find out if cancer cells have spread within the breast or to other parts of the body. This process is called staging. Whether the cancer is only in the breast, is found in lymph nodes under your arm, or has spread outside the breast determines your stage of breast cancer. The type and stage of breast cancer tell doctors what kind of treatment you need.

How Is Breast Cancer Treated?

Breast cancer is treated in several ways. It depends on the kind of breast cancer and how far it has spread. People with breast cancer often get more than one kind of treatment.

- **Surgery.** An operation where doctors cut out cancer tissue.

- **Chemotherapy.** Using special medicines to shrink or kill cancer. The drugs can be pills you take or medicines given in your veins, or sometimes both.

- **Hormonal therapy**. Blocks cancer cells from getting the hormones they need to grow.

- **Biological therapy**. Works with your body's immune system to help it fight cancer or to control side effects from other cancer treatments. Side effects are how your body reacts to drugs or other treatments.

- **Radiation therapy**. Using high-energy rays (similar to X-rays) to kill cancer.

Doctors from different specialties often work together to treat breast cancer. Surgeons are doctors who perform operations. Medical oncologists are doctors who treat cancer with medicine. Radiation oncologists are doctors who treat cancer with radiation.

Which Treatment Is Right for Me?

Choosing the treatment that is right for you may be hard. Talk to your cancer doctor about the treatment options available for your type and stage of cancer. Your doctor can explain the risks and benefits of each treatment and their side effects.

Sometimes people get an opinion from more than one cancer doctor. This is called a "second opinion." Getting a second opinion may help you choose the treatment that is right for you.

Complementary and Alternative Medicine

Complementary and alternative medicine are medicines and health practices that are not standard cancer treatments. Complementary medicine is used in addition to standard treatments, and alternative medicine is used instead of standard treatments. Meditation, yoga, and supplements like vitamins and herbs are some examples.

Many kinds of complementary and alternative medicine have not been tested scientifically and may not be safe. Talk to your doctor before you start any kind of complementary or alternative medicine.

Chapter 4

Breast Cancer in Various Populations

Chapter Contents

Section 4.1

Breast Cancer in Young Women

This section includes text excerpted from "Cancer Prevention and Control—Breast Cancer in Young Women," Centers for Disease Control and Prevention (CDC), October 1, 2018.

"Breast cancer doesn't just happen to someone that's 75 years old," says breast cancer survivor Charity. When she was diagnosed with breast cancer at age 27, she made a series of decisions to be proactive about her health.

"You need to take your health seriously. Talk to your doctor. There isn't just one face to breast cancer."

Most breast cancers are found in women who are 50 years old or older, but breast cancer also affects younger women. About 10 percent of all new cases of breast cancer in the United States are found in women younger than 45 years of age. Knowing your risk of breast cancer can empower you to take action to manage it.

Who Has a Higher Risk for Breast Cancer?

Some young women are at a higher risk for getting breast cancer at an early age compared with other women their age. If you are a woman under age 45, you may have a higher risk if you have:

- Close relatives who were diagnosed with breast or ovarian cancer when they were younger than 45, especially if more than one relative was diagnosed or if a male relative had breast cancer

- Changes in your *BRCA1* or *BRCA2* genes, or close relatives with these changes

- An Ashkenazi Jewish heritage

- Been treated with radiation therapy to the breast or chest during childhood or early adulthood

- Had breast cancer or certain other breast-health problems

- Been told that you have dense breasts on a mammogram

What Can You Do to Lower Your Risk of Breast Cancer?

It is important that you:

- **Know how your breasts normally look and feel.** If you notice a change in the size or shape of your breast, feel pain in your breast, have nipple discharge other than breast milk (including blood), or other symptoms, talk to a doctor right away.

- **Make healthy choices.** Keeping a healthy weight, getting enough physical activity and sleep, and breastfeeding your babies can help lower your overall risk. If you are taking, or have been told to take, hormone replacement therapy (HRT) or oral contraceptives (OC) (birth control pills), ask your doctor about the risks.

- **Talk to your doctor about your risk.** If your risk is high, your doctor may talk to you about getting mammograms earlier and more often than other women, whether other screening tests might be right for you, and medicines or surgeries that can lower your risk. Your doctor may also suggest that you get genetic counseling to determine if you should be tested for changes in your *BRCA1*, *BRCA2*, and other genes related to breast cancer.

Section 4.2

Breast Cancer in Young African American Women

This section includes text excerpted from "Breast Cancer in Young African American Women," Centers for Disease Control and Prevention (CDC), September 15, 2017.

Every year, 24,000 women under the age of 45 are diagnosed with breast cancer; and 3,000 will die as a result. Young African American women under the age of 35 have breast cancer rates that are two times higher than Caucasian women of the same age. Furthermore, young African American women are three times as likely to die from breast cancer as Caucasian women of the same age. Once diagnosed, young African American women face unique challenges that are either not present or are less severe for older women. Having a breast health course of action and discussing the significant implications of a breast-cancer diagnosis is essential for young African American women in taking care of their health.

Risks of Breast Cancer for Younger Women

Younger women tend to face more-aggressive breast cancers, are diagnosed at later stages and as a result, have lower survival rates. Women aged 45 and younger are more likely to have higher-grade tumors, larger tumor sizes, and a higher comorbidity of lymph-node involvement than women over 65. The relative 5-year breast-cancer survival rate is lower in women diagnosed with breast cancer before the age of 40 (82%) compared to women diagnosed with breast cancer at the age of 40 or older (89%). Being aware of risk factors and consulting a doctor about breast health is important for young African American women to mitigate and manage their risk.

The lack of awareness among young African American women on their risk for breast cancer is often a factor into why they have more harsh outcomes. Approximately 40 percent of young women with breast cancer had no idea a young woman could get breast cancer prior to their own diagnosis. Fear and stigma are commonly cited reasons for not getting a mammogram. Unfortunately, cultural barriers like fear and stigma associated with illness and poverty deter African American women from getting breast-cancer screenings, which results in a late-stage diagnosis. Lack of dialogue among families about generational health and increased risks are key barriers to women taking the steps to minimize their risk of breast cancer.

Young women under the age 45 have a higher risk for breast cancer if:

- A close relative (parent, sibling, or child) was diagnosed with breast or ovarian cancer at an age younger than 45

- They have other breast-health problems or were treated with radiation therapy to the breast or chest during childhood or early adulthood

- They have changes in certain breast-cancer genes (*BRCA1* and *BRCA2*) or have close relatives with these changes

Prevention Strategies for Young African American Women

Reducing Risk

Unfortunately, there is no effective method of screening for young women. Young African American women should be familiar with how their breasts normally look and feel and be aware of the signs of abnormal breast health in order to take the proper steps to manage their risk. Knowing the signs of breast malignancy can save lives. Eighty percent of young women ultimately diagnosed with breast cancer find their breast abnormality themselves and the earlier the abnormality is found, the greater the survival rate. More importantly, African American women need to feel comfortable and even encouraged to talk about their bodies. Recognizing the signs of abnormal breast health and consulting a doctor to assess concerns if any known symptoms appear is important to reduce the risk of breast cancer in young African American women.

Knowing Symptoms

Symptoms include:

- Change in shape or size of the breast
- Pain in the breast
- A liquid discharge other than breast milk

Women who are at higher risk for breast cancer at a young age should consult their doctor to learn more about how to manage their risk.

After Diagnosis

Young women face unique challenges upon being diagnosed with breast cancer, including:

- The possibility of early menopause caused by chemotherapy
- Effects on fertility
- Psychological distress including concerns about body image
- Disruption of employment (both voluntary and involuntary) and challenges to financial stability. A breast-cancer diagnosis in young women interferes at a transition point in their lives. Treatment for breast cancer has the potential to impact the life

of a young woman in ways that are less pertinent or less severe to older women. Once diagnosed, it is important that young women consult with their healthcare team to understand the impact breast-cancer treatment can have on their lives.

Section 4.3

Breast Cancer in Men

This section includes text excerpted from "Male Breast Cancer Treatment (PDQ®)—Patient Version," National Cancer Institute (NCI), December 28, 2018.

Men and Breast Cancer: Facts

Male breast cancer is a disease in which malignant (cancer) cells form in the tissues of the breast. Breast cancer may occur in men. Breast cancer may occur in men at any age, but it usually occurs in men between 60 and 70 years of age. Male breast cancer makes up less than 1 percent of all cases of breast cancer.

Types of Breast Cancer Found in Men

The following types of breast cancer are found in men:

- **Infiltrating ductal carcinoma (IDC).** It is a cancer that has spread beyond the cells lining ducts in the breast. This is the most common type of breast cancer in men.

- **Ductal carcinoma *in situ* (DCIS).** Abnormal cells that are found in the lining of a duct; also called "intraductal carcinoma."

- **Inflammatory breast cancer.** It is a type of cancer in which the breast looks red and swollen and feels warm.

- **Paget disease of the nipple.** It is a tumor that has grown from ducts beneath the nipple onto the surface of the nipple.

Lobular carcinoma *in situ* (LCIS) (abnormal cells found in one of the lobes or sections of the breast), which sometimes occurs in women, has not been seen in men.

Risk Factors for Breast Cancer in Men

Anything that increases your risk of getting a disease is called a risk factor. Having a risk factor does not mean that you will get cancer; not having risk factors doesn't mean that you will not get cancer. Talk to your doctor if you think you may be at risk. Risk factors for breast cancer in men may include the following:

- Treatment with radiation therapy to your breast/chest

- Having a disease linked to high levels of estrogen in the body, such as cirrhosis (liver disease) or Klinefelter syndrome (KS) (a genetic disorder)

- Having one or more female relatives who have had breast cancer

- Having mutations (changes) in genes such as *BRCA2*

Genetics Can Be a Cause

The genes in cells carry the hereditary information that is received from a person's parents. Hereditary breast cancer makes up about 5 to 10 percent of all breast cancer. Some mutated genes related to breast cancer, such as *BRCA2*, are more common in certain ethnic groups. Men who have a mutated gene related to breast cancer have an increased risk of this disease.

There are tests that can detect (find) mutated genes. These genetic tests are sometimes done for members of families with a high risk of cancer.

Signs and Symptoms of Breast Cancer in Men

Men with breast cancer usually have lumps that can be felt. Lumps and other signs may be caused by male breast cancer or by other conditions. Check with your doctor if you have any of the following:

- A lump or thickening in or near the breast or in the underarm area

- A change in the size or shape of the breast

- A dimple or puckering in the skin of the breast

- A nipple turned inward into the breast

- Fluid from the nipple, especially if it's bloody

- Scaly, red, or swollen skin on the breast, nipple, or areola (the dark area of skin around the nipple)

- Dimples in the breast that look like the skin of an orange, called peau d'orange

Survival for Men with Breast Cancer

Survival for men with breast cancer is similar to that for women with breast cancer when their stage at diagnosis is the same. Breast cancer in men, however, is often diagnosed at a later stage. Cancer found at a later stage may be less likely to be cured.

Chapter 5

Statistics on Breast Cancer in the United States

Breast Cancer Incidence and Mortality

Breast cancer is the most common noncutaneous cancer in United States women, with an estimated 266,120 cases of invasive disease, 63,960 cases of *in situ* disease, and 40,920 deaths expected in 2018. Women with inherited risk, especially *BRCA1* and *BRCA2* gene carriers, comprise no more than 10 percent of breast-cancer cases. Males account for 1 percent of breast-cancer cases and breast-cancer deaths.

The biggest risk factor for breast cancer is being female, followed by advancing age. Other risk factors include hormonal aspects (such as early menarche, late menopause, nulliparity, late first pregnancy, and postmenopausal hormone therapy (PMHT)), alcohol consumption, and exposure to ionizing radiation.

Breast-cancer incidence in white women is higher than in black women, who also have a lower survival rate for every stage when diagnosed. This may reflect differences in screening behavior and access to

This chapter contains text excerpted from the following sources: Text under the heading "Breast Cancer Incidence and Mortality" is excerpted from "Breast Cancer Screening (PDQ®)—Health Professional Version," National Cancer Institute (NCI), October 8, 2018; Text beginning with the heading "Statistics at a Glance" is excerpted from "Cancer Stat Facts: Female Breast Cancer," Surveillance, Epidemiology and End Results Program (SEER), National Cancer Institute (NCI), April 16, 2018.

healthcare. Hispanic and Asian Pacific Islanders have lower incidence of mortality rate than whites or blacks.

Breast-cancer incidence depends on reproductive issues (such as early versus late pregnancy, multiparity, and breastfeeding), participation in screening, and postmenopausal hormone usage. The incidence of breast cancer (especially ductal carcinoma *in situ* (DCIS)) increased dramatically after mammography was widely adopted in the United States and the United Kingdom. Widespread use of postmenopausal hormone therapy was associated with a dramatic increase in breast-cancer incidence, a trend that reversed when its use decreased.

In any population, the adoption of screening is not followed by a decline in the incidence of advanced-stage cancer.

Statistics at a Glance
Number of New Cases and Deaths per 100,000

The number of new cases of female breast cancer was 126.0 per 100,000 women per year. The number of deaths was 20.9 per 100,000 women per year. These rates are age-adjusted and based on 2011 to 2015 cases and deaths.

Lifetime Risk of Developing Cancer

Approximately 12.4 percent of women will be diagnosed with female breast cancer at some point during their lifetime, based on 2013 to 2015 data.

Prevalence of Breast Cancer

In 2015, there were an estimated 3,418,124 women living with female breast cancer in the United States.

Table 5.1. Estimated New Cases and Deaths in 2018

At a Glance	
Estimated new cases in 2018	266,120
Percent of all new cancer cases	15.30%
Estimated deaths in 2018	40,920
Percent of all cancer deaths	6.70%
Percent surviving 5 years (2008 to 2014)	0.897

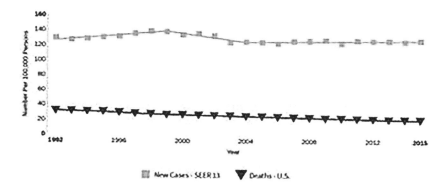

Figure 5.1. *Data of Estimated New Cases and Deaths in 2018*

Modeled trend lines were calculated from the underlying rates using the Joinpoint Trend Analysis Software

Survival Statistics
How Many People Survive Five Years or More after Being Diagnosed with Female Breast Cancer?

Relative survival statistics compare the survival of patients diagnosed with cancer with the survival of people in the general population who are the same age, race, and sex and who have not been diagnosed with cancer. Because survival statistics are based on large groups of people, they cannot be used to predict exactly what will happen to an individual patient. No two patients are entirely alike, and treatment and responses to treatment can vary greatly.

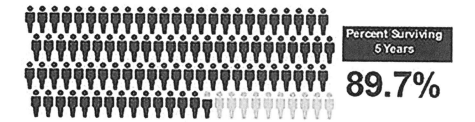

Figure 5.2. *Number of Patients Surviving More than Five Years*

Based on data from SEER 18 2008 to 2014.

41

Survival by Stage

Cancer stage at diagnosis, which refers to extent of a cancer in the body, determines treatment options and has a strong influence on the length of survival. In general, if the cancer is found only in the part of the body where it started it is localized (sometimes referred to as stage 1). If it has spread to a different part of the body, the stage is regional or distant. The earlier female breast cancer is caught, the better chance a person has of surviving five years after being diagnosed. For female breast cancer, 62.1 percent are diagnosed at the local stage. The 5-year survival for localized female breast cancer is 98.7 percent.

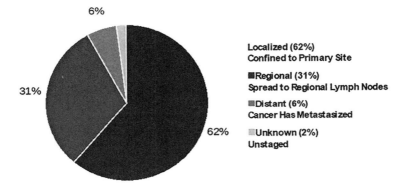

Figure 5.3. *Percent of Cases by Stage*

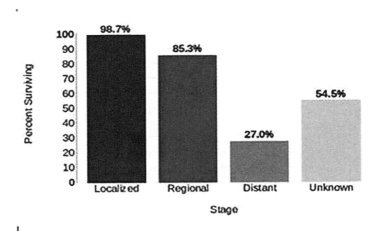

Figure 5.4. *Five-Year Relative Survival*

Number of New Cases and Deaths due to Breast Cancer

How Common Is This Cancer?

Compared to other cancers, female breast cancer is fairly common.

Table 5.2. Number of New Cases and Deaths

S.No	Common Types of Cancer	Estimated New Cases 2018	Estimated Deaths 2018
1	Breast Cancer (Female)	266,120	40,920
2	Lung and Bronchus Cancer	234,030	154,050
3	Prostate Cancer	164,690	29,430
4	Colorectal Cancer	140,250	50,630
5	Melanoma of the Skin	91,270	9,320
6	Bladder Cancer	81,190	17,240
7	Non-Hodgkin Lymphoma	74,680	19,910
8	Kidney and Renal Pelvis Cancer	65,340	14,970
9	Uterine Cancer	63,230	11,350
10	Leukemia	60,300	24,370

Female breast cancer represents 15.3 percent of all new cancer cases in the United States

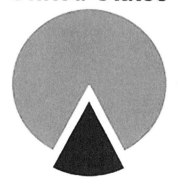

Figure 5.5. *New Cancer Cases in the United States*

In 2018, it is estimated that there will be 266,120 new cases of female breast cancer and an estimated 40,920 people will die of this disease.

Who Gets This Cancer?

Female breast cancer is most common in middle-aged and older women. Although rare, men can develop breast cancer as well. The number of new cases of female breast cancer was 126.0 per 100,000 women per year based on 2011 to 2015 cases.

Table 5.3. Number of New Cases per 100,000 Persons by Race/Ethnicity: Female Breast Cancer

Females	
All Races	126
White	128.6
Black	126.9
Asian/Pacific Islander	100.6
American Indian/Alaska Native	82.6
Hispanic	93.7
Non-Hispanic	131.6

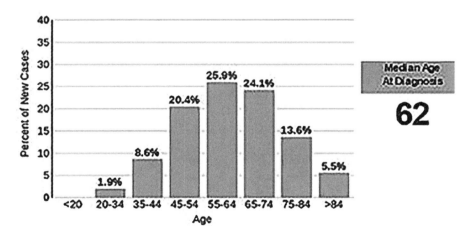

Figure 5.6. *Percent of New Cases by Age Group: Female Breast Cancer*

Female breast cancer is most frequently diagnosed among women aged 55 to 64.

Who Dies from This Cancer?

Overall, female breast cancer survival is good. However, women who are diagnosed at an advanced age may be more likely than younger women to die of the disease. Female breast cancer is the fourth leading cause of cancer death in the United States. The number of deaths was 20.9 per 100,000 women per year based on 2011 to 2015.

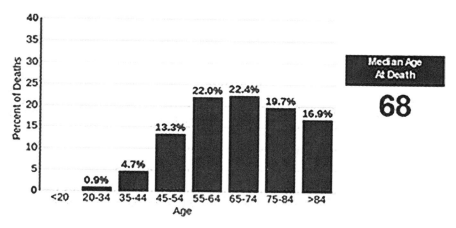

Figure 5.7. *Percent of Deaths by Age Group: Female Breast Cancer*

The percent of female breast-cancer deaths is highest among women aged 65 to 74.

Trends in Breast-Cancer Rates
Changes over Time

Keeping track of the number of new cases, deaths, and survival over time (trends) can help scientists understand whether progress is being made and where additional research is needed to address challenges, such as improving screening or finding better treatments.

Using statistical models for analysis, rates for new female breast cancer cases have been rising on average 0.3 percent each year over the last 10 years. Death rates have been falling on average 1.8 percent each year over 2006 to 2015. Five-year survival trends are shown below.

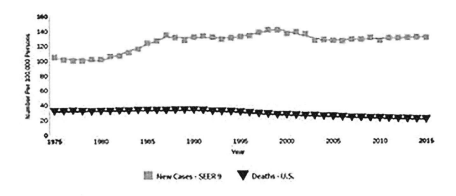

Figure 5.8. *New Cases, Deaths and Five-Year Relative Survival*

New cases come from SEER 9 Incidence. Deaths come from U.S. mortality. 1975 to 2015, All races females. Rates are age-adjusted.

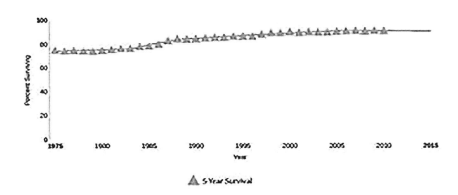

Figure 5.9. *New Cases, Deaths and Five-Year Relative Survival*

SEER 9 Incidence. Five-year relative survival percentage from 1975 to 2010, All races females.

46

Chapter 6

Decrease in Breast-Cancer Deaths

Nowadays, fewer American women are dying from breast cancer. In the past 10 years, the death rates from breast cancer have dropped an average of 1.9 percent per year, while the rate of breast-cancer diagnoses has been stable. Federally funded research increased screening, and new and improved treatments have saved lives and improved women's quality of life (QOL) when they are confronted with a breast-cancer diagnosis.

Breast-Cancer Status

Breast cancer thirty years ago:

- Breast-cancer death rates for all women peaked in 1985 at 32.98 per 100,000 women.

- Mastectomy (surgery to remove the breast) was the commonly accepted surgical option for breast-cancer treatment.

- Scientists began studying hormonal treatments (called selective estrogen receptor modulators, or SERMs) after breast-cancer surgery.

This chapter includes text excerpted from "Decrease in Breast Cancer Deaths," Office on Women's Health (OWH), U.S. Department of Health and Human Services (HHS), March 14, 2018.

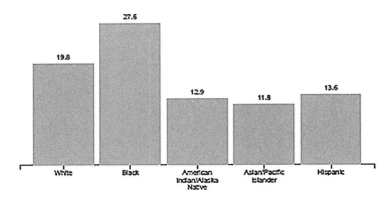

Figure 6.1. *Rate of Cancer Deaths by Race/Ethnicity, Female in 2015* (Source: "Rate of Cancer Deaths—Female Breast, United States, 2015," Centers for Disease Control and Prevention (CDC).)

Female breast death rate per 100,000 women

- Not much was known about which genetic factors increase a woman's risk for breast cancer.

- Prevention of breast cancer seemed unlikely.

Breast cancer as of in 2018:

- Thanks to new cancer treatments and screening that finds cancer earlier, the breast-cancer death rate for all women continues to decline and is currently at 21.92 per 100,000 women.

- Breast-conserving surgery (lumpectomy) and radiation treatment have replaced mastectomy for the treatment of early-stage breast cancer.

- Hormonal medications (like tamoxifen) are now standard for estrogen receptor-positive (ER+) breast cancer, both as an additional treatment before or after surgery and in treating inoperable breast cancer.

- Much is now known regarding several genetic mutations (changes to genes) that can lead to breast cancer, including *BRCA1, BRCA2, TP53,* and *PTEN/MMAC1.*

- Women who are at high risk because of a breast cancer gene (or other family histories) now have medical and surgical options to help prevent breast cancer. And all women can take steps, such as eating right and exercising, to help reduce their risk for breast cancer.

48

Part Two

Types of Breast Cancer

Chapter 7

Ductal Carcinoma in Situ

What Is Ductal Carcinoma in Situ*?*

Ductal carcinoma *in situ* (DCIS) is a noninvasive condition that can be associated with, or evolve into, invasive cancer, with variable frequency and time course. Some researchers include DCIS with invasive breast-cancer statistics, but others argue that it would be better if the term were replaced with ductal intraepithelial neoplasia (DIN), similar to the terminology used for cervical and prostate precursor lesions, and that excluding DCIS from breast-cancer statistics should be considered.

How Is Ductal Carcinoma in Situ *Diagnosed?*

DCIS is most often diagnosed by mammography. In the United States, only 4,900 women were diagnosed with DCIS in 1983 before the adoption of mammography screening, compared with approximately 63,960 women who are expected to be diagnosed in 2018. The Canadian National Breast Screening Study-2 (CNBSS-2), which evaluated

This chapter contains text excerpted from the following sources: Text beginning with the heading "What Is Ductal Carcinoma *in Situ*?" is excerpted from "Breast Cancer Screening (PDQ®)—Health Professional Version," National Cancer Institute (NCI), October 8, 2018; Text under the heading "Risk of Death due to Breast Cancer is Low after a Diagnosis of Ductal Carcinoma *in Situ*" is excerpted from "Risk of Breast Cancer Death Is Low after a Diagnosis of Ductal Carcinoma *in Situ*," National Cancer Institute (NCI), August 26, 2015. Reviewed February 2019.

women aged 50 to 59 years, found a fourfold increase in DCIS cases in women screened by clinical breast examination (CBE) plus mammography compared with those screened by CBE alone, with no difference in breast-cancer mortality.

The natural history of DCIS is poorly understood because nearly all DCIS cases are detected by screening and nearly all are treated. Development of breast cancer after treatment of DCIS depends on the pathologic characteristics of the lesion and on the treatment. In a randomized trial, 13.4 percent of women whose DCIS was excised by lumpectomy developed ipsilateral invasive breast cancer within 90 months, compared with 3.9 percent of those treated by both lumpectomy and radiation. Among women diagnosed and treated for DCIS, the percentage of women who died of breast cancer is lower than that for the age-matched population at large. This favorable outcome may reflect the benign nature of the condition, the benefits of treatment, or the volunteer effect (i.e., women who undergo breast-cancer screening are generally healthier than those who do not do so).

Risk of Death due to Breast Cancer Is Low after a Diagnosis of Ductal Carcinoma in Situ

A study suggests that women who are diagnosed with DCIS—generally have a low risk of dying from breast cancer. In addition, treating these lesions may help prevent a recurrence in the breast but does not appear to decrease the already-low risk of dying from the disease, even after 20 years of follow up.

The findings, from an observational study involving more than 100,000 women, were published in *JAMA Oncology*. Steven A. Narod, M.D., of the Women's College Hospital, Toronto, and his colleagues used data from National Cancer Institute's (NCI) Surveillance, Epidemiology and End Results (SEER) program to estimate the death rate from breast cancer among women diagnosed with DCIS.

In the study, most women received either a lumpectomy (with or without radiation therapy) or a single or double mastectomy. The overall death rate from breast cancer at 20 years after diagnosis was 3.3 percent, a rate similar to that of the general population. The death rates did not vary with the type of treatment used, the researchers noted.

"DCIS has extremely favorable outcomes irrespective of the type of therapy used," said Barry Kramer, M.D., Director of NCI's Division of Cancer Prevention (DCP), who was not involved in the study. He noted that treatments for DCIS are associated with potential harms. For instance, exposure to radiation therapy increases the risk of developing secondary cancers in the future, and mastectomy can cause serious health problems as well.

Some women with DCIS may be at an increased risk of dying from breast cancer, including those diagnosed at a younger age and African Americans, the study showed. Death rates were higher for women diagnosed before age 35 than for older women (7.8% versus 3.2%) and higher for African Americans than for Caucasians (7% versus 3%).

The mean age at diagnosis among women in the study was 54 years old, and less than 1.5 percent of the women with DCIS were under age 35. The authors of an accompanying editorial said the study's large numbers and long-term follow up provide a compelling case to reconsider how DCIS is treated.

"Given the low breast-cancer mortality risk, we should stop telling women that DCIS is an emergency and that they should schedule definitive surgery within two weeks of diagnosis," wrote Laura Esserman, M.D., and Christina Yau, Ph.D., of the University of California, San Francisco.

The finding of greatest clinical importance, the study authors noted, was the observation that preventing the development of invasive-breast cancer in women diagnosed with DCIS did not reduce the chances of dying from breast cancer. For example, among women who had a lumpectomy, radiation therapy reduced the risk of a recurrence in the same breast compared with women not treated with radiation (2.5% versus 4.9%), but it did not reduce the risk of death from breast cancer 10 years later (0.8% versus 0.9%).

"The study showed that even though a lumpectomy can reduce the risk of a recurrence developing in the same breast, it does not change the risk of dying from the disease," said Dr. Kramer. "This suggests that what you do locally to treat DCIS may not affect the risk of dying, which is the most important outcome." This observation, Dr. Kramer added, "gives us important insights into the biology of DCIS."

In another finding, 517 women diagnosed with DCIS died of breast cancer without ever developing invasive cancer in the same or another breast prior to death. Some cases of DCIS may have "an inherent potential" to spread to other parts of the body, the study authors wrote.

The finding, Drs. Esserman and Yau concluded, suggests that "our current approach of surgical removal and radiation therapy may not suffice for the rare cases that lead to breast-cancer mortality and thus new approaches are needed."

Chapter 8

Lobular Carcinoma in Situ

Lobular carcinoma *in situ* (LCIS) describes abnormal cell growth that occurs in the lobules, which are tiny milk-producing glands located at the ends of milk ducts in the breasts. Although the term "carcinoma" refers to cancer in the lining of an organ, LCIS is not technically considered a form of cancer. Left untreated, LCIS does not spread beyond the lobules to surrounding tissues to become invasive carcinoma. As a result, some healthcare professionals prefer the term "lobular neoplasia," which refers to a group of abnormal cells in the lobules. "*In situ*" means that the abnormal cells are confined to the area where they originally began growing, as is generally found in the earliest forms of breast cancer.

Although LCIS is not considered precancer, studies have shown that women diagnosed with LCIS have an increased risk of developing invasive breast cancer later in life. LCIS is thus viewed as a marker or indicator of higher-than-average breast-cancer risk. While the average woman faces an approximately 12.5 percent risk of developing invasive breast cancer in her lifetime, a woman with LCIS is estimated to have a 30 to 40 percent lifetime risk. Other studies suggest the risk is 7 to 11 times higher for women with LCIS. When women with LCIS develop breast cancer, however, it typically occurs years or even decades later. The invasive cancer is equally likely to develop in the breast with LCIS or the other breast.

"Lobular Carcinoma *in Situ* (LCIS)," © 2016 Omnigraphics. Reviewed February 2019.

Diagnosis of Lobular Carcinoma in Situ

LCIS can be difficult to diagnose because it does not usually present any obvious symptoms, such as a lump or visible change to the breast. In addition, LCIS may not appear on a mammogram because the abnormal cells often lack microcalcifications, the tiny specks of calcium that form within most breast-cancer cells. As a result, experts believe that many cases of LCIS are never diagnosed and never cause any problems.

When LCIS is diagnosed, it usually occurs through a biopsy that is performed to diagnose a different breast problem, such as an abnormal mammogram result or a suspicious lump. A biopsy is a procedure used to remove samples of tissue for examination under a microscope by a pathologist. In a fine needle aspiration biopsy, a small, hollow needle is inserted into the breast tissue to remove a sample of suspicious cells. In an incisional biopsy, a surgeon makes an incision to remove a small piece of tissue for further examination. In an excisional biopsy, the entire lump or abnormal area is removed from the breast.

A challenge for the pathologist examining cell samples is to differentiate between LCIS and ductal carcinoma *in situ* (DCIS), which is found in the milk ducts rather than the lobules. Although they may appear similar, DCIS is considered to be cancer and can spread without treatment. More than half of women diagnosed with LCIS will have abnormal cell growth in multiple lobules, while about one-third of women will have both breasts affected by LCIS.

Some factors that increase a woman's likelihood of being diagnosed with LCIS include having a history of breast cancer in her immediate family, having taken hormone replacement therapy for menopausal symptoms, and being in her early forties. LCIS is most commonly found in women between the ages of 40 and 50 who have not yet undergone menopause.

Treatment Options for Lobular Carcinoma in Situ

Since LCIS does not become invasive, it does not require traditional cancer treatments, such as chemotherapy and radiation therapy. In some cases, doctors may recommend removing the abnormal cells with an excisional biopsy. In most cases, however, the main forms of treatment for women who are diagnosed with LCIS involve strategies to reduce the risk of developing invasive breast cancer in the future.

One option is to monitor for signs of breast cancer through careful observation. This treatment approach typically includes adhering to a schedule of frequent breast self-examinations, biannual clinical examinations, annual mammograms, and other imaging techniques if there is a family history or additional risk factors to consider. The goal of careful observation is to find and treat invasive breast cancer before it spreads.

A second treatment option involves taking medication to reduce the risk of developing breast cancer. Hormonal therapy drugs like Tamoxifen and Raloxifene (Evista) block estrogen receptors in breast tissue, which helps prevent cancer cells from receiving the estrogen they need to grow. Studies have shown that these medications can reduce a woman's risk of developing breast cancer by 50 percent. However, they are not recommended for women who have heart disease or multiple risk factors for heart disease because they increase the risk of stroke. Another option for postmenopausal women is exemestane (Aromasin), which reduces the risk of breast cancer in high-risk women by decreasing the production of estrogen in the body.

Finally, some women opt for preventative surgery to eliminate the risk of developing invasive breast cancer. Prophylactic mastectomy involves the surgical removal of both breasts. It is considered as an option for women who have LCIS as well as other factors that increase their risk of breast cancer, such as a strong family history or a *BRCA* gene mutation.

References

1. "LCIS—Lobular Carcinoma *in Situ*," BreastCancer.org, February 18, 2016.

2. "Lobular Carcinoma *in Situ*," American Cancer Society (ACS), June 10, 2015.

3. "Lobular Carcinoma *in Situ* (LCIS)," Mayo Clinic, 2016.

Chapter 9

Invasive Carcinoma of the Breast

Chapter Contents

Section 9.1

Understanding Invasive Breast Cancer

This section contains text excerpted from the following sources: Text under the heading "What Is Invasive Breast Cancer?" is excerpted from "A Randomized Trial of Chemotherapy in Surgical Patients with Infiltrating Ductal Carcinoma of Breast (COC-IDCP)," ClinicalTrials. gov, National Institutes of Health (NIH), March 9, 2018; Text under the heading "Changing Patterns in Survival for U.S. Women with Invasive Breast Cancer" is excerpted from "Changing Patterns in Survival for U.S. Women with Invasive Breast Cancer," National Cancer Institute (NCI), July 20, 2015. Reviewed February 2019; Text under the heading "Role of Cancer Genome Atlas in Invasive Breast Cancer" is excerpted from "The Cancer Genome Atlas (TCGA): An Immeasurable Source of Knowledge," National Center for Biotechnology Information (NCBI), January 20, 2015. Reviewed February 2019.

What Is Invasive Breast Cancer?

Invasive breast cancer is cancer that has spread from where it began in the breast to surrounding normal tissue. There are two types:

- The most common type of invasive breast cancer is invasive ductal carcinoma, which begins in the lining of the milk ducts (thin tubes that carry milk from the lobules of the breast to the nipple). Once found, invasive ductal carcinoma (IDC) usually has already broken through the wall of the milk duct and begun to invade the tissues of the breast. Over time, IDC can spread to the lymph nodes and possibly to other areas of the body with high frequency.

- Another type is invasive lobular carcinoma, which begins in the lobules (milk glands) of the breast. Invasive breast cancer can spread through the blood and lymph systems to other parts of the body. Also called "infiltrating breast cancer."

- About 80 percent of all breast cancers are IDCs. According to the statistics of the American Cancer Society, more than 180,000 women in the United States are diagnosed with IDC each year. Although IDC can affect women at any age, it is more common as they grow older, and approximately two-thirds of women are 55 or older when they are diagnosed with IDC.

Treatments for Invasive Ductal Carcinoma

The treatments for invasive ductal carcinoma fall into two broad categories.

- Local treatments for IDC, including surgery and radiation, which treat the primary tumor and surrounding areas, such as the chest and lymph nodes

- Systemic treatments for IDC, including chemotherapy, hormone therapy, and targeted therapy, which deliver cytotoxicity throughout the body in an effort in an effort to eliminate any cancer cells that have left the primary site and to minimize the risk of recurrent disease

Changing Patterns in Survival for U.S. Women with Invasive Breast Cancer

Breast-cancer mortality rates have been declining among women in many Western countries since the 1970s. Overall, breast-cancer survival rates following diagnosis have improved for all women diagnosed with local and regional (the area around the tumor) disease. Women diagnosed before age 70 have experienced lower short-term (less than 5 years) death rates, even for metastatic disease. And the long-term death rates (survival beyond the first 5 years) have improved among those with the local and regional disease in all age groups.

Tumor size at diagnosis has shrunk since the 1980s, but new evidence shows that changes in tumor size within each stage at diagnosis explain only a small proportion of the improvement in breast-cancer mortality in women under the age of 70. However, changes in tumor size account for about half of the improvements for women diagnosed with local or regional breast cancer at age 70 and older. This conclusion comes from an analysis of data from the National Cancer Institute's Surveillance, Epidemiology, and End Results (SEER) database. The study also found that changes in estrogen-receptor (ER) status explains little of the improvement after adjustment for tumor size, except for women age 70 and older within 5 years after diagnosis. Experts have established that rates of harder to treat estrogen receptor-negative tumors have been declining since 1990. Some of the stage-specific survival improvements may also be due to changes in diagnostic procedures over time that tend to increase the proportion of women with more favorable prognoses within each stage. Findings from this large-scale study help clarify factors associated with breast-cancer survival in women of all ages, according to the investigators.

Role of Cancer Genome Atlas in Invasive Breast Cancer

The Cancer Genome Atlas (TCGA) is a publicly funded project that aims to catalog and discover major cancer-causing genomic alterations to create a comprehensive "atlas" of cancer genomic profiles. Cancer is considered the most complex disease that humankind has to face. The demand for better diagnosis, treatment, and prevention of cancer is ongoing and strongly correlates with a better understanding of genetic changes in the tumor. Progress in the technological development of genome-wide sequencing and bioinformatics has shed new light on the cancer genome. The Cancer Genome Atlas (TCGA) was launched in 2005, and the International Cancer Genome Consortium (ICGC) was launched in 2008 as the two main projects accelerating the comprehensive understanding of the genetics of cancer through innovative genome analysis technologies. This work helps to generate new cancer therapies, diagnostic methods, and preventive strategies.

The TCGA program focuses mostly on two types of invasive breast cancer: ductal carcinoma and lobular carcinoma. Invasive ductal carcinoma is the most common type of breast cancer. It comprises about 65 to 85 percent of all breast cancer and develops in the milk-producing lobules or glands. About 10 percent of all cases of advanced breast cancer are invasive lobular breast carcinoma.

What Have the Cancer Genome Atlas Researchers Learned about Breast Cancer?*

TCGA researchers have:

- Described new integrated insights into the four standard molecular subtypes of breast cancer: HER2-enriched, Luminal A, Luminal B, and basal-like

- Identified mutated genes that are specific to each subtype

- Found that the basal-like subtype shares many genetic features with high-grade serous ovarian cancer, suggesting that the cancers have a common molecular origin and may share therapeutic opportunities

- Performed computational analyses that suggest that basal-like breast cancer and serous ovarian cancer might both be susceptible to two types of cancer treatment

- Identified a drug that inhibits blood vessel growth, cutting off the blood supply to the tumor

- Developed bioreductive drugs, which are inactive drugs that become toxic to cancer cells under low oxygen conditions

* Excerpted from "Breast Ductal Carcinoma," The Cancer Genome Atlas (TCGA), National Cancer Institute (NCI), October 12, 2012. Reviewed February 2019.

Section 9.2

Invasive Lobular Carcinoma

"Invasive Lobular Carcinoma,"
© 2019 Omnigraphics. Reviewed February 2019.

What Is Invasive Lobular Carcinoma?

Cancer that spreads from breast tissue to the surrounding normal tissue is called "invasive lobular carcinoma." It consists of two types:

- Invasive ductal carcinoma (IDC)
- Invasive lobular carcinoma (ILC)

ILC starts in the lobules/milk glands of the breast and spreads to the surrounding tissues. It spreads to the other parts of the body through blood and lymph nodes. ILC is also called "infiltrating lobular carcinoma." About 10 percent of breast cancers are ILCs.

What Are the Symptoms of Invasive Lobular Carcinoma?

Women who develop ILC may notice some of the following changes while doing their self-breast examination:

- Thickening of the breasts
- Changes in the appearance of skin on the breasts or nipples such as scaling, reddening, dimpling, or puckering
- Changes in size and shape of the breasts
- Colorless or blood-stained discharge from the nipple
- Changes in nipple position, such as inversion

What Are the Factors That Increase the Risk of Invasive Lobular Carcinoma?

Some of the factors that may put you in the high-risk category for developing ILC include:

- **Age**—Older women are at higher risk. Only 10 percent of women under 45 years of age are diagnosed with ILC.

- **Family history of breast cancer**—If you have a positive family history, especially maternally, with one or more relatives having had a history of breast cancer, then you are at higher risk.

- **Race**—ILC is more commonly diagnosed in white women than in Black, Asian, or Hispanic women.

- **Weight**—If you are obese, or if your breasts are dense, then you are at higher risk.

- **Pregnancy after 35**—If you became pregnant after the age of 35, then you are at higher risk.

How Is Invasive Lobular Carcinoma Diagnosed?

ILC can be diagnosed with the help of tumor grading, receptor testing, and gene testing.

- **Tumor grading**: After surgical removal of the tumor, it will be sent to a pathology laboratory for grading. A grade will be assigned to the tumor based on how closely the cancer cells resemble normal cells when viewed under a microscope.

- **Low-grade** means the tumor looks similar to normal breast cells.

- **High-grade** means it looks less similar, which means that the cancer is aggressive.

- **Receptor testing**: This will show if the female hormones estrogen and progesterone influence the cancer cells. If your result is positive, then it means your hormones contribute to the growth of cancer cells. If this is the case, hormone suppression or blockage may help treat your cancer.

- **HER2 gene test**: This test will also be done and, if you are positive, then Herceptin (a drug used to treat *HER2*-positive cancers) will be given as additional drug therapy.

How Is Invasive Lobular Carcinoma Treated?

After a firm diagnosis has been made, healthcare providers may decide suitable treatment options for you. Some of them are:

- **Surgical Intervention**—There are two interventional methods:

  - **Lumpectomy**: Removal of the lump (cancer) and some healthy tissue around it (surrounding margin) by a surgeon

  - **Mastectomy**: Removal of the entire breast (performed after chemotherapy trials)

- **Drug Trials**—Also called "chemotherapy." These drugs are given before the surgery, in order to shrink the cancer cells and make them operable. Chemotherapy is also given after the surgery to prevent reoccurrence of cancer cells.

- **Radiation therapy**—Is given usually after surgical removal of cancer cells along with chemotherapy to prevent the growth of cancer cells.

- **Hormone therapy**—Certain drugs are given if the cancer cells are found to have positive hormone receptors.

- **Targeted therapy**—If cancer cells are found to have the genes *HER2*, then treatment with specific drugs such as Herceptin is given as an additional drug.

- **Clinical trials**—Test new treatment options on patients using a combination of new drugs. The trials help healthcare providers and scientists determine safe and effective therapies with improved outcomes. You can choose whether or not to be a part of a clinical trial. Patients who undergo clinical trials may benefit by receiving treatment that is not yet available in the usual healthcare setting. BreastCancerTrials.org, an online resource, provides details about clinical trials and provides a clinical trial–matching service for all breast-cancer patients.

The Cancer Genome Atlas Study Identifies Genomic Features of Invasive Lobular Carcinoma

Investigators in the Cancer Genome Atlas (TCGA) research network have identified molecular characteristics of ILC that distinguish it from IDC. Researchers analyzed the genomes of 817 breast tumors to understand the genetic drivers of ILC. Understanding the genomic differences between ILC and IDC may enable healthcare providers to treat breast cancer more effectively.

ILC is said to be the second-most-common subtype of invasive breast cancer, and it is caused by hallmark loss of protein E-cadherin, which leads to a lack of cell-to-cell adhesion. The mutated genes and signaling activity of AKT (protein kinase B, PKB is also called as AKT, which is an enzyme that helps to transfer signals inside the cells) affect cell growth. *FOXA1* gene mutations are found more frequently in ILC than IDC tumors, whereas *GATA3* mutations are more common in IDC. *GATA3* proteins, as well as the FOXA1, are said to be the key regulators of estrogen-receptor function. ILC tumors show greater AKT signaling pathway activity, and less expression of the tumor suppressor protein PTEN, which suggests that these ILC tumors may be more sensitive to AKT pathway-blocking drugs. Researchers further identified three subtypes of ILC—reactive-like, immune-related, and proliferative.

References

1. "Invasive Breast Cancer: Symptoms, Treatments, Prognosis," WebMD, August 1, 2017.

2. Tomczak, Katarzyna; Czerwinska, Patrycja; Wiznerowicz, Maciej, "The Cancer Genome Atlas (TCGA): An Immeasurable Source of Knowledge," National Center for Biotechnology Information, U.S. National Library of Medicine (NLM), PubMed Central, January 20, 2015.

3. National Cancer Institute (NCI). "TCGA Study Identifies Genomic Features of Invasive Lobular Breast Carcinoma," National Institutes of Health (NIH), October 8, 2015.

Chapter 10

Inflammatory Breast Cancer

What Is Inflammatory Breast Cancer?

Inflammatory breast cancer (IBC) is a rare and very aggressive disease in which cancer cells block lymph vessels in the skin of the breast. This type of breast cancer is called "inflammatory" because the breast often looks swollen and red, or inflamed.

IBC is rare, accounting for one to five percent of all breast cancers diagnosed in the United States. Most IBCs are invasive-ductal carcinomas (IDC), which means they developed from cells that line the milk ducts of the breast and then spread beyond the ducts.

IBC progresses rapidly, often in a matter of weeks or months. At diagnosis, IBC is either stage III or IV disease, depending on whether cancer cells have spread only to nearby lymph nodes or to other tissues as well.

Additional features of IBC include the following:

- Compared with other types of breast cancer, IBC tends to be diagnosed at younger ages.

- IBC is more common and diagnosed at younger ages in African American women than in white women.

- Inflammatory breast tumors are frequently hormone receptor negative, which means they cannot be treated with hormone

This chapter includes text excerpted from "Inflammatory Breast Cancer," National Cancer Institute (NCI), January 6, 2016.

therapies (HT), such as tamoxifen, that interferes with the growth of cancer cells fueled by estrogen.

- IBC is more common in obese women than in women of normal weight.

Like other types of breast cancer, IBC can occur in men, but usually at an older age than in women.

What Are the Symptoms of Inflammatory Breast Cancer?

Symptoms of IBC include swelling (edema) and redness (erythema) that affect a third or more of the breast. The skin of the breast may also appear pink, reddish purple, or bruised. In addition, the skin may have ridges or appear pitted, like the skin of an orange (called peau d'orange). These symptoms are caused by the buildup of fluid (lymph) in the skin of the breast. This fluid buildup occurs because cancer cells have blocked lymph vessels in the skin, preventing the normal flow of lymph through the tissue. Sometimes the breast may contain a solid tumor that can be felt during a physical exam, but more often a tumor cannot be felt.

Other symptoms of IBC include a rapid increase in breast size; sensations of heaviness, burning, or tenderness in the breast; or a nipple that is inverted (facing inward). Swollen lymph nodes may also be present under the arm, near the collarbone, or both.

It is important to note that these symptoms may also be signs of other diseases or conditions, such as an infection, injury, or another type of breast cancer that is locally advanced. For this reason, women with IBC often have a delayed diagnosis of their disease.

How Is Inflammatory Breast Cancer Diagnosed?

IBC can be difficult to diagnose. Often, there is no lump that can be felt during a physical exam or seen in a screening mammogram. In addition, most women diagnosed with IBC have dense breast tissue, which makes cancer detection in a screening mammogram more difficult. Also, because IBC is so aggressive, it can arise between scheduled screening mammograms and progress quickly. The symptoms of IBC may be mistaken for those of mastitis, which is an infection of the breast, or another form of locally advanced breast cancer.

To help prevent delays in diagnosis and in choosing the best course of treatment, an international panel of experts published guidelines on how doctors can diagnose and stage IBC correctly. Their recommendations are summarized below.

Minimum criteria for a diagnosis of IBC include the following:

- A rapid onset of erythema (redness), edema (swelling), and a peau d'orange appearance (ridged or pitted skin) and/or abnormal breast warmth, with or without a lump that can be felt

- The above-mentioned symptoms have been present for less than six months

- The erythema covers at least a third of the breast

- Initial biopsy samples from the affected breast show invasive carcinoma

Further examination of tissue from the affected breast should include testing to see if the cancer cells have hormone receptors (estrogen and progesterone receptors) or if they have greater than normal amounts of the *HER2* gene and/or the HER2 protein (HER2-positive breast cancer).

Imaging and staging tests include the following:

- A diagnostic mammogram and an ultrasound of the breast and regional (nearby) lymph nodes

- A positron emission tomography (PET) scan or computed tomography (CT) scan and a bone scan to see if cancer has spread to other parts of the body

Proper diagnosis and staging of IBC help doctors develop the best treatment plan and estimate the likely outcome of the disease. Patients diagnosed with IBC may want to consult a doctor who specializes in this disease.

How Is Inflammatory Breast Cancer Treated?

IBC is generally treated first with systemic chemotherapy to help shrink the tumor, then with surgery to remove the tumor, followed by radiation therapy. This approach to treatment is called a "multimodal approach." Studies have found that women with IBC who are treated with a multimodal approach have better responses to therapy and longer survival. Treatments used in a multimodal approach may include those described below.

- **Neoadjuvant chemotherapy.** This type of chemotherapy is given before surgery and usually includes both anthracycline and taxane drugs. Doctors generally recommend that at least six cycles of neoadjuvant chemotherapy be given over the course of four to six months before the tumor is removed unless the disease continues to progress during this time and doctors decide that surgery should not be delayed.

- **Targeted therapy.** IBC often produce greater than normal amounts of the HER2 protein, which means that drugs such as trastuzumab (Herceptin) that target this protein may be used to treat them. Anti-HER2 therapy can be given both as part of neoadjuvant therapy and after surgery (adjuvant therapy).

- **Hormone therapy.** If the cells of a woman's IBC contain hormone receptors, HT is another treatment option. Drugs such as tamoxifen, which prevent estrogen from binding to its receptor, and aromatase inhibitors such as letrozole, which block the body's ability to make estrogen, can cause estrogen-dependent cancer cells to stop growing and die.

- **Surgery.** The standard surgery for IBC is a modified radical mastectomy (MRM). This surgery involves removal of the entire affected breast and most or all of the lymph nodes under the adjacent arm. Often, the lining over the underlying chest muscles is also removed, but the chest muscles are preserved. Sometimes, however, the smaller chest muscle (pectoralis minor) may be removed, too.

- **Radiation therapy.** Postmastectomy radiation therapy (PMRT) to the chest wall under the breast that was removed is a standard part of multimodal therapy (MMT) for IBC. If a woman received trastuzumab before surgery, she may continue to receive it during postoperative radiation therapy (PORT). Breast reconstruction can be performed in women with IBC, but, due to the importance of radiation therapy in treating this disease, experts generally recommend delayed reconstruction.

- **Adjuvant therapy.** Adjuvant systemic therapy may be given after surgery to reduce the chance of cancer recurrence. This therapy may include additional chemotherapy, HT, targeted therapy (such as trastuzumab), or some combination of these treatments.

What Is the Prognosis of Patients with Inflammatory Breast Cancer?

The prognosis, or likely outcome, for a patient diagnosed with cancer is often viewed as the chance that cancer will be treated successfully and that the patient will recover completely. Many factors can influence a cancer patient's prognosis, including the type and location of cancer, the stage of the disease, the patient's age and overall general health, and the extent to which the patient's disease responds to treatment. Because IBC usually develops quickly and spreads aggressively to other parts of the body, women diagnosed with this disease, in general, do not survive as long as women diagnosed with other types of breast cancer.

It is important to keep in mind, however, that survival statistics are based on large numbers of patients and that an individual woman's prognosis could be better or worse, depending on her tumor characteristics and medical history. Women who have IBC are encouraged to talk with their doctor about their prognosis, given their particular situation.

Ongoing research, especially at the molecular level, will increase in understanding of how IBC begins and progresses. This knowledge should enable the development of new treatments and more accurate prognoses for women diagnosed with this disease. It is important, therefore, that women who are diagnosed with IBC talk with their doctor about the option of participating in a clinical trial.

Chapter 11

Paget Disease of the Breast

What Is Paget Disease of the Breast?

Paget disease (PD) of the breast (also known as Paget disease of the nipple and mammary Paget disease) is a rare type of cancer involving the skin of the nipple and, usually, the darker circle of skin around it, which is called the "areola." Most people with PD of the breast also have one or more tumors inside the same breast. These breast tumors are either ductal carcinoma *in situ* (DCIS) or invasive breast cancer (IBC).

PD of the breast is named after the nineteenth-century British doctor Sir James Paget, who, in 1874, noted a relationship between changes in the nipple and breast cancer. (Several other diseases are named after Sir James Paget, including PD of bone and extramammary PD (EMPD), which includes PD of the vulva and PD of the penis. These other diseases are not related to PD of the breast.)

Malignant cells known as "Paget cells" are a telltale sign of PD of the breast. These cells are found in the epidermis (surface layer) of the skin of the nipple and the areola. Paget cells often have a large, round appearance under a microscope; they may be found as single cells or as small groups of cells within the epidermis.

This chapter includes text excerpted from "Paget Disease of the Breast," National Cancer Institute (NCI), April 10, 2012. Reviewed February 2019.

Who Gets Paget Disease of the Breast

PD of the breast occurs in both women and men, but most cases occur in women. Approximately 1 to 4 percent of all cases of breast cancer also involve PD of the breast. The average age at diagnosis is 57 years, but the disease has been found in adolescents and in people in their late eighties.

What Causes Paget Disease of the Breast

Doctors do not fully understand what causes PD of the breast. The most widely accepted theory is that cancer cells from a tumor inside the breast travel through the milk ducts to the nipple and areola. This would explain why PD of the breast and tumors inside the same breast are almost always found together.

A second theory is that cells in the nipple or areola become cancerous on their own. This would explain why a few people develop PD of the breast without having a tumor inside the same breast. Moreover, it may be possible for PD of the breast and tumors inside the same breast to develop independently.

What Are the Symptoms of Paget Disease of the Breast?

The symptoms of PD of the breast are often mistaken for those of some benign skin conditions, such as dermatitis or eczema. These symptoms may include the following:

- Itching, tingling, or redness in the nipple and/or areola
- Flaking, crusty, or thickened skin on or around the nipple
- A flattened nipple
- Discharge from the nipple that may be yellowish or bloody

Because the early symptoms of PD of the breast may suggest a benign skin condition, and because the disease is rare, it may be misdiagnosed at first. People with PD of the breast have often had symptoms for several months before being correctly diagnosed.

How Is Paget Disease of the Breast Diagnosed?

A nipple biopsy allows doctors to correctly diagnose PD of the breast. There are several types of nipple biopsy, including the procedures described below.

- **Surface biopsy.** It is a type of biopsy where a glass slide or other tool is used to gently scrape cells from the surface of the skin.

- **Shave biopsy.** It is a type of biopsy where a razor-like tool is used to remove the top layer of skin.

- **Punch biopsy.** It is a type of biopsy where a circular cutting tool, called a "punch," is used to remove a disk-shaped piece of tissue.

- **Wedge biopsy.** It is a type of biopsy where a scalpel is used to remove a small wedge of tissue.

In some cases, doctors may remove the entire nipple. A pathologist then examines the cells or tissue under a microscope to look for Paget cells.

Most people who have PD of the breast also have one or more tumors inside the same breast. In addition to ordering a nipple biopsy, the doctor should perform a clinical breast exam (CBE) to check for lumps or other breast changes. As many as 50 percent of people who have PD of the breast have a breast lump that can be felt in a CBE. The doctor may order additional diagnostic tests, such as a diagnostic mammogram, an ultrasound exam, or a magnetic resonance imaging (MRI) scan to look for possible tumors.

How Is Paget Disease of the Breast Treated?

For many years, mastectomy, with or without the removal of lymph nodes under the arm on the same side of the chest (known as "axillary lymph node dissection" (ALND)), was regarded as the standard surgery for PD of the breast. This type of surgery was done because patients with PD of the breast were almost always found to have one or more tumors inside the same breast. Even if only one tumor was present, that tumor could be located several centimeters away from the nipple and areola and would not be removed by surgery on the nipple and areola alone.

Studies have shown, however, that breast-conserving surgery that includes removal of the nipple and areola, followed by whole-breast radiation therapy (WBRT), is a safe option for people with PD of the breast who do not have a palpable lump in their breast and whose mammograms do not reveal a tumor.

People with PD of the breast who have a breast tumor and are having a mastectomy should be offered sentinel lymph node biopsy

(SLNB) to see whether cancer has spread to the axillary lymph nodes. If cancer cells are found in the sentinel lymph node(s), more extensive axillary lymph node surgery may be needed. Depending on the stage and other features of the underlying breast tumor (for example, the presence or absence of lymph node involvement, estrogen receptors (ER) and progesterone receptors (PR) in the tumor cells, and HER2 protein overexpression in the tumor cells), adjuvant therapy, consisting of chemotherapy and/or hormonal therapy (HT), may also be recommended.

What Is the Prognosis for People with Paget Disease of the Breast?

The prognosis, or outlook, for people with PD of the breast, depends on a variety of factors, including the following:

- Whether or not a tumor is present in the affected breast

- If one or more tumors are present in the affected breast, whether those tumors are ductal carcinoma *in situ* or invasive breast cancer

- If invasive breast cancer is present in the affected breast, the stage of that cancer

The presence of invasive cancer in the affected breast and the spread of cancer to nearby lymph nodes are associated with reduced survival.

According to the National Cancer Institute's (NCI) Surveillance, Epidemiology, and End Results (SEER) program, the 5-year relative survival for all women in the United States. who were diagnosed with PD of the breast between 1988 and 2001 was 82.6 percent. This compares with a 5-year relative survival of 87.1 percent for women diagnosed with any type of breast cancer. For women with both PD of the breast and invasive cancer in the same breast, the 5-year relative survival declined with increasing stage of the cancer (stage I, 95.8%; stage II, 77.7%; stage III, 46.3%; stage IV, 14.3%).

Chapter 12

Triple-Negative
Breast Cancer

Triple-negative breast cancer is a relatively rare form of the disease in which the cancer cells test negative for the three most common types of receptors that promote tumor growth: estrogen receptors, progesterone receptors, and hormone epidermal growth factor receptor 2 (HER-2). Receptors are proteins that are found both on the surface and inside of cells throughout the body. They enable cells to receive the chemical messages that control their growth and function.

All three types of receptors are normally present in healthy breast cells, and they can be found in most breast-cancer cells as well. Estrogen and progesterone support the growth of more than 60 percent of breast cancer tumors, while 20 to 30 percent of tumors have an excess of HER-2 receptors, which stimulates the cancer cells to divide and grow quickly. Only 10 to 20 percent of breast cancer cases are diagnosed as triple negative.

Since triple-negative tumor cells lack estrogen, progesterone, and HER-2 receptors, they do not respond to many common treatments—like hormone therapy—that interfere with the receptors' work in order to slow the growth of the cancer cells. Chemotherapy has proven effective in treating triple-negative breast cancer, however, and research is underway to find new treatment methods and medications.

"Triple-Negative Breast Cancer," © 2016 Omnigraphics. Reviewed February 2019.

Risks of Triple-Negative Breast Cancer

Unlike most other types of breast cancer, which primarily affect older women, triple-negative breast cancer is more likely to occur before age 40 to 50. It is most common among African American women, who are three times more likely to be affected than white women. Hispanic women also have an elevated risk of developing triple-negative breast cancer compared to white women and Asian women. Although anyone can develop triple-negative breast cancer, it is also the type of cancer that usually affects people with an inherited *BRCA1* genetic mutation, especially if they develop breast cancer before age 50.

Studies have shown that triple-negative breast cancer tends to be more aggressive than other types of breast cancer. It is more likely to recur following treatment and to spread beyond the breast to other parts of the body. These risks are highest within the first three years after treatment, however, and decline to the same rates as other types of breast cancer after that time. Similarly, the five-year survival rates for women with triple-negative breast cancer are lower, at 77 percent, than for women with other types of breast cancer, at 93 percent. But this increased risk of death only pertains for the first five years following diagnosis and then begins to decline.

Triple-negative breast cancer also tends to be a higher grade at diagnosis than other types of breast cancer. The grade of the tumor refers to the degree to which its cells resemble healthy cells, with a higher grade having less resemblance. Finally, triple-negative breast-cancer cells are often a specific subtype called basal-like, meaning that they resemble the basal cells that line the breast ducts. Basal-like cancers are more likely to be aggressive, higher-grade varieties.

Treatment of Triple-Negative Breast Cancer

Since triple-negative breast-cancer cells are not fueled by hormones, this type of cancer does not typically respond well to hormone therapy. The drugs commonly used in hormone therapy—such as tamoxifen, Arimidex (anastrozole), Aromasin (exemestane), Faslodex (fulvestrant), and Femara (letrozole)—are designed to alter the levels of estrogen and progesterone in the body or interfere with the action of receptors in the cells. Likewise, patients with triple-negative breast cancer are not good candidates for medications like Herceptin (trastuzumab) or Tykerb (lapatinib) that target HER-2.

The main forms of treatment for triple-negative breast cancer include surgery, chemotherapy, and radiation therapy. On the plus side, research suggests that breast cancers that test negative for hormone receptors may respond better to chemotherapy than other types of breast cancer. Some studies have also shown positive results for women with triple-negative breast cancer who have neoadjuvant therapy, which involves undergoing chemotherapy prior to surgery. The results indicated that two-thirds of patients with locally advanced triple-negative tumors had no evidence of disease following the initial chemotherapy. In addition, their survival rates were similar to those of women with other types of breast cancer.

Research is ongoing to find new and better approaches to treating triple-negative breast cancer. Clinical trials of some targeted therapies have shown promising results. Unlike traditional therapies such as radiation and chemotherapy that affect all fast-growing cells—both healthy cells and cancer cells—targeted therapies are designed to interfere with a specific process that fuels the growth of cancer cells without affecting healthy cells. Although hormone therapy is not effective for triple-negative breast cancer, some of the other targeted therapies that are under development include:

- **Poly ADP-ribose polymerase (PARP) inhibitors.** PARP is an enzyme that repairs damage to DNA in cells. By interfering with this process, PARP inhibitors make it more difficult for cancer cells to repair the damage done by chemotherapy drugs, thus making the treatment more effective. Research suggests that women with advanced triple-negative breast cancer may benefit from taking PARP inhibitors such as iniparib or olaparib in combination with chemotherapy.

- **Vascular endothelial growth factor (VEGF) inhibitors.** VEGF is a protein that stimulates the creation of new blood vessels—a process known as "angiogenesis." Cancer tumors rely on angiogenesis to obtain the oxygen and nutrients they need to grow. VEGF inhibitors like Avastin (bevacizumab) and Sutent (sunitinib) block the interaction between VEGF and receptors on blood vessels, thus preventing angiogenesis and tumor growth.

- **Epidermal growth factor receptor (EGFR) therapies.** EGFR is a protein that receives signals that stimulate cell growth. An excess of EGFRs is typical of triple-negative breast-cancer cells. Treatments that target EGFRs, such as Erbitux (cetuximab), attach to the receptors and prevent growth signals from reaching the cancer cells.

Since new medications are still being developed for triple-negative breast cancer, it is important to seek opinions from several doctors and compare their recommendations before choosing a course of treatment.

References

1. "Triple-Negative Breast Cancer," BreastCancer.org, October 23, 2015.

2. "Triple-Negative Breast Cancer," National Breast Cancer Foundation (NBCF), 2015.

Chapter 13

Rare Types of Breast Cancer

Chapter Contents

81

Section 13.1

Familial Breast Cancer

This section includes text excerpted from "Familial Breast Cancer," Genetic and Rare Diseases Information Center (GARD), National Center for Advancing Translational Sciences (NCATS), August 30, 2017.

Familial breast cancer is a cluster of breast cancer within a family. Most cases of breast cancer occur sporadically in people with little to no family history of the condition. Approximately 5 to 10 percent of breast cancer is considered "hereditary" and is thought to be caused by an inherited predisposition to breast cancer that is passed down through a family in an autosomal dominant manner. In some of these families, the underlying genetic cause is not known; however, many of these cases are caused by changes (mutations) in the *BRCA1*, *BRCA2*, *PTEN*, *TP53*, *CDH1*, or *STK11* genes (which are each associated with a unique hereditary cancer syndrome). Additional genes, such as *CHEK2*, *BRIP1*, *RAD51*, and *ATM*, are associated with breast and/or gynecologic cancers in some cases. About 15 to 20 percent of women diagnosed with breast cancer have a significant family history of breast cancer (two or more first-degree or second-degree relatives with breast cancer) but have no identifiable mutation in a gene known to cause a hereditary predisposition to breast cancer. These clusters of breast cancer are likely due to a combination of gene(s) and other shared factors such as environment and lifestyle.

High-risk cancer screening and other preventative measures such as chemoprevention and/or prophylactic surgeries are typically recommended in women who have an increased risk for breast cancer based on their personal and/or family histories.

Causes of Familial Breast Cancer

Most cases of breast cancer occur sporadically in people with little to no family history of the condition. They are due to random changes (mutations) that occur only in the cells of the breast. These mutations (called "somatic mutations") accumulate during a person's lifetime and are not inherited or passed on to future generations.

Approximately 15 to 20 percent of women diagnosed with breast cancer have a significant family history of breast cancer (two or more first-degree or second-degree relatives with breast cancer) but have no identifiable mutation in a gene known to cause a hereditary predisposition to breast cancer. These clusters of breast cancer are likely due to a combination of gene(s) and other shared factors such as environment and lifestyle.

An additional 5 to 10 percent of breast cancer is considered "hereditary." These cases are thought to be caused by an inherited predisposition to breast cancer that is passed down through a family in an autosomal dominant manner. In some of these families, the underlying genetic cause is not known. However, many of these cases are part of a hereditary cancer syndrome. The following cancer syndromes are associated with an increased risk of breast cancer and several other types of cancer:

- Hereditary breast and ovarian cancer syndrome due to mutations in the *BRCA1* or *BRCA2* gene is the commonly known cause of hereditary breast cancer.

- Cowden syndrome is caused by mutations in *PTEN* gene.

- Li Fraumeni syndrome (LFS) is caused by mutations in the *TP53* gene.

- Hereditary Diffuse Gastric Cancer is caused by mutations in the *CDH1* gene.

- Peutz-Jeghers syndrome (PJS) is caused by mutations in the *STK11* gene.

Of note, some research suggests that inherited mutations in several other genes (including *CHEK2*, *BRIP1*, *ATM*, *PALB2*, *RAD51*, *BARD1*, *MRE11A*, *NBN*, and *RAD50*) may also be associated with an increased risk for breast cancer. However, the risk associated with many of these genes is not well understood. Most are termed "moderate- or low-penetrant" genes which mean that, on their own, they would be expected to have a relatively small effect on breast-cancer risk. However, in combination with other genes and/or environmental factors, these genes may lead to a significant risk of breast cancer.

Inheritance of Familial Breast Cancer

Most cases of breast cancer occur sporadically in people with little to no family history of the condition. However, approximately 5 to 10 percent is thought to be inherited in an autosomal dominant manner. In these cases, a person is born with a mutation in a gene known to cause a hereditary predisposition to breast cancer and has a 50 percent chance with each pregnancy of passing along the mutated gene to his or her child. A person only needs a mutation in one copy of the responsible gene in each cell to have an increased risk for breast cancer. In some cases, a person with familial breast cancer inherits the mutation from a parent who has had or has familial breast cancer. Other cases may result from new (*de novo*) mutations in the gene.

An additional 15 to 20 percent of women who are diagnosed with breast cancer have a significant family history of breast cancer (two or more first-degree or second-degree relatives who have or have had breast cancer) but the cancer follows no clear pattern of inheritance. These cases of breast cancer may be due to inherited gene(s), shared factors such as environment and lifestyle, or a combination of all these factors.

Treatment of Familial Breast Cancer

Management of familial breast cancer is generally focused on high-risk cancer screening to allow for early detection and treatment of cancer. In general, the National Comprehensive Cancer Network (NCCN) recommends high-risk breast-cancer screening for women who have:

- A personal and family history suggestive of a hereditary cancer syndrome that is associated with breast cancer, or

- A greater than 20 percent risk of developing breast cancer in their lifetime based largely on family history

The recommended screening protocol includes:

- Breast awareness and breast self-exams

- Clinical breast exams (CBE) every 6 to 12 months beginning at age 30 or individualized based on the earliest breast-cancer diagnosis in the family

- Annual mammogram and breast magnetic resonance imaging (MRI) beginning at age 30 or individualized based on the earliest breast-cancer diagnosis in the family

- Discussion of other risk reduction strategies such as chemoprevention and/or prophylactic surgeries

If the familial breast cancer is part of a known hereditary cancer syndrome, management will also include screening for the other associated cancers.

Section 13.2

Phyllodes Tumor of the Breast

This section includes text excerpted from "Phyllodes
Tumor of the Breast," Genetic and Rare Diseases Information
Center (GARD), National Center for Advancing
Translational Sciences (NCATS), July 4, 2016.

Phyllodes tumors of the breast are rare tumors that start in the connective (stromal) tissue of the breast. They get their name from the leaf-like pattern in which they grow (phyllodes means leaf-like in Greek). They are most common in women in their thirties and forties, although women of any age can be affected. These tumors, which are usually painless, tend to grow quickly, but rarely spread outside of the breast. Most phyllodes tumors are benign. About 1 in 10 are cancerous. The underlying cause of these tumors is unknown. Surgery is the main treatment. Because the tumors can reoccur if they are not removed with enough surrounding tissue, the tumor and at least 1 cm of tissue should be removed. Cancerous phyllodes tumors are often treated with mastectomy. Close follow-up with frequent breast examinations is recommended after surgery.

Other Names: Phyllodes breast tumor; Cystosarcoma phyllodes; Phylloides tumor

Treatment of Phyllodes Tumor of the Breast

Surgery is the main treatment for phyllodes tumors of the breast. This is the case regardless of whether they are benign or malignant. Because these tumors can come back if enough normal tissue is not removed, surgery should involve removing the tumor and at least 1 cm of the surrounding tissue. Some doctors feel that an even wider margin of healthy tissue should be removed (wide excision). Malignant phyllodes tumors may be treated more aggressively, with removal of wider margins of tissue or removal of part or all of the breast (partial or total mastectomy). Because spread to the underarm lymph nodes is rare, it is usually not necessary to remove them.

Phyllodes tumors of the breast do not respond to hormone therapy. Radiation and chemotherapy are not typically used as there is little evidence that these methods are effective for phyllodes tumors.

Because phyllodes tumors can come back, close follow-up with frequent breast examinations and imaging are recommended following surgery. This may include self and clinical breast exams, mammograms, ultrasound of the breast, magnetic resonance imaging (MRI) of the breast, and/or computerized tomography (CT) scans of the chest and abdomen (especially in malignant or metastatic cases).

Prognosis for Phyllodes Tumor of the Breast

Phyllodes tumors that are benign have an excellent prognosis following surgery. However, local recurrence is possible. If the tumor recurs locally, further surgery, including local excision or partial or total mastectomy typically results in a good outcome. The SArcoma and PHYllode Restrospective (SAPHYR) Study reported a three-year survival rate for benign and borderline phyllodes tumors of 100 percent. Other studies have reported similar findings. Malignant tumors have a higher chance of coming back. If the tumor metasticizes, common locations include the lung, mediastinum, and skeleton. The five-year survival rate for malignant phyllodes tumors has been reported to be 60 to 80 percent.

Section 13.3

Other Types of Rare Breast Cancer

This section contains text excerpted from the following sources:
Text under the heading "BRCA2 Hereditary Breast and Ovarian
Cancer Syndrome" is excerpted from "BRCA2 Hereditary Breast and
Ovarian Cancer Syndrome," Genetic and Rare Diseases Information
Center (GARD), National Center for Advancing Translational
Sciences (NCATS), March 10, 2015. Reviewed February 2019;
Text under the heading "Metaplastic Carcinoma of the Breast" is
excerpted from "Metaplastic Carcinoma of the Breast," Genetic
and Rare Diseases Information Center (GARD), National Center
for Advancing Translational Sciences (NCATS), June 22, 2011.
Reviewed February 2019; Text under the heading "Secretory Breast
Carcinoma" is excerpted from "Secretory Breast Carcinoma," Genetic
and Rare Diseases Information Center (GARD), National Center for
Advancing Translational Sciences (NCATS), March 28, 2018.

BRCA2 *Hereditary Breast and Ovarian Cancer Syndrome*

BRCA2 hereditary breast and ovarian cancer syndrome (BRCA2 HBOC) is an inherited condition that is characterized by an increased risk for a variety of different cancers. Women with this condition have a 49 to 55 percent risk of developing breast cancer, a 16 to 18 percent risk of developing ovarian cancer, and a 62 percent risk of developing contralateral breast cancer by age 70. Men have a 6 percent lifetime risk of breast cancer and an increased risk for prostate cancer. Both men and women with BRCA2 HBOC have an elevated risk for pancreatic cancer. BRCA2 HBOC may also be associated with cancers of the stomach, gallbladder, bile duct, esophagus, stomach, fallopian tube, primary peritoneum, and skin; however, these risks are not well defined. This condition is caused by changes (mutations) in the *BRCA2* gene and is inherited in an autosomal dominant manner. Management may include high-risk cancer screening, chemoprevention, and/or prophylactic surgeries.

Other Names: HBOC; Familial susceptibility to breast-ovarian cancer 2; BROVCA2

Metaplastic Carcinoma of the Breast

Metaplastic carcinoma of the breast is a rare form of breast cancer. The exact prevalence is not known. While estimates vary, it is thought to account for less than one percent of all breast cancers. In the broad sense, metaplastic carcinoma of the breast is also genetic. All cancers involve genetic changes in affected cells. Currently, no inherited genetic predisposing risk factors have been identified. The underlying cause of this cancer is unknown.

The tumor cells differ in type from that of the typical ductal or lobular breast cancers. The cells look like skin cells or cells that make bone. Some women experience no early signs or symptoms, while others experience general symptoms of breast cancers, such as new breast lumps. Treatment of metaplastic carcinoma of the breast is similar to that of invasive ductal cancer.

Other Names: Metaplastic breast cancer

Secretory Breast Carcinoma

Secretory breast carcinoma (SBC) is a very rare, slow-growing type of breast cancer. It was originally referred to as "juvenile breast carcinoma" because it was first recognized in children and adolescents. However, many cases reported in the last several decades have occurred in adults of all ages. SBC may occur in males or females but, like other types of breast cancer, it is much more common in females. Signs and symptoms of SBC most commonly include a painless, firm mass in the breast, which may move when palpated. Some people with SBC also have nipple discharge. There is currently no consensus regarding treatment for SBC, and treatment options may depend on the person's age and the size of the tumor. Options may include surgery to remove the tumor or breast (mastectomy), surgery to also remove nearby lymph nodes, radiotherapy, and chemotherapy. SBC may recur in some cases, but when this happens, it is often in the same area of the breast and after a long period of time (called a late "local recurrence"). SBC is usually associated with an excellent prognosis (prolonged survival), even when it spreads (metastasizes) to the lymph nodes. The risk for SBC to spread to other parts of the body is thought to be extremely low.

Other Names: SBC; Juvenile breast carcinoma (formerly); Juvenile breast cancer (formerly); Secretory carcinoma of the breast.

Part Three

Risk Factors, Symptoms, and Prevention of Breast Cancer

Chapter 14

An Overview on Risk Factors and Symptoms of Breast Cancer

Chapter Contents

Section 14.1

Risk Factors of Breast Cancer

This section includes text excerpted from "What Are the
Risk Factors for Breast Cancer?" Centers for Disease
Control and Prevention (CDC), September 11, 2018.

Breast cancer is a disease in which malignant (cancer) cells form in
the tissues of the breast. Studies have shown that your risk for breast
cancer is due to a combination of factors. The main factors that influence your risk include being a woman and getting older. Most breast
cancers are found in women who are 50 years old or older.

Some women will get breast cancer even without any other risk factors that they know of. Having a risk factor does not mean you will get
the disease, and not all risk factors have the same effect. Most women
have some risk factors, but most women do not get breast cancer. If
you have breast-cancer risk factors, talk with your doctor about ways
you can lower your risk and about screening for breast cancer.

Risk Factors You Cannot Change

There are certain risk factors that you cannot change. It include:

- **Getting older.** The risk for breast cancer increases with age;
  most breast cancers are diagnosed after age 50.

- **Genetic mutations.** Inherited changes (mutations) to certain
  genes, such as *BRCA1* and *BRCA2*. Women who have inherited
  these genetic changes are at higher risk of breast and ovarian
  cancer.

- **Reproductive history**. Early menstrual periods before age 12
  and starting menopause after age 55 expose women to hormones
  longer, raising their risk of getting breast cancer.

- **Having-dense breasts.** Dense breasts have more connective
  tissue than fatty tissue, which can sometimes make it hard to
  see tumors on a mammogram. Women with dense breasts are
  more likely to get breast cancer.

- **Personal history of breast cancer or certain
  noncancerous breast diseases.** Women who have had breast
  cancer are more likely to get breast cancer a second time. Some
  noncancerous breast diseases such as atypical hyperplasia or

lobular carcinoma *in situ* (LCIS) are associated with a higher risk of getting breast cancer.

- **Family history of breast cancer.** A woman's risk for breast cancer is higher if she has a mother, sister, or daughter (first-degree relative) or multiple family members on either her mother's or father's side of the family who has had breast cancer. Having a first-degree male relative with breast cancer also raises a woman's risk.

- **Previous treatment using radiation therapy.** Women who had radiation therapy to the chest or breasts (for treatment of Hodgkin lymphoma (HL) before age 30, etc.) have a higher risk of getting breast cancer later in life.

- Women who took the drug diethylstilbestrol (DES), which was given to some pregnant women in the United States between 1940 and 1971 to prevent miscarriage, have a higher risk. Women whose mothers took DES while pregnant with them are also at risk.

Risk Factors You Can Change

There are certain risk factors that you can change. It includes:

- **Not being physically active.** Women who are not physically active have a higher risk of getting breast cancer.

- **Being overweight or obese after menopause.** Older women who are overweight or obese have a higher risk of getting breast cancer than those at a normal weight.

- **Taking hormones.** Some forms of hormone-replacement therapy (HRT) (those that include both estrogen and progesterone) taken during menopause can raise risk for breast cancer when taken for more than five years. Certain oral contraceptives (OCs) (birth control pills) also have been found to raise breast-cancer risk.

- **Reproductive history.** Having the first pregnancy after age 30, not breastfeeding, and never having a full-term pregnancy can raise breast-cancer risk.

- **Drinking alcohol.** Studies show that a woman's risk for breast cancer increases the more alcohol she drinks.

Research suggests that other factors such as smoking, being exposed to chemicals that can cause cancer, and changes in other hormones due to night shift working also may increase breast-cancer risk.

Section 14.2

Symptoms of Breast Cancer

This section includes text excerpted from "What Are the Symptoms of
Breast Cancer?" Centers for Disease Control and Prevention (CDC),
September 11, 2018.

What Are the Symptoms of Breast Cancer?

Different people have different symptoms of breast cancer. Some
people do not have any signs or symptoms at all.

Some warning signs of breast cancer are:

- New lump in the breast or underarm (armpit)

- Thickening or swelling of part of the breast

- Irritation or dimpling of breast skin

- Redness or flaky skin in the nipple area or the breast

- Pulling in of the nipple or pain in the nipple area

- Nipple discharge other than breast milk, including blood

- Any change in the size or the shape of the breast

- Pain in any area of the breast

Breast pain can be a symptom of cancer.

Keep in mind that these symptoms can happen with other conditions that are not cancer. If you have any symptoms that worry you,
be sure to see your doctor right away.

What Is a Normal Breast?

No breast is typical. What is normal for you may not be normal for
another woman. Most women say their breasts feel lumpy or uneven.
The way your breasts look and feel can be affected by getting your
period, having children, losing or gaining weight, and taking certain
medications. Breasts also tend to change as you age.

What Do Lumps in Your Breast Mean?

Many conditions can cause lumps in the breast, including cancer.
But most breast lumps are caused by other medical conditions. The

two most common causes of breast lumps are fibrocystic breast condition and cysts. The fibrocystic condition causes noncancerous changes in the breast that can make them lumpy, tender, and sore. Cysts are small fluid-filled sacs that can develop in the breast.

Chapter 15

Family History and Risk of Breast Cancer

If you have close relatives with breast, you may be at higher risk for developing these diseases. Does your family health history put you at higher risk? Would you benefit from cancer genetic counseling and testing?

Each year, about 242,000 women in the United States are diagnosed with breast cancer. About 3 percent of breast cancers (about 7,300 women per year) result from inherited mutations (changes) in the *BRCA1* and *BRCA2* genes that are passed on in families. Inherited mutations in other genes can also cause breast, but *BRCA1* and *BRCA2* are the genes most commonly affected. Although breast cancer is much more common in women, men with *BRCA1* or *BRCA2* mutations are more likely to get breast cancer than other men. *BRCA* mutations also increase the likelihood of getting pancreatic cancer and, in men, high-grade prostate cancer. Knowing your family health history can help you find out if you could be more likely to develop breast and other cancers. If so, you can take steps to prevent cancer or to detect it earlier when it may be more treatable.

This chapter includes text excerpted from "Does Breast or Ovarian Cancer Run in Your Family?" Centers for Disease Control and Prevention (CDC), October 16, 2018.

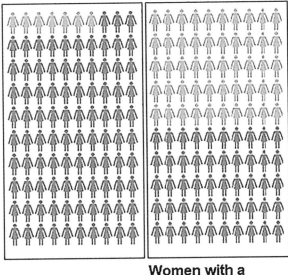

Women in the U.S. General Population

Women with a BRCA1 or BRCA2 Mutation

Figure 15.1. *Breast-Cancer Risk*

Does Your Family Health History Put You at Risk?

Collect your family health history of breast and other cancers and share this information with your doctor. You can inherit *BRCA* and other mutations from your mother or your father, so be sure to include information from both sides of your family. Include your close relatives: parents, sisters, brothers, children, grandparents, aunts, uncles, nieces, nephews, and grandchildren. If you have had breast or other cancers, make sure that your family members know about your diagnosis.

Tell your doctor if you have a personal or family health history of any of the following:

- Breast cancer, especially at a younger age (age 50 or younger)

- Triple-negative breast cancer (TNBC) at age 60 or younger in women (Triple-negative cancers are a type of breast cancer that lack estrogen receptors (ER), progesterone receptors (PR) and human epidermal growth factor receptor 2 (HER2))

- Cancer in both breasts

- Breast cancer in a male relative

- Ovarian, fallopian tube, or primary peritoneal cancer (PPC)

- Pancreatic cancer or high-grade prostate cancer

- Breast, ovarian, pancreatic, or high-grade prostate cancer among multiple blood relatives

- Ashkenazi (Eastern European) Jewish ancestry

- A known *BRCA* mutation in the family

You can use the *Know: BRCA tool* to collect your family health-history information, assess your risk for *BRCA* mutations, and share this information with your doctor. Update your family health history on a regular basis and let your doctor know if any new cases of breast cancer occur.

Cancer Risks for Women with **BRCA1 / BRCA2** Mutations

Women who inherit a mutation in the *BRCA1 or BRCA2* gene have a much higher risk of developing breast cancer. But, important steps can be taken to help lower the risk of cancer in these women. It's important to know that not everyone who inherits a *BRCA1 or BRCA2* mutation will get breast cancer and that not all inherited forms of breast cancer are due to mutations in *BRCA1* and *BRCA2*.

Table 15.1. Breast-Cancer Risk

Women in the U.S. General Population	Women with a *BRCA1* or *BRCA2* Mutation
About 7 out of 100 women in the U.S. general population will get breast cancer by age 70.	About 50 out of 100 women with a *BRCA1* or *BRCA2* mutation will get breast cancer by age 70.
About 93 out of 100 of these women will NOT get breast cancer by age 70.	About 50 out of 100 of these women will NOT get breast cancer by age 70.

What Can You Do If You Are Concerned about Your Risk?

If your doctor decides that your family health history makes you more likely to get breast, ovarian, and other cancers, he or she may refer you for genetic counseling. Even if your doctor doesn't recommend genetic testing and counseling, your family health history of breast cancer can affect when you start mammography screening. If you are a woman with a parent, sibling, or child with breast cancer, you are at higher risk for breast cancer. Based on current recommendations, you should consider talking to your doctor about starting mammography screening in your forties.

The genetic counselor can use your family health-history information to determine your possible cancer risks and whether you might consider *BRCA genetic testing* to find out if you have a *BRCA1* or *BRCA2* mutation. Genetic testing is most useful if first performed on someone in your family who has had breast cancer. If this relative has a *BRCA1* or *BRCA2* mutation, then her close relatives can be offered to test for that mutation. If she does not have a *BRCA1* or *BRCA2* mutation, then her relatives may not need to be tested. Remember that most breast cancer is not caused by *BRCA* mutations so most women don't need *BRCA* genetic testing.

The genetic counselor can discuss the pros and cons of testing and what possible test results could mean for you and your family. It is important to note that genetic testing for *BRCA* mutations will not find all the causes of hereditary breast cancer. In some cases, the genetic counselor might recommend genetic testing using a panel that looks for mutations in several genes in addition to *BRCA1* and *BRCA2*. *BRCA* genetic counseling and testing is often, but not always, covered without cost sharing by many health plans under the Affordable Care Act (ACA).

Chapter 16

Women with Inherited Breast-Cancer Risk Face Numerous Challenges

As genetic testing for hereditary cancer has become more widespread, researchers are grappling with questions about the impact this information will have on individuals, their families and the healthcare system. Will individuals understand their genetic test results, particularly if the results are not definitive? Will the information affect how individuals manage their health? Are healthcare professionals ready to help at-risk individuals make informed choices about their care? How will an already overburdened healthcare system incorporate this information into the standard of care?

This chapter spotlights a Swiss study on women who are at increased risk for inherited breast cancer and the long-term challenges they face in managing their care. It also identifies some of the challenges of providing care to at-risk individuals and highlights opportunities for improved models of care.

According to a study published in *Genetics in Medicine*, Maria Caiata-Zufferey, Ph.D. at the University of Geneva in Switzerland and a team of Swiss researchers from four different genetic-counseling

This chapter includes text excerpted from "Women with Inherited Breast Cancer Risk Face Numerous Challenges," National Human Genome Research Institute (NHGRI), November 2, 2015. Reviewed February 2019.

centers interviewed a group of 32 French- and Italian- speaking women who carried the breast-cancer genes 1 and 2 (*BRCA1/BRCA2*). The study's supporting statistics state that a woman carrying *BRCA1* and *BRCA2* mutations has a significant probability of developing breast or ovarian cancer (as high as 75%) within her lifetime, and these mutations account for 20 to 25 percent of all inherited breast cancers.

Researchers interviewed women, ages 26 to 60, who were unaffected by disease and had known of their positive mutation status for at least 3 years. Participants generally viewed the recommended health guidelines in two ways: as a rational and moral responsibility (i.e., something they were obligated to follow) or as a questionable option (i.e., something ambiguous and uncertain at times).

The Swiss guidelines for managing health and minimizing breast or ovarian cancer in at-risk individuals include:

- Breast exams and breast magnetic resonance imaging (MRI)

- Mammograms

- Transvaginal ultrasounds and blood tests

- Removal of the fallopian tubes and ovaries

- Removal of the breasts

Women who felt strongly that they should adhere to the medical guidelines were influenced by a number of psychosocial factors, including: pressure from healthcare providers to minimize their cancer risk; a duty to stay healthy for their families; the desire to be a role model to family members who may have inherited the same mutations; and a personal desire to overcome their genetic risk.

At the same time, these women felt confused about the appropriate way to deal with genetic risk for several reasons:

- Contradictory views of healthcare professionals who were part of the care team (gynecologists, radiologists, surgeons and medical geneticists in collaboration with a primary care physician)

- Poorly informed specialists or physicians who developed their own interpretation of the care guidelines

- The possible impact on life events such as maternity and breastfeeding

- No guarantee that the recommended care would reduce the risk of developing breast cancer

Participants found it difficult to actively pursue their health programs for several other reasons. Because the women weren't sick, it was up to them to organize their medical exams and decide how to proceed, sometimes without adequate input from their physicians. Because of the personal nature of the disease, the women found it difficult to connect and share information with others undergoing the same experience. And because the women weren't sick, healthcare professionals classified them as "not urgent cases" for appointments or feedback on screening results.

Other studies have noted that primary care physicians have the greatest contact with patients and are likely to be the first provider asked about genetic testing. However, most primary care physicians are not trained in medical genetics, diagnostic testing, and genetic counseling. Thus, it's important that healthcare professionals are educated in the scientific, interpersonal and ethical issues related to genetic testing; improve communication with at-risk individuals; and apply evidence-based care guidelines consistently, the Swiss researchers wrote. Women with the *BRCA1/BRCA2* mutation would also benefit from multi-disciplinary hereditary cancer clinics that could provide specialized information, emotional support and knowledge from women with similar conditions, concluded the researchers.

Chapter 17

Reproductive History and Breast-Cancer Risk

Is There a Relationship between Pregnancy and Breast-Cancer Risk?

Studies have shown that a woman's risk of developing breast cancer is related to her exposure to hormones that are produced by her ovaries (endogenous estrogen (ER) and progesterone (PR)). Reproductive factors that increase the duration and/or levels of exposure to ovarian hormones, which stimulate cell growth, have been associated with an increase in breast-cancer risk. These factors include early onset of menstruation, late onset of menopause, and factors that may allow breast tissue to be exposed to high levels of hormones for longer periods of time, such as later age at first pregnancy and never having given birth.

Conversely, pregnancy and breastfeeding, which both reduce a woman's lifetime number of menstrual cycles and thus her cumulative exposure to endogenous hormones, are associated with a decrease in breast-cancer risk. In addition, pregnancy and breastfeeding have direct effects on breast cells, causing them to differentiate, or mature, so they can produce milk. Some researchers hypothesize that these differentiated cells are more resistant to becoming transformed into cancer cells than cells that have not undergone differentiation.

This chapter includes text excerpted from "Reproductive History and Cancer Risk," National Cancer Institute (NCI), November 9, 2016.

105

Are Any Pregnancy-Related Factors Associated with a Lower Risk of Breast Cancer?

Some pregnancy-related factors have been associated with a reduced risk of developing breast cancer later in life. These factors include:

- **Early age at first full-term pregnancy.** Women who have their first full-term pregnancy at an early age have a decreased risk of developing breast cancer later in life. For example, in women who have a first full-term pregnancy before age 20, the risk of developing breast cancer is about half that of women whose first full-term pregnancy occurs after the age of 30. This risk reduction is limited to hormone receptor-positive breast cancer; age at first full-term pregnancy does not appear to affect the risk of hormone receptor-negative breast cancer.

- **Increasing number of births.** The risk of breast cancer declines with the number of children born. Women who have given birth to five or more children have half the breast-cancer risk of women who have not given birth. Some evidence indicates that the reduced risk associated with a higher number of births may be limited to hormone receptor-positive breast cancer.

- **History of preeclampsia.** Women who have had preeclampsia may have a decreased risk of developing breast cancer. Preeclampsia is a complication of pregnancy in which a woman develops high blood pressure and excess amounts of protein in her urine. Scientists are studying whether certain hormones and proteins associated with preeclampsia may affect breast-cancer risk.

- **Longer duration of breastfeeding.** Breastfeeding for an extended period (at least a year) is associated with decreased risks of both hormone receptor–positive and hormone receptor-negative breast cancers.

Are Any Pregnancy-Related Factors Associated with an Increase in Breast-Cancer Risk?

Some factors related to pregnancy may increase the risk of breast cancer. These factors include:

- **Older age at birth of first child.** The older a woman is when she has her first full-term pregnancy, the higher her risk of breast cancer. Women who are older than 30 when they give birth to their first child have a higher risk of breast cancer than women who have never given birth.

- **Recent childbirth.** Women who have recently given birth have a short-term increase in breast-cancer risk that declines after about 10 years. The reason for this temporary increase is not known, but some researchers believe that it may be due to the effect of high levels of hormones on the development of cancers or to the rapid growth of breast cells during pregnancy.

- **Taking diethylstilbestrol (DES) during pregnancy.** DES is a synthetic form of estrogen that was used between the early 1940s and 1971 to prevent miscarriages and other pregnancy problems. Women who took DES during pregnancy may have a slightly higher risk of developing breast cancer than women who did not take DES during pregnancy. Some studies have shown that daughters of women who took DES during pregnancy may also have a slightly higher risk of developing breast cancer after age 40 than women who were not exposed to DES while in the womb, but the evidence is inconsistent.

Is Abortion Linked to Breast-Cancer Risk?

A few retrospective (case-control) studies reported in the mid-1990s suggested that induced abortion (the deliberate ending of a pregnancy) was associated with an increased risk of breast cancer. However, these studies had important design limitations that could have affected the results. A key limitation was their reliance on self-reporting of medical history information by the study participants, which can introduce bias. Prospective studies, which are more rigorous in design and unaffected by such bias, have consistently shown no association between induced abortion and breast-cancer risk. Moreover, the Committee on Gynecologic Practice of the American College of Obstetricians and Gynecologists (ACOG) concluded that "more rigorous studies demonstrate no causal relationship between induced abortion and a subsequent increase in breast-cancer risk." Major findings from these studies include:

- Women who have had an induced abortion have the same risk of breast cancer as other women

- Women who have had a spontaneous abortion (miscarriage) have the same risk of breast cancer as other women

• Cancers other than breast cancer also appear to be unrelated to a history of induced or spontaneous abortion

Does Fertility Treatment Affect the Risk of Breast Cancers?

Women who have difficulty becoming pregnant or carrying a pregnancy to term may receive fertility treatment. Such treatment can include surgery (to repair diseased, damaged, or blocked fallopian tubes or to remove uterine fibroids, patches of endometriosis, or adhesions); medications to stimulate ovulation, and assisted reproductive technology (ART).

Ovarian stimulation and some assisted reproductive technologies involve treatments that temporarily change the levels of estrogen and progesterone in a woman's body. For example, women undergoing in vitro fertilization (IVF) receive multiple rounds of hormone treatment to first suppress ovulation until the developing eggs are ready, then stimulate the development of multiple eggs, and finally promote maturation of the eggs. The use of hormones in some fertility treatments has raised concerns about possible increased risks of cancer, particularly cancers that are linked to elevated levels of these hormones.

Many studies have examined possible associations between the use of fertility drugs or IVF and the risks of breast, ovarian, and endometrial cancers. The results of such studies can be hard to interpret because infertility itself is linked to increased risks of these cancers (that is, compared with fertile women, infertile women are at higher risk of these cancers even if they do not use fertility drugs). Also, these cancers are relatively rare and tend to develop years after treatment for infertility, which can make it difficult to link their occurrence to past use of fertility drugs.

The bulk of the evidence is consistent with no increased risk of breast cancer associated with the use of fertility drugs or IVF.

Chapter 18

The Role of Estrogen in Breast-Cancer Development

Estrogen refers to three related hormones—estrone, estradiol, and estriol—that are primarily responsible for female sexual and reproductive development. Like all hormones, estrogen is a chemical substance that circulates in the bloodstream, binds to receptors on certain cells, and carries messages that influence the growth and function of organs and tissues. In women, estrogen is produced in the ovaries, adrenal glands, liver, and fat tissues. Estrogen plays an important role in breast development, menstruation, pregnancy, lactation, bone growth, and many other processes. Although males do produce some estrogen, its role in the male body is not well understood.

Importance of Estrogen

The role of estrogen in the female body changes throughout the lifespan. Estradiol is mainly produced in the ovaries and is the dominant form of estrogen during the reproductive years. Estriol is produced by the placenta during pregnancy and controls many of the bodily changes that support childbearing. Estrone becomes the most abundant form of estrogen in the bodies of women who have reached menopause when

"The Role of Estrogen in Breast-Cancer Development," © 2016 Omnigraphics. Reviewed February 2019.

menstruation stops and estrogen production declines. Some of the major functions of estrogen include:

- Developing breasts and other secondary sex characteristics at the onset of puberty

- Regulating the menstrual cycle (the ovaries produce estrogen during the first part of the cycle to prepare the lining of the uterus to receive a fertilized egg; if fertilization does not occur, estrogen levels drop sharply, causing the uterine lining to break down and menstruation to occur)

- Controlling lactation and other changes to the breasts during pregnancy

- Breaking down and rebuilding bones

- Maintaining vaginal lubrication and the strength and thickness of the vaginal wall

- Regulating brain chemistry that affects mood and helping to control inflammation in the brain that leads to neurodegenerative disorders

- Affecting blood clotting and cholesterol levels

Changes in Estrogen Levels

Estrogen levels in the bloodstream change naturally over time. They increase at puberty and during pregnancy, for instance, and they decrease while breastfeeding and after menopause. The decline in estrogen production that occurs with menopause can cause a variety of symptoms, including:

- Irregular menstrual cycles

- Hot flashes and night sweats

- Vaginal dryness

- Loss of sex drive

- Bone loss (osteoporosis)

- Trouble sleeping

- Anxiety and mood swings

Declining estrogen levels can also result from other health conditions besides menopause, such as diminished function of the ovaries (hypogonadism), polycystic ovary syndrome, nonalcoholic fatty liver disease, or anorexia nervosa.

Estrogen Therapy

Estrogen is used in a number of different medications. It can be found in most oral contraceptives, for instance, because maintaining steady estrogen levels throughout the menstrual cycle prevents ovulation from occurring. Birth control pills containing estrogen are also prescribed to help regulate menstrual cycles and relieve menstrual cramps. Estrogen hormone therapy is also used to treat the delayed onset of puberty, and to help transgender women achieve the physical changes that are important in the transition from male to female.

Hormone-replacement therapy (HRT) was once used extensively to relieve the symptoms of menopause and reduce the risk of chronic health conditions related to decreasing estrogen levels, such as osteoporosis and heart disease. In the early 2000s, however, studies showed that HRT led to an increased risk of breast cancer, stroke, and blood clots. The U.S. Food and Drug Administration (FDA) responded by changing its guidelines regarding HRT. Doctors are now encouraged to prescribe estrogen at the lowest possible dose and for the shortest possible length of time to achieve treatment goals.

Experts saw a significant drop in cases of breast cancer in postmenopausal women over age 50 as soon as the new guidelines went into effect. They attributed the change to the role of estrogen in breast-cancer development. Like many other cells, some potentially cancerous cells contain estrogen receptors. When estrogen circulating through the bloodstream attaches to these cells, it causes them to divide and grow. Without estrogen, the cells would stop growing and eventually die.

Estrogen and Breast Cancer

Since the majority of breast cancers are estrogen-receptor positive (ER+), researchers believe that increasing estrogen levels through HRT may promote tumor growth. Conversely, treatments aimed at blocking estrogen production or reducing estrogen levels may help slow the progression of breast cancer or prevent recurrence following surgery.

Given the relationship between estrogen and breast cancer, doctors have identified a number of circumstances that tend to raise estrogen levels or extend exposure to estrogen over the lifespan, and thus may increase the risk of developing breast cancer. Some of these circumstances include:

- Early onset of menstruation (before age 12)

- Taking oral contraceptives

- Never becoming pregnant, or giving birth to a first child after age 35

- Not breastfeeding

- Late onset of menopause (after age 55)

- Using HRT during menopause

- Being overweight, especially after menopause

- Exposure to synthetic estrogens in the environment, through absorption of chemicals found in some plastics, cleaning products, pesticides, herbicides, skin creams, and sunscreens

References

1. Bradford, Alina. "What Is Estrogen?" Live Science, March 29, 2016.

2. "Estrogen and Breast Cancer," Cancer Compass, 2016.

3. Manson, Joann E. "Estrogen," HealthyWomen, July 28, 2015.

Chapter 19

Diethylstilbestrol and Breast-Cancer Risk

Diethylstilbestrol (DES) is a synthetic form of the female hormone estrogen. It was prescribed to pregnant women between 1940 and 1971 to prevent miscarriage, premature labor, and related complications of pregnancy. The use of DES declined after studies in the 1950s showed that it was not effective in preventing these problems.

In 1971, researchers linked prenatal (before birth) DES exposure to a type of cancer of the cervix and vagina called clear cell adenocarcinoma in a small group of women. Soon after, the U.S. Food and Drug Administration (FDA) notified physicians throughout the country that DES should not be prescribed to pregnant women. The drug continued to be prescribed to pregnant women in Europe until 1978.

DES is now known to be an endocrine-disrupting chemical, one of a number of substances that interfere with the endocrine system to cause cancer, birth defects, and other developmental abnormalities. The effects of endocrine-disrupting chemicals are most severe when exposure occurs during fetal development.

This chapter includes text excerpted from "Diethylstilbestrol (DES) and Cancer," National Cancer Institute (NCI), October 5, 2011. Reviewed February 2019.

Cancer Risk among Women Who Were Exposed to Diethylstilbestrol before Birth

The daughters of women who used DES while pregnant—commonly called "DES daughters"—have about 40 times the risk of developing clear cell adenocarcinoma of the lower genital tract than unexposed women. However, this type of cancer is still rare; approximately 1 in 1,000 DES daughters develops it.

The first DES daughters who were diagnosed with clear cell adeno-carcinoma were very young at the time of their diagnoses. Subsequent research has shown that the risk of developing this disease remains elevated as women age into their forties.

DES daughters have an increased risk of developing abnormal cells in the cervix and the vagina that are precursors of cancer (dysplasia, cervical intraepithelial neoplasia (CIN), and squamous intraepithelial lesions). These abnormal cells resemble cancer cells, but they do not invade nearby healthy tissue and are not cancer. They may develop into cancer, however, if left untreated. Scientists estimated that DES-exposed daughters were 2.2 times more likely to have these abnormal cell changes in the cervix than unexposed women. Approximately four percent of DES daughters developed these conditions because of their exposure. It has been recommended that DES daughters have a yearly Papanicolaou (Pap) test and pelvic exam to check for abnormal cells.

DES daughters may also have a slightly increased risk of breast cancer after age 40. A study from the United States suggested that, overall, breast-cancer risk is not increased in DES daughters, but that, after age 40, DES daughters have approximately twice the risk of breast cancer as unexposed women of the same age and with similar risk factors. However, another study from Europe found no difference in breast-cancer risk between DES daughters and unexposed women and no difference in overall cancer risk. A 2011 study found that about two percent of a large cohort of DES daughters has developed breast cancer due to their exposure.

DES daughters should be aware of these health risks, share their medical history with their doctors, and get regular physical examinations.

Health Problems Women Who Took Diethylstilbestrol during Pregnancy Might Have

Women who used DES may have a slight increase in the risk of developing and dying from breast cancer compared with women who did not use DES. No evidence exists to suggest that women who took DES are at higher risk for any other type of cancer.

What Diethylstilbestrol-Exposed Daughters Should Do

Women who know or believe they were exposed to DES before birth should be aware of the health effects of DES and inform their doctor about their possible exposure. It has been recommended that exposed women have an annual medical examination to check for the adverse health effects of DES. A thorough examination may include the following:

- **Pelvic examination**
- **Pap test and colposcopy.** A routine cervical Pap test is not adequate for DES daughters. The Pap test must gather cells from the cervix and the vagina. It is also good for a clinician to see the cervix and vaginal walls. They may use a colposcope to follow up if there are any abnormal findings.
- **Biopsy—breast examinations.** It is recommended that DES daughters continue to rigorously follow the routine breast-cancer screening recommendations for their age group.

What Diethylstilbestrol-Exposed Mothers Should Do

A woman who took DES while pregnant or who suspects she may have taken it should inform her doctor. She should try to learn the dosage, when the medication was started, and how it was used. She also should inform her children who were exposed before birth so that this information can be included in their medical records.

It is recommended that DES-exposed mothers have regular breast-cancer screenings and yearly medical check-ups that include a pelvic examination and a Pap test.

Chapter 20

Oral Contraceptives and Breast-Cancer Risk

What Are Oral Contraceptives?

Oral contraceptives (OC) (birth control pills) are hormone-containing medications that are taken by mouth to prevent pregnancy. They prevent pregnancy by inhibiting ovulation and also by preventing sperm from penetrating through the cervix.

By far the most commonly prescribed type of OC in the United States contains synthetic versions of the natural female hormones estrogen and progesterone. This type of birth control pill is often called a "combined oral contraceptive (COC)." Another type of OC, sometimes called the "mini-pill," contains only progestin, which is a human-made version of progesterone.

What Is Known about the Relationship between Oral Contraceptive Use and Breast Cancer?

Nearly all the research on the link between OCs and cancer risk comes from observational studies, both large prospective cohort studies, and population-based case-control studies. Data from observational studies cannot definitively establish that an exposure—in

This chapter includes text excerpted from "Oral Contraceptives and Cancer Risk," National Cancer Institute (NCI), February 22, 2018.

this case, OCs—causes (or prevents) cancer. That is because women who take OCs may differ from those who don't take them in ways other than their OC use, and it is possible that these other differences—rather than OC use—are what explains their different cancer risk.

Overall, however, these studies have provided consistent evidence that the risks of breast and cervical cancers are increased in women who use OCs.

An analysis of data from more than 150,000 women who participated in 54 epidemiologic studies showed that, overall, women who had ever used OCs had a slight (7%) increase in the relative risk of breast cancer compared with women who had never used OCs. Women who were currently using OCs had a 24 percent increase in risk that did not increase with the duration of use. Risk declined after use of OCs stopped, and no risk increase was evident by 10 years after use had stopped.

A 2010 analysis of data from the Nurses' Health Study (NHS), which has been following more than 116,000 female nurses who were 24- to 43- years old when they enrolled in the study in 1989, also found that participants who used OCs had a slight increase in breast-cancer risk. However, nearly all of the increased risk was seen among women who took a specific type of OC, a "triphasic" pill, in which the dose of hormones is changed in 3 stages over the course of a woman's monthly cycle. An elevated risk associated with specific triphasic formulations was also reported in a nested case-control (NCC) study that used electronic medical records to verify OC use.

In 2017, a large prospective Danish study reported breast cancer risks associated with formulations of OCs. Overall, women who were using or had stopped using oral combined hormone contraceptives (CHC) had a modest (about 20%) increase in the relative risk of breast cancer compared with women who had never used OCs. The risk increase varied from 0 to 60 percent, depending on the specific type of oral CHC. The risk of breast cancer also increased the longer OCs were used.

How Could Oral Contraceptives Influence Breast-Cancer Risk?

Naturally occurring estrogen and progesterone stimulate the development and growth of some cancers (e.g., cancers that express receptors for these hormones, such as breast cancer). Because birth control pills contain synthetic versions of these female hormones, they could potentially also increase cancer risk.

Chapter 21

Menopausal Hormone Therapy and Breast-Cancer Risk

What Is Menopausal Hormone Therapy?

Menopausal hormone therapy (MHT)—also called "postmenopausal hormone therapy" and "hormone-replacement therapy"—is a treatment that doctors may recommend to relieve common symptoms of menopause and to address long-term biological changes, such as bone loss, that result from declining levels of the natural hormones estrogen and progesterone in a woman's body during and after menopause.

MHT usually involves treatment with estrogen alone or estrogen plus progestin, a synthetic hormone whose effects are similar to those of progesterone.

Women who have a uterus—that is, who have not had a hysterectomy—are generally prescribed estrogen plus progestin for MHT. This is because estrogen alone is associated with an increased risk of endometrial cancer, but estrogen plus progestin is not. Estrogen is used alone only in women who have had a hysterectomy.

This chapter includes text excerpted from "Menopausal Hormone Therapy and Cancer," National Cancer Institute (NCI), July 17, 2018.

What Are the Health Effects of Menopausal Hormone Therapy?

Women who took estrogen alone had a lower risk of breast cancer than women who took placebo. After nearly 11 years of follow-up, the risk of breast cancer among women who took estrogen alone remained lower than that among women who took placebo.

Women who took estrogen plus progestin were more likely to be diagnosed with breast cancer than women who took placebo. The breast cancers in these women were larger and more likely to have spread to the lymph nodes by the time they were diagnosed. The risk of breast cancer was greater the longer women took the combined hormone therapy, but it decreased markedly when hormone use stopped.

These studies also showed that both combination and estrogen-alone hormone use made mammography less effective for the early detection of breast cancer. Women taking hormones needed more repeat mammograms to check on abnormalities found in a screening mammogram and more breast biopsies to determine whether abnormalities detected in mammograms were cancer.

An ancillary study of the Women's Health Initiative (WHI) showed that use of combination hormone therapy was associated with increases in the amount of dense breast tissue seen on a mammogram. Dense breasts are a risk factor for breast cancer. The results of a case-control study nested within the WHI showed that the increase in mammographic density in the first year after women started taking estrogen plus progestin accounted for all of the subsequent increase in their breast-cancer risk.

There were more deaths from breast cancer, as well as from all causes, following a diagnosis of breast cancer among women who took estrogen plus progestin than among women who took placebo. During 18 years of follow up, there were more breast-cancer deaths among women who took combined hormone therapy, and fewer breast-cancer deaths among women who took estrogen alone, compared with women who took placebo.

Is It Safe for Women Who Have Had a Breast-Cancer Diagnosis to Take Menopausal Hormone Therapy?

One of the roles of naturally occurring estrogen is to promote the normal growth of cells in the breast and uterus. Some cancers also use estrogen to promote their growth. Thus, it is generally believed that

MHT may promote further tumor growth in women who have already been diagnosed with breast cancer. However, studies of MHT use in breast-cancer survivors have produced conflicting results, with some studies showing an increased risk of breast-cancer recurrence and others showing no increased risk of recurrence.

Chapter 22

Dense Breasts and Risk of Breast Cancer

Frequently Asked Questions on Dense Breasts and Risk of Breast Cancer
What Are Dense Breasts?

Breasts contain glandular, connective, and fat tissue. Breast density is a term that describes the relative amount of these different types of breast tissue as seen on a mammogram. Dense breasts have relatively high amounts of glandular tissue and fibrous connective tissue and relatively low amounts of fatty breast tissue.

How Do You Know If You Have Dense Breasts?

Only a mammogram can show if a woman has dense breasts. Dense breast tissue cannot be felt in a clinical breast exam (CBE) or in a breast self-exam. For this reason, dense breasts are sometimes referred to as "mammographically dense breasts."

How Common Are Dense Breasts?

Nearly half of all women age 40 and older who get mammograms are found to have dense breasts. Breast density is often inherited, but

This chapter includes text excerpted from "Dense Breasts: Answers to Commonly Asked Questions," National Cancer Institute (NCI), September 7, 2018.

other factors can influence it. Factors associated with lower breast density include increasing age, having children, and using tamoxifen. Factors associated with higher breast density include using postmenopausal hormone-replacement therapy (PMHRT) and having a low body mass index (BMI).

How Is Breast Density Categorized?

Doctors use the Breast Imaging Reporting and Data System, called "BI-RADS," to group different types of breast density. This system, developed by the American College of Radiology (ACR), helps doctors to interpret and report back mammogram findings. Doctors who review mammograms are called "radiologists." BI-RADS classifies breast density into four categories, as follows:

- Almost entirely fatty breast tissue, found in about 10 percent of women

- Scattered areas of dense glandular tissue and fibrous connective tissue (scattered fibroglandular breast tissue) found in about 40 percent of women

- Heterogeneously dense breast tissue with many areas of glandular tissue and fibrous connective tissue, found in about 40 percent of women

- Extremely dense breast tissue, found in about 10 percent of women

If you are told that you have dense breasts, it means that you have either "heterogeneously dense" or "extremely dense" breasts.

Does Having Dense Breast Tissue Affect a Woman's Mammogram?

Dense breast tissue appears white on a mammogram, as do some abnormal breast changes, such as calcifications and tumors. This can make a mammogram harder to read and may make it more difficult to find breast cancer in women with dense breasts. Women with dense breasts may be called back for follow-up tests more often than women with fatty breasts.

Are Dense Breasts a Risk Factor for Breast Cancer?

Yes, women with dense breasts have a higher risk of breast cancer than women with fatty breasts, and the risk increases with increasing breast density. This increased risk is separate from the effect of dense breasts on the ability to read a mammogram.

Are Breast Cancer Patients with Dense Breasts More Likely to Die from Breast Cancer?

No. Research has found that breast cancer patients who have dense breasts are no more likely to die from breast cancer than breast-cancer patients who have fatty breasts, after accounting for other health factors and tumor characteristics.

Should Women with Dense Breasts Have Additional Screening for Breast Cancer?

In some states, mammography providers are required to inform women who have a mammogram about breast density in general or about whether they have dense breasts. Many states now require that women with dense breasts be covered by insurance for supplemental imaging tests.

Nevertheless, the value of supplemental, or additional, screening tests such as ultrasound or magnetic resonance imaging (MRI) for women with dense breasts is not yet clear, according to the *Final Recommendation Statement on Breast Cancer Screening* by the U.S. Preventive Services Task Force (USPSTF). Ongoing clinical trials are evaluating the role of supplemental imaging tests in women with dense breasts. Research has suggested that for women with dense breasts, a screening strategy that also takes into account a woman's risk factors and protective factors may be the best predictor of whether a woman will develop breast cancer after a normal mammogram and before her next scheduled mammogram.

As you talk with your doctor about your personal risk for breast cancer, keep in mind that:

- Risk factors increase your chance of breast cancer
- Protective factors lower your chance of breast cancer

It may help to ask your doctor these questions, to put your risk for breast cancer into context:

- What are the findings of my recent mammogram?
- Are other additional screening or diagnostic tests recommended?
- What are my personal risk factors for breast cancer? Protective factors for breast cancer?
- What steps can I take to lower my risk of breast cancer?

Chapter 23

Obesity and Breast-Cancer Risk

Obesity is a condition in which a person has an unhealthy amount and/or distribution of body fat.

To measure obesity, researchers commonly use a scale known as the body mass index (BMI). BMI is calculated by dividing a person's weight (in kilograms) by their height (in meters) squared (commonly expressed as kg/m^2). BMI provides a more accurate measure of obesity than weight alone, and for most people, it is a fairly good (although indirect) indicator of body fatness.

Other measurements that reflect the distribution of body fat—that is, whether more fat is carried around the hips or the abdomen—are increasingly being used along with BMI as indicators of obesity and disease risks. These measurements include waist circumference and the waist-to-hip ratio (the waist circumference divided by the hip circumference).

What Is Known about the Relationship between Obesity and Breast Cancer?

Nearly all of the evidence linking obesity to cancer risk comes from large cohort studies, a type of observational study. However,

This chapter includes text excerpted from "Obesity and Cancer," National Cancer Institute (NCI), January 17, 2017.

data from observational studies can be difficult to interpret and cannot definitively establish that obesity causes cancer. That is because obese or overweight people may differ from lean people in ways other than their body fat, and it is possible that these other differences— rather than their body fat—are what explains their different cancer risk.

Despite the limitations of the study designs, there is consistent evidence that higher amounts of body fat are associated with increased risks of a number of cancers, including breast cancer.

Many studies have shown that, in postmenopausal women (PMW), a higher BMI is associated with a modest increase in the risk of breast cancer. For example, a 5-unit increase in BMI is associated with a 12 percent increase in risk. Among postmenopausal women, those who are obese have a 20 to 40 percent increase in the risk of developing breast cancer compared with normal-weight women. The higher risks are seen mainly in women who have never used menopausal hormone therapy (MHT) and for tumors that express hormone receptors. Obesity is also a risk factor for breast cancer in men.

In premenopausal women, by contrast, overweight and obesity have been found to be associated with a 20 percent decreased the risk of breast tumors that express hormone receptors.

How Might Obesity Increase the Risk of Breast Cancer?

Several possible mechanisms have been suggested to explain how obesity might increase the risks of some cancers. Fat tissue (also called "adipose tissue") produces excess amounts of estrogen, high levels of which have been associated with increased risks of breast, endometrial, ovarian, and some other cancers. Other possible mechanisms by which obesity could affect cancer risk include changes in the mechanical properties of the scaffolding that surrounds breast cells and altered immune responses, effects on the nuclear factor kappa beta system, and oxidative stress.

Does Avoiding Weight Gain or Losing Weight Decrease the Risk of Breast Cancer?

Many observational studies have provided consistent evidence that people who have lower weight gain during adulthood have lower risks of colon cancer, kidney cancer, and—for postmenopausal women— breast, endometrial, and ovarian cancers.

Fewer studies have examined possible associations between weight loss and cancer risk. Some of these have found decreased risks of breast, endometrial, colon, and prostate cancers among people who have lost weight. However, most of these studies were not able to evaluate whether the weight loss was intentional or unintentional (and possibly related to underlying health problems).

Stronger evidence for a relationship between weight loss and cancer risk comes from studies of people who have undergone bariatric surgery (surgery performed on the stomach or intestines to induce weight loss). Obese people who have bariatric surgery appear to have lower risks of obesity-related cancers than obese people who do not have bariatric surgery. Nevertheless, the follow-up study of weight and breast cancer in the Women's Health Initiative (WHI) found that for women who were already overweight or obese at baseline, weight change (either gain or loss) was not associated with breast-cancer risk during follow up. However, for women who were of normal weight at baseline, gaining more than five percent of body weight was associated with increased breast-cancer risk.

How Does Obesity Affect Breast-Cancer Survivorship?

Most of the evidence about obesity in cancer survivors come from people who were diagnosed with breast, prostate, or colorectal cancer. Research indicates that obesity may worsen several aspects of cancer survivorship, including quality of life (QOL), cancer recurrence, cancer progression, and prognosis (survival). For example, obesity is associated with increased risks of treatment-related lymphedema in breast-cancer survivors.

Several randomized clinical trials in breast-cancer survivors have reported weight-loss interventions that resulted in both weight loss and beneficial changes in biomarkers that have been linked to the association between obesity and prognosis. However, there is little evidence about whether weight loss improves cancer recurrence or prognosis.

Chapter 24

Alcohol Consumption and Breast-Cancer Risk

Alcohol is the common term for ethanol or ethyl alcohol, a chemical substance found in alcoholic beverages such as beer, hard cider, malt liquor, wines, and distilled spirits (liquor). Alcohol is produced by the fermentation of sugars and starches by yeast. Alcohol is also found in some medicines, mouthwashes, and household products (including vanilla extract and other flavorings).

According to the National Institute on Alcohol Abuse and Alcoholism (NIAAA), a standard alcoholic drink in the United States contains 14.0 grams (0.6 ounces) of pure alcohol. Generally, this amount of pure alcohol is found in:

- 12 ounces of beer

- 8 to 9 ounces of malt liquor

- 5 ounces of wine

- 1.5 ounces, or a "shot," of 80-proof distilled spirits (liquor)

These amounts are used by public-health experts in developing health guidelines about alcohol consumption and to provide a way for people to compare the amounts of alcohol they consume. However,

This chapter includes text excerpted from "Alcohol and Cancer Risk," National Cancer Institute (NCI), September 13, 2018.

they may not reflect the typical serving sizes people may encounter in daily life.

According to the federal government's *Dietary Guidelines for Americans 2015–2020*, individuals who do not drink alcohol should not start drinking for any reason. It recommends that if alcohol is consumed, it should be done in moderation and defines **moderate alcohol drinking** as "up to one drink per day for women and up to two drinks per day for men." **Heavy alcohol drinking** is defined as "having 4 or more drinks on any day or 8 or more drinks per week for women and 5 or more drinks on any day or 15 or more drinks per week for men." **Binge drinking** is defined as "consuming 4 or more drinks for women and 5 or more drinks for men in one sitting (typically in about 2 hours)."

Alcohol May Increase the Risk of Breast Cancer

Researchers have hypothesized that alcohol may increase the risk of breast cancer. It increases blood levels of estrogen, a sex hormone linked to the risk of breast cancer.

Alcohol Drinking Can Cause Breast Cancer

There is a strong scientific consensus that alcohol drinking can cause several types of cancer. In its *Report on Carcinogens*, the National Toxicology Program (NTP) of the U.S. Department of Health and Human Services (HHS) lists consumption of alcoholic beverages as a known human carcinogen. The evidence indicates that the more alcohol a person drinks—particularly the more alcohol a person drinks regularly over time—the higher her or his risk of developing alcohol-associated cancer.

Clear patterns have emerged between alcohol consumption and the development of breast cancer. Epidemiologic studies have consistently found an increased risk of breast cancer with increasing alcohol intake. Pooled data from 118 individual studies indicate that light drinkers have a slightly increased (1.04-fold higher) risk of breast cancer, compared with nondrinkers. The risk increase is greater in moderate drinkers (1.23-fold higher) and heavy drinkers (1.6-fold higher). An analysis of prospective data for 88,000 women participating in two cohort studies concluded that for women who have never smoked, light to moderate drinking was associated with a 1.13-fold increased risk of alcohol-related cancers (mostly breast cancer)

Alcohol consumption may also be associated with an increased risk of second primary cancers. It is less clear whether alcohol consumption increases the risk of second primary cancers at other sites, such as the breast.

Chapter 25

Environmental Factors and Breast-Cancer Risk

About 12 percent, or 1 in 8, women in the United States will develop breast cancer during their lifetime. It is the second most common cancer among U.S. women, behind skin cancer. Breast cancer occurs mostly in women, but men can also develop the disease.

Breast cancer starts when cells begin to grow out of control. These cells normally form a tumor. If the cancerous cells spread to other parts of the body, it is called "metastatic breast cancer."

Although scientists have identified many risk factors that increase a woman's chance of developing breast cancer, they do not yet know what causes normal cells to become cancerous. Most experts agree that breast cancer is caused by a combination of genetic, hormonal, and environmental factors.

However, most women who develop breast cancer have no family history of the disease, suggesting an environmental link. Since environmental factors can sometimes be identified, and lifestyles modified to avoid them, National Institute of Environmental Health Sciences

This chapter contains text excerpted from the following sources: Text in this chapter begins with excerpts from "Breast Cancer," National Institute of Environmental Health Sciences (NIEHS), December 28, 2018; Text under the heading "How Environment Is Linked with Breast Cancer" is excerpted from "Breast Cancer Link to Environment Highlighted at Symposium," National Institute of Environmental Health Sciences (NIEHS), April 2018.

(NIEHS) scientists and other experts in the field believe that prevention strategies are the best way to try to stop breast cancer before it starts.

How Environment Is Linked with Breast Cancer

Researchers supported by NIEHS are working to gain a deeper understanding of environmental factors with potential links to breast cancer. They and others spoke, during "Breast Cancer and the Environment," a symposium sponsored by the Duke University Program in Environmental Health and Toxicology and the Duke Superfund Research Center.

Joel Meyer, Ph.D., Director of Graduate Studies in Duke's Nicholas School of the Environment, led the symposium.

"Twin studies and other evidence have indicated that genetics alone account for approximately 15 percent of breast-cancer cases," he said, explaining the choice of topics for the annual symposium.

"The speakers in our symposium did a wonderful job of covering research from mechanistic laboratory work to three-generation epidemiological studies that cast light on the contribution of environmental exposures to breast cancer," Meyer added.

Sensitive to Endocrine Disruptors

Sue Fenton, Ph.D., Head of the National Toxicology Program (NTP) Reproductive Endocrinology Group, spoke about her lab's research on mammary-gland development. The mammary gland can be a sensitive target for endocrine-disrupting chemicals (EDC), she said. Endocrine disruptors are compounds that can interfere with hormones in the body.

Early life exposure to bisphenol A (BPA) resulted in mammary gland tumors and increased sensitivity to estrogens in rodents studied by Fenton and her colleagues. BPA is widely used in manufacturing plastics and other products. The team also studied several replacement chemicals for BPA, including bisphenol AF (BPAF) and bisphenol S (BPS).

According to Fenton, these replacements may not be any less risky than BPA when it comes to breast cancer. "The worst part about these chemicals is they're either more or equally active as BPA in terms of their estrogenicity," she reported.

Mammary glands are targets for other chemicals as well, Fenton explained. For example, early life exposure of mice to perfluorooctanoic acid, or PFOA, which was previously used to manufacture nonstick coatings, led to later life deficits in mammary-gland development.

Better Research Methods

Melissa Troester, Ph.D., a lead researcher at the University of North Carolina at Chapel Hill Breast Cancer and the Environment Research Program (ERP), described her work to develop an atlas for precancer states of the breast. She said that studying the breast's susceptibility to environmental exposures calls for understanding how exposures in early life, such as before birth and in early childhood, can affect breast-cancer risk later on.

Mammographic density (MD), which refers to the appearance of breast tissue on a mammogram, is another area of Troester's research.

"Mammographic density is one of the strongest risk factors for breast cancer, and it isn't fully understood why that's the case," Troester said. Combining mammographic density (MD) with precancer breast tissue samples may help researchers develop new biomarkers for studying the environment's role in the disease.

Air Pollution and Breast Cancer

Alexandra White, Ph.D., a postdoctoral fellow in the NIEHS Epidemiology Branch, highlighted airborne metals as a potential risk factor. White began by explaining that rare genetic mutations such as the *BRCA1* gene are responsible for only five to ten percent of breast-cancer cases. "Genetics is important, but we've long known that environment and lifestyle risks are also important for breast cancer," she said.

According to White, environmental risk factors of breast cancer are understudied, including air pollution. So she decided to look at participants in the NIEHS Sister Study, which collects data on more than 50,000 women with sisters who have breast cancer.

By comparing air pollutants near the homes of women who had later breast-cancer diagnoses, White and colleagues found associations between airborne metals such as lead and cadmium and postmenopausal-breast cancer.

Windows of Susceptibility

A theme in many of the talks was that the timing of environmental exposure plays a large role in breast-cancer outcomes. Time periods during gestation, before puberty, and during pregnancy are critical windows for exposure, according to Barbara Cohn, Ph.D., from the Public Health Institute (PHI).

"Because of the timing of the development of the breast, if you insult it at one point in life, you may get a specific outcome," she said, pointing to early puberty and altered lactation as two examples.

Chapter 26

Antiperspirants/Deodorants and Breast-Cancer Risk

Several scientists and others have suggested a possible connection between their use and breast cancer since underarm antiperspirants or deodorants are applied near the breast and contain potentially harmful ingredients. However, no scientific evidence links the use of these products to the development of breast cancer.

What Is Known about the Ingredients in Antiperspirants and Deodorants?

Aluminum-based compounds are used as the active ingredient in antiperspirants. These compounds form a temporary "plug" within the sweat duct that stops the flow of sweat to the skin's surface. Some research suggests that aluminum-containing underarm antiperspirants, which are applied frequently and left on the skin near the breast, may be absorbed by the skin and have estrogen-like (hormonal) effects.

Because estrogen can promote the growth of breast-cancer cells, some scientists have suggested that the aluminum-based compounds in antiperspirants may contribute to the development of breast cancer. In addition, it has been suggested that aluminum may have direct activity in breast tissue. However, no studies to date have confirmed

This chapter includes text excerpted from "Antiperspirants/Deodorants and Breast Cancer," National Cancer Institute (NCI), August 9, 2016.

any substantial adverse effects of aluminum that could contribute to increased breast-cancer risks. A 2014 review concluded there was no clear evidence showing that the use of aluminum-containing underarm antiperspirants or cosmetics increases the risk of breast cancer.

Some research has focused on parabens, which are preservatives used in some deodorants and antiperspirants that have been shown to mimic the activity of estrogen in the body's cells. It has been reported that parabens are found in breast tumors, but there is no evidence that they cause breast cancer. Although parabens are used in many cosmetic, food, and pharmaceutical products, most deodorants and antiperspirants in the United States do not currently contain parabens. The National Library of Medicine's (NLM) Household Products Database (www.householdproducts.nlm.nih.gov) has information about the ingredients used in most major brands of deodorants and antiperspirants.

What Is Known about the Relationship between Antiperspirants or Deodorants and Breast Cancer?

Only a few studies have investigated a possible relationship between breast cancer and underarm antiperspirants/deodorants. One study did not show any increase in risk for breast cancer among women who reported using an underarm antiperspirant or deodorant. The results also showed no increase in breast-cancer risk among women who reported using a blade (nonelectric) razor and an underarm antiperspirant or deodorant, or among women who reported using an underarm antiperspirant or deodorant within 1 hour of shaving with a blade razor. These conclusions were based on interviews with 813 women with breast cancer and 793 women with no history of breast cancer.

A subsequent study also found no association between antiperspirant use and breast-cancer risk, although it included only 54 women with breast cancer and 50 women without breast cancer.

A retrospective cohort study examining the frequency of underarm shaving and antiperspirant/deodorant use among 437 breast-cancer survivors reported younger age at breast-cancer diagnosis for women who used antiperspirants/deodorants frequently or who started using them together with shaving at an earlier age. Because of the retrospective nature of the study, the results are not conclusive.

Because studies of antiperspirants and deodorants and breast cancer have provided conflicting results, additional research would be needed to determine whether a relationship exists.

Chapter 27

Breast Cancer Genetic Testing: Understanding BRCA1 *and* BRCA2

What Are BRCA1 *and* BRCA2*?*

BRCA1 and *BRCA2* are human genes that produce tumor suppressor proteins. These proteins help repair damaged deoxyribonucleic acid (DNA) and, therefore, play a role in ensuring the stability of each cell's genetic material. When either of these genes is mutated or altered, such that its protein product is not made or does not function correctly, DNA damage may not be repaired properly. As a result, cells are more likely to develop additional genetic alterations that can lead to cancer.

Specific inherited mutations in *BRCA1* and *BRCA2* most notably increase the risk of female breast cancer, but they have also been associated with increased risks of several additional types of cancer. People who have inherited mutations in *BRCA1* and *BRCA2* tend to develop breast cancer at younger ages than people who do not have these mutations.

A harmful *BRCA1* or *BRCA2* mutation can be inherited from a person's mother or father. Each child of a parent who carries a mutation in one of these genes has a 50 percent chance (or 1 chance in 2)

This chapter includes text excerpted from "*BRCA* Mutations: Cancer Risk and Genetic Testing," National Cancer Institute (NCI), January 30, 2018.

141

of inheriting the mutation. The effects of mutations in *BRCA1* and *BRCA2* are seen even when a person's second copy of the gene is normal.

How Much Does Having a BRCA1 or BRCA2 Gene Mutation Increase a Woman's Risk of Breast Cancer?

A woman's lifetime risk of developing breast cancer is greatly increased if she inherits a harmful mutation in *BRCA1* or *BRCA2*.

About 12 percent of women in the general population will develop breast cancer sometime during their lives. By contrast, a large study estimated that about 72 percent of women who inherit a harmful *BRCA1* mutation and about 69 percent of women who inherit a harmful *BRCA2* mutation will develop breast cancer by the age of 80.

Like women from the general population, those with harmful *BRCA1* or *BRCA2* mutations also have a high risk of developing a new primary cancer in the opposite (contralateral) breast in the years following a breast-cancer diagnosis. It has been estimated that, by 20 years after first breast-cancer diagnosis, about 40 percent of women who inherit a harmful *BRCA1* mutation and about 26 percent of women who inherit a harmful *BRCA2* mutation will develop cancer in their other breast.

Are Mutations in BRCA1 and BRCA2 More Common in Certain Racial/Ethnic Populations Than Others?

Yes. For example, people of Ashkenazi Jewish descent have a higher prevalence of harmful *BRCA1* and *BRCA2* mutations than people in the general United States population. Other ethnic and geographic populations around the world, such as the Norwegian, Dutch, and Icelandic peoples, also have a higher prevalence of specific harmful *BRCA1* and *BRCA2* mutations.

In addition, the prevalence of specific harmful *BRCA1* and *BRCA2* mutations may vary among individual racial and ethnic groups in the United States, including African Americans, Hispanics, Asian Americans, and non-Hispanic whites.

This question is under intensive study, since identifying population-specific mutations in these genes can greatly simplify the genetic testing for *BRCA1* and *BRCA2* mutations.

Are Genetic Tests Available to Detect BRCA1 *and* BRCA2 *Mutations?*

Yes, several different tests are available. Some tests look for a specific harmful *BRCA1* or *BRCA2* gene mutation that has already been identified in another family member. Other tests check for all of the known harmful mutations in both genes. Multigene (panel) testing uses next-generation sequencing to look for harmful mutations in many genes that are associated with an increased risk of breast cancer, including *BRCA1* and *BRCA2*, at the same time.

DNA (usually from a blood or saliva sample) is needed for all of these tests. The sample is sent to a laboratory for analysis. It usually takes about a month to get the test results.

Who Should Consider Genetic Testing for BRCA1 *and* BRCA2 *Mutations?*

Because harmful *BRCA1* and *BRCA2* gene mutations are relatively rare in the general population, most experts agree that mutation testing of individuals who do not have cancer should be performed only when the person's individual or family history suggests the possible presence of a harmful mutation in *BRCA1* or *BRCA2*.

The United States Preventive Services Task Force (USPSTF) recommends that women who have family members with breast, ovarian, fallopian tube, or peritoneal cancer be evaluated to see if they have a family history that is associated with an increased risk of a harmful mutation in one of these genes.

Several screening tools are available to help healthcare providers with this evaluation. These tools assess personal or family history factors that are associated with an increased likelihood of having a harmful mutation in *BRCA1* or *BRCA2*, such as:

- Breast cancer diagnosed before age 50 years

- Cancer in both breasts in the same woman

- Breast cancer in either the same woman or the same family

- Multiple-breast cancers in the family

- Two or more primary types of *BRCA1* or *BRCA2*-related cancers in a single family member

- Cases of male breast cancer

- Ashkenazi Jewish ethnicity

143

When an individual has a family history that is suggestive of the presence of a *BRCA1* or *BRCA2* mutation, it may be most informative to first test a family member who has cancer, if that person is still alive and willing to be tested. If that person has a harmful *BRCA1* or *BRCA2* mutation, then other family members may want to consider genetic counseling to learn more about their potential risks and whether genetic testing for mutations in *BRCA1* and *BRCA2* might be appropriate for them.

If it can't be determined whether the family member with cancer has a harmful *BRCA1* or *BRCA2* mutation, members of a family whose history is suggestive of the presence of a *BRCA1* or *BRCA2* gene mutation may still want to consider genetic counseling for possible testing.

Some individuals—for example, those who were adopted at birth—may not know their family history. If a woman with an unknown-family history has early-onset breast cancer or a man with an unknown-family history is diagnosed with breast cancer, that individual may want to consider genetic counseling and testing for a *BRCA1* or *BRCA2* mutation.

Professional societies do not recommend that children under age 18, even those with a family history suggestive of a harmful *BRCA1* or *BRCA2* mutation, undergo genetic testing for *BRCA1* or *BRCA2*. This is because there are no risk-reduction strategies that are specifically meant for children, and children's risks of developing a cancer type associated with a *BRCA1* or *BRCA2* mutation are extremely low.

Should People Considering Genetic Testing for BRCA1 *and* BRCA2 *Mutations Talk with a Genetic Counselor?*

Genetic counseling is generally recommended before and after any genetic test for an inherited cancer syndrome. This counseling should be performed by a healthcare professional who is experienced in cancer genetics. Genetic counseling usually covers many aspects of the testing process, including:

- A hereditary cancer-risk assessment (HCRA) based on an individual's personal- and family-medical history

- Discussion of:

  - The appropriateness of genetic testing

  - The medical implications of a positive or negative test result

- The possibility that a test result might not be informative (that is, it might find an alteration whose effect on cancer risk is not known)

- The psychological risks and benefits of genetic test results

- The risk of passing a mutation to children

- Explanation of the specific test(s) that might be used and the technical accuracy of the test(s)

Does Health Insurance Cover the Cost of BRCA1 *and* BRCA2 *Mutation Testing?*

People considering *BRCA1* and *BRCA2* mutation testing may want to confirm their insurance coverage for genetic counseling and testing.

The Affordable Care Act (ACA) considers genetic counseling and *BRCA1* and *BRCA2* mutation testing a covered preventive service for women who have not already been diagnosed with cancer-related to a mutation in *BRCA1* or *BRCA2* and who meet the U.S. Preventive Services Task Force (USPSTF) recommendations for testing.

Medicare covers *BRCA1* and *BRCA2* mutation testing for women who have signs and symptoms of breast or other cancers that are related to mutations in *BRCA1* and *BRCA2* but not for unaffected women.

Some of the genetic testing companies that offer to test for *BRCA1* and *BRCA2* mutations may offer testing at no charge to patients who lack insurance and meet specific financial and medical criteria.

What Do BRCA1 *or* BRCA2 *Genetic Test Results Mean?*

BRCA1 and *BRCA2* gene mutation testing can give several possible results: a positive result, a negative result, or an ambiguous or uncertain result.

Positive result. A positive test result indicates that a person has inherited a known harmful mutation in *BRCA1* or *BRCA2* and, therefore, has an increased risk of developing certain cancers. However, a positive test result cannot tell whether or when an individual will actually develop cancer. Some women who inherit a harmful *BRCA1* or *BRCA2* mutation never develop breast cancer.

A positive test result may also have important implications for family members, including future generations.

- Both men and women who inherit a harmful *BRCA1* or *BRCA2* mutation, whether or not they develop cancer themselves, may pass the mutation on to their sons and daughters. Each child has a 50 percent chance of inheriting a parent's mutation.

- If a person learns that he or she has inherited a harmful *BRCA1* or *BRCA2* mutation, this will mean that each of his or her full siblings has a 50 percent chance of having inherited the mutation as well.

Negative result. A negative test result can be more difficult to understand that a positive result because what the result means depends in part on an individual's family history of cancer and whether a *BRCA1* or *BRCA2* mutation has been identified in a blood relative.

If a close (first- or second-degree) relative of the tested person is known to carry a harmful *BRCA1* or *BRCA2* mutation, a negative test result is clear: it means that a person does not carry the harmful mutation that is responsible for their family's cancer risk, and thus cannot pass it on to their children. Such a test result is called a true negative. A person with such a test result is currently thought to have the same risk of cancer as someone in the general population.

If the tested person has a family history that suggests the possibility of having a harmful mutation in *BRCA1* or *BRCA2* but complete gene testing identifies no such mutation in the family, a negative result is less clear. The likelihood that genetic testing will miss a known harmful *BRCA1* or *BRCA2* mutation is very low, but it could happen. Moreover, scientists continue to discover new *BRCA1* and *BRCA2* mutations and have not yet identified all potentially harmful ones. Therefore, it is possible that a person in this scenario with a "negative" test result may actually have a harmful *BRCA1* or *BRCA2* mutation that has not previously been identified.

It is also possible for people to have a mutation in a gene other than *BRCA1* or *BRCA2* that increases their cancer risk but is not detectable by the test used. It is important that people considering genetic testing for *BRCA1* and *BRCA2* mutations discuss these potential uncertainties with a genetic counselor before undergoing testing.

Ambiguous or uncertain result. Sometimes, a genetic test finds a change in *BRCA1* or *BRCA2* that has not been previously associated with cancer. This type of test result may be described as "ambiguous" (often referred to as "a genetic variant of uncertain significance") because it isn't known whether this specific genetic change is harmful. One study found that ten percent of women who underwent *BRCA1* and *BRCA2* mutation testing had this type of ambiguous result.

As more research is conducted and more people are tested for *BRCA1* and *BRCA2* mutations, scientists will learn more about these changes and cancer risk. Genetic counseling can help a person understand what an ambiguous change in *BRCA1* or *BRCA2* may mean in terms of cancer risk. Over time, additional studies of variants of uncertain significance may result in a specific mutation being reclassified as either clearly harmful or clearly not harmful.

How Can a Person Who Has a Harmful BRCA1 or BRCA2 *Gene Mutation Manage Their Risk of Cancer?*

Several options are available for managing cancer risk in individuals who have a known harmful *BRCA1* or *BRCA2* mutation. These include enhanced screening, prophylactic (risk-reducing) surgery, and chemoprevention.

Enhanced screening. Some women who test positive for *BRCA1* and *BRCA2* mutations may choose to start breast-cancer screening at younger ages, and/or have more frequent screening, than women at average risk of breast cancer. For example, some experts recommend that women who carry a harmful *BRCA1* or *BRCA2* mutation undergo clinical breast examinations beginning at age 25 to 35 years. And some expert groups recommend that women who carry such a mutation have a mammogram every year, beginning at age 25 to 35 years.

Enhanced screening may increase the chance of detecting breast cancer at an early stage, when it may have a better chance of being treated successfully. Studies have shown that magnetic resonance imaging (MRI) may be better able than mammography to find tumors, particularly in younger women at high risk of breast cancer. However, mammography can also identify some breast cancers that are not identified by MRI. Also, MRI may be less specific (that is, lead to more false-positive results) than mammography.

Several organizations, such as the American Cancer Society (ACS) and the National Comprehensive Cancer Network (NCCN), now recommend annual screening with both mammography and MRI for women who have a high risk of breast cancer. Women who test positive for a *BRCA1* or *BRCA2* mutation should ask their healthcare provider about the possible harms of diagnostic tests that involve radiation (mammograms or X-rays).

The benefits of screening for breast and other cancers in men who carry harmful mutations in *BRCA1* or *BRCA2* are also not known, but some expert groups recommend that men who are known to carry a harmful mutation undergo regular breast exams as well as testing for prostate cancer.

Prophylactic (risk-reducing) surgery. Prophylactic surgery involves removing as much of the "at-risk" tissue as possible. Women may choose to have both breasts removed (bilateral prophylactic mastectomy) to reduce their risk of breast cancer. Surgery to remove a woman's ovaries and fallopian tubes (bilateral prophylactic salpingo-oophorectomy) can help reduce her risk of ovarian cancer. (Ovarian cancers often originate in the fallopian tubes, so it is essential that they are removed along with the ovaries.) Removing the ovaries may also reduce the risk of breast cancer in premenopausal women by eliminating a source of hormones that can fuel the growth of some types of breast cancer.

Whether bilateral prophylactic mastectomy reduces breast-cancer risk in men with a harmful *BRCA1* or *BRCA2* mutation or a family history of breast cancer isn't known. Therefore, bilateral prophylactic mastectomy for men at high risk of breast cancer is considered an experimental procedure, and insurance companies will not normally cover it.

Prophylactic surgery does not guarantee that cancer will not develop because not all at-risk tissue can be removed by these procedures. That is why these surgical procedures are often described as "risk-reducing" rather than "preventive." Some women have developed breast cancer, ovarian cancer, or primary peritoneal carcinomatosis (PPC) (a type of cancer similar to ovarian cancer) even after risk-reducing surgery (RRS). Nevertheless, these surgical procedures confer substantial benefits. For example, research demonstrates that women who underwent bilateral prophylactic salpingo-oophorectomy had a nearly 80 percent reduction in risk of dying from ovarian cancer, a 56 percent reduction in risk of dying from breast cancer, and a 77 percent reduction in risk of dying from any cause during the studies' follow-up periods.

The reduction in breast-cancer risk from the removal of the ovaries and fallopian tubes appears to be similar for carriers of *BRCA1* and *BRCA2* mutations.

Chemoprevention. Chemoprevention is the use of medicines to try to reduce the risk of cancer. Although two chemopreventive drugs (tamoxifen and raloxifene) have been approved by the U.S. Food and Drug Administration (FDA) to reduce the risk of breast cancer in women at increased risk, the role of these drugs in women with harmful *BRCA1* or *BRCA2* mutations is not yet clear. However, these medications may be an option for women who don't choose, or can't undergo, surgery.

Data from three studies suggest that tamoxifen may be able to help lower the risk of breast cancer in women who carry harmful mutations in *BRCA2*, as well as the risk of cancer in the opposite breast among *BRCA1* and *BRCA2* mutation carriers previously diagnosed with breast cancer. Studies have not examined the effectiveness of raloxifene in *BRCA1* and *BRCA2* mutation carriers specifically.

What Are Some of the Benefits of Genetic Testing for Breast-Cancer Risk?

There can be benefits to genetic testing, regardless of whether a person receives a positive or a negative result.

The potential benefits of a true negative result include a sense of relief regarding the future risk of cancer, learning that one's children are not at risk of inheriting the family's cancer susceptibility, and the possibility that special checkups, tests, or preventive surgeries may not be needed.

A positive test result may bring relief by resolving uncertainty regarding future cancer risk and may allow people to make informed decisions about their future healthcare, including taking steps to reduce their cancer risk. In addition, people who have a positive test result may choose to participate in medical research that could, in the long run, help reduce deaths from hereditary breast cancer.

What Are Some of the Possible Harms of Genetic Testing for BRCA Gene Mutations?

The direct medical harms of genetic testing are minimal, but knowledge of test results may have harmful effects on a person's emotions, social relationships, finances, and medical choices.

People who receive a positive test result may feel anxious, depressed, or angry, particularly immediately after they learn the result. People who learn that they carry a *BRCA* mutation may have difficulty making choices about whether to have preventive surgery or about which surgery to have.

People who receive a negative test result may experience "survivor guilt," caused by the knowledge that they likely do not have an increased risk of developing a disease that affects one or more loved ones.

Because genetic testing can reveal information about more than one family member, the emotions caused by test results can create tension within families. Test results can also affect personal life choices, such as decisions about career, marriage, and childbearing.

Violations of privacy and of the confidentiality of genetic test results are additional potential risks. However, the federal Health Insurance Portability and Accountability Act (HIPAA) and various state laws protect the privacy of a person's genetic information. Moreover, the federal Genetic Information Nondiscrimination Act (GINA), along with many state laws, prohibits discrimination based on genetic information in relation to health insurance and employment, although it does not cover life insurance, disability insurance, or long-term care insurance.

Finally, there is a small chance that test results may not be accurate, leading people to make medical decisions based on incorrect information. Although it is rare that results are inaccurate, people with these concerns should address them during genetic counseling.

What Are the Implications of Having a Harmful BRCA1 or BRCA2 Mutation for Breast-Cancer Prognosis and Treatment?

Some studies have investigated whether there are clinical differences between breast and ovarian cancers that are associated with harmful *BRCA1* or *BRCA2* mutations and cancers that are not associated with these mutations.

- There is evidence that, over the long term, women who carry these mutations are more likely to develop second cancer in either the same (ipsilateral) breast or the opposite (contralateral) breast than women who do not carry these mutations. Thus, some women with a harmful *BRCA1* or *BRCA2* mutation who develop breast cancer in one breast opt for a bilateral mastectomy (BMX), even if they would otherwise be candidates for breast-conserving surgery. Because of the increased risk of second breast cancer among *BRCA1* and *BRCA2* mutation carriers, some doctors recommend that women with early-onset breast cancer and those whose family history is consistent with a mutation in one of these genes have genetic testing when breast cancer is diagnosed.

- Breast cancers in women with a harmful *BRCA1* mutation tend to be "triple-negative breast cancers (TNBC)" (that is, the breast cancer cells do not have estrogen receptors, progesterone receptors, or large amounts of HER2/neu protein), which generally have a poorer prognosis than other breast cancers.

- Because the *BRCA1* and *BRCA2* genes are involved in DNA repair, some investigators have suggested that cancer cells with a harmful mutation in either of these genes may be more sensitive to anticancer agents that act by damaging DNA, such as cisplatin. A class of drugs called poly ADP ribose polymerase (PARP) inhibitors, which block the repair of DNA damage, have been found to arrest the growth of cancer cells that have *BRCA1* or *BRCA2* mutations. Olaparib is also approved for the treatment of human epidermal growth factor receptor 2 (HER2)-negative metastatic breast cancers in women with a *BRCA1* or *BRCA2* mutation.

Do Inherited Mutations in Other Genes Increase the Risk of Breast Tumors?

Yes. Although harmful mutations in *BRCA1* and *BRCA2* are responsible for the disease in nearly half of families with multiple cases of breast cancer and up to 90 percent of families with both breast cancer, mutations in a number of other genes have been associated with increased risks of breast cancer. These other genes include several that are associated with the inherited disorders Cowden syndrome (CS), Peutz-Jeghers syndrome (PJS), Li-Fraumeni syndrome (LFS), and Fanconi anemia (FA), which increase the risk of many cancer types.

Most mutations in these other genes do not increase breast-cancer risk to the same extent as mutations in *BRCA1* and *BRCA2*. However, researchers have reported that inherited mutations in the *PALB2* gene are associated with a risk of breast cancer nearly as high as that associated with inherited *BRCA1* and *BR*

CA2 mutations. They estimated that 33 percent of women who inherit a harmful mutation in *PALB2* will develop breast cancer by age 70 years.

Mutations in other genes that increase breast-cancer risk have been identified. These include mutations in the genes *TP53, CDH1,* and *CHEK2*, which increase the risk of breast cancer. Genetic testing for these other mutations is available as part of multigene (panel) testing. However, expert groups have not yet developed specific guidelines for who should be tested, or for the management of breast-cancer risk in people with these other high-risk mutations.

Chapter 28

Preventing Breast Cancer in People Who Are Susceptible

Chapter Contents

153

Section 28.1

Overview of Protective Factors and Interventions

This section includes text excerpted from "Breast Cancer Prevention (PDQ®)—Patient Version," National Cancer Institute (NCI), October 19, 2018.

Avoiding Risk Factors and Increasing Protective Factors May Help Prevent Breast Cancer

Avoiding cancer risk factors may help prevent certain cancers. Risk factors include smoking, being overweight, and not getting enough exercise. Increasing protective factors such as quitting smoking and exercising may also help prevent some cancers. Talk to your doctor or other healthcare professional about how you might lower your risk of cancer.

The National Cancer Institute's (NCI) Breast Cancer Risk Assessment Tool (www.bcrisktool.cancer.gov) uses a woman's risk factors to estimate her risk for breast cancer during the next 5 years and up to age 90. This online tool is meant to be used by a healthcare provider. For more information on breast-cancer risk, call 800-422-6237.

Protective Factors for Breast Cancer

The following are protective factors for breast cancer:

Less exposure of breast tissue to estrogen made by the body. Decreasing the length of time, a woman's breast tissue is exposed to estrogen, may help prevent breast cancer. Exposure to estrogen is reduced in the following ways:

- **Early pregnancy.** Estrogen levels are lower during pregnancy. Women who have a full-term pregnancy before age 20 have a lower risk of breast cancer than women who have not had children or who give birth to their first child after age 35.

- **Breastfeeding.** Estrogen levels may remain lower while a woman is breastfeeding. Women who breastfed have a lower risk of breast cancer than women who have had children but did not breastfeed.

Taking estrogen-only hormone therapy after hysterectomy, selective estrogen receptor modulators, or aromatase inhibitors and inactivators.

- **Estrogen-only hormone therapy after hysterectomy.** Hormone therapy with estrogen only may be given to women who have had a hysterectomy. In these women, estrogen-only therapy after menopause may decrease the risk of breast cancer. There is an increased risk of stroke and heart and blood vessel disease in postmenopausal women who take estrogen after a hysterectomy.

- **Selective estrogen receptor modulators.** Tamoxifen and raloxifene belong to the family of drugs called "selective estrogen receptor modulators (SERMs)." SERMs act like estrogen on some tissues in the body but block the effect of estrogen on other tissues.

Treatment with tamoxifen lowers the risk of estrogen receptor-positive (ER-positive) breast cancer and ductal carcinoma *in situ* (DCIS) in premenopausal and postmenopausal women at high risk. Treatment with raloxifene also lowers the risk of breast cancer in postmenopausal women. With either drug, the reduced risk lasts for several years or longer after treatment is stopped. Lower rates of broken bones have been noted in patients taking raloxifene.

Taking tamoxifen increases the risk of hot flashes, endometrial cancer, stroke, cataracts, and blood clots (especially in the lungs and legs). The risk of having these problems increases markedly in women older than 50 years compared with younger women. Women younger than 50 years who have a high risk of breast cancer may benefit the most from taking tamoxifen. The risk of having these problems decreases after tamoxifen is stopped. Talk with your doctor about the risks and benefits of taking this drug.

Taking raloxifene increases the risk of blood clots in the lungs and legs, but does not appear to increase the risk of endometrial cancer. In postmenopausal women with osteoporosis (decreased-bone density), raloxifene lowers the risk of breast cancer for women who have a high or low risk of breast cancer. It is not known if raloxifene would have the same effect in women who do not have osteoporosis. Talk with your doctor about the risks and benefits of taking this drug.

Other SERMs are being studied in clinical trials.

- **Aromatase inhibitors and inactivators.** Aromatase inhibitors (anastrozole, letrozole) and inactivators (exemestane) lower the risk of recurrence and of new breast cancers in women who have a history of breast cancer. Aromatase inhibitors also decrease the risk of breast cancer in women with the following conditions:

- Postmenopausal women with a personal history of breast cancer

- Women with no personal history of breast cancer who are 60 years and older, have a history of DCIS with mastectomy or have a high risk of breast cancer based on the Gail model tool (a tool used to estimate the risk of breast cancer)

In women with an increased risk of breast cancer, taking aromatase inhibitors decreases the amount of estrogen made by the body. Before menopause, estrogen is made by the ovaries and other tissues in a woman's body, including the brain, fat tissue, and skin. After menopause, the ovaries stop making estrogen, but the other tissues do not. Aromatase inhibitors block the action of an enzyme called "aromatase," which is used to make all of the body's estrogen. Aromatase inactivators stop the enzyme from working.

Possible harms from taking aromatase inhibitors include muscle and joint pain, osteoporosis, hot flashes, and feeling very tired.

- **Risk-reducing mastectomy.** Some women who have a high risk of breast cancer may choose to have a risk-reducing mastectomy (the removal of both breasts when there are no signs of cancer). The risk of breast cancer is much lower in these women and most feel less anxious about their risk of breast cancer. However, it is very important to have a cancer-risk assessment and counseling about the different ways to prevent breast cancer before making this decision.

- **Ovarian ablation.** The ovaries make most of the estrogen that is made by the body. Treatments that stop or lower the amount of estrogen made by the ovaries include surgery to remove the ovaries, radiation therapy, or taking certain drugs. This is called "ovarian ablation."

Premenopausal women who have a high risk of breast cancer due to certain changes in the *BRCA1* and *BRCA2* genes may choose to have a risk-reducing oophorectomy (the removal of both ovaries when there are no signs of cancer). This decreases the amount of estrogen made by the body and lowers the risk of breast cancer. Risk-reducing oophorectomy also lowers the risk of breast cancer in normal premenopausal women and in women with an increased risk of breast cancer due to radiation to the chest. However, it is very important to have a cancer risk assessment and counseling before making this decision. The sudden drop in estrogen levels may cause the symptoms of menopause to begin. These include hot flashes, trouble sleeping, anxiety, and depression. Long-term effects include decreased sex drive, vaginal dryness, and decreased bone density.

- **Getting enough exercise.** Women who exercise four or more hours a week have a lower risk of breast cancer. The effect of exercise on breast-cancer risk may be greatest in premenopausal women who have normal or low body weight.

Section 28.2

What You Can Do to Reduce Your Risk of Breast Cancer

This section includes text excerpted from "What Are the Risk Factors for Breast Cancer?" Centers for Disease Control and Prevention (CDC), September 11, 2018.

Studies have shown that your risk for breast cancer is due to a combination of factors. The main factors that influence your risk include being a woman and getting older. Most breast cancers are found in women who are 50 years old or older.

Some women will get breast cancer even without any other risk factors that they know of. Having a risk factor does not mean you will get the disease, and not all risk factors have the same effect. Most women have some risk factors, but most women do not get breast cancer. If you have breast-cancer risk factors, talk with your doctor about ways you can lower your risk and about screening for breast cancer.

There are certain risk factors that you cannot change and there are some you change.

Risk factors you cannot change include:

- Getting older

- Genetic mutations
- Reproductive history
- Having dense breasts
- Personal history of breast cancer or certain noncancerous breast diseases
- Family history of breast cancer
- Previous treatment using radiation therapy
- Women who took the drug diethylstilbestrol (DES)

  Risk factors you can change include:
- Not being physically active
- Being overweight or obese after menopause
- Taking hormones
- Reproductive history
- Drinking alcohol

What Can You Do to Reduce Your Risk of Breast Cancer?

Many factors over the course of a lifetime can influence your breast-cancer risk. You can't change some factors, such as getting older or your family history, but you can help lower your risk of breast cancer by taking care of your health in the following ways:

- Keep a healthy weight
- Exercise regularly
- Don't drink alcohol, or limit alcoholic drinks to no more than one per day
- If you are taking, or have been told to take, hormone-replacement therapy or oral contraceptives (birth control pills), ask your doctor about the risks and find out if it is right for you
- Breastfeed your children, if possible
- If you have a family history of breast cancer or inherited changes in your *BRCA1* and *BRCA2* genes, talk to your doctor about other ways to lower your risk.

Staying healthy throughout your life will lower your risk of developing cancer, and improve your chances of surviving cancer if it occurs.

Section 28.3

Surgery to Reduce the Risk of Breast Cancer

This section includes text excerpted from "Surgery to Reduce the Risk of Breast Cancer," National Cancer Institute (NCI), August 12, 2013. Reviewed February 2019.

What Kinds of Surgery Can Reduce the Risk of Breast Cancer?

Two kinds of surgery can be performed to reduce the risk of breast cancer in a woman who has never been diagnosed with breast cancer but is known to be at very high risk of the disease.

A woman can be at very high risk of developing breast cancer if she has a strong family history of breast and/or ovarian cancer, a deleterious (disease-causing) mutation in the *BRCA1* gene or the *BRCA2* gene, or a high-penetrance mutation in one of several other genes associated with breast-cancer risk, such as *TP53* or *PTEN*.

The most common risk-reducing surgery is bilateral prophylactic mastectomy (also called "bilateral risk-reducing mastectomy"). Bilateral prophylactic mastectomy may involve complete removal of both breasts, including the nipples (total mastectomy), or it may involve removal of as much breast tissue as possible while leaving the nipples intact (subcutaneous or nipple-sparing mastectomy). Subcutaneous mastectomies preserve the nipple and allow for more natural-looking breasts if a woman chooses to have breast reconstruction surgery afterward. However, total mastectomy provides the greatest breast-cancer risk reduction because more breast tissue is removed in this procedure than in a subcutaneous mastectomy.

Even with total mastectomy, not all breast tissue that may be at risk of becoming cancerous in the future can be removed. The chest wall, which is not typically removed during a mastectomy, may contain some breast tissue, and breast tissue can sometimes be found in the armpit, above the collarbone, and as far down as the abdomen—and it is impossible for a surgeon to remove all of this tissue.

The other kind of risk-reducing surgery is bilateral prophylactic salpingo-oophorectomy, which is sometimes called "prophylactic oophorectomy." This surgery involves removal of the ovaries and fallopian tubes and may be done alone or along with bilateral prophylactic mastectomy in premenopausal women who are at very high risk of breast cancer. Removing the ovaries in premenopausal women reduces the amount of estrogen that is produced by the body. Because estrogen promotes the growth of some breast cancers, reducing the amount of this hormone in the body by removing the ovaries may slow the growth of those breast cancers.

How Effective Are Risk-Reducing Surgeries?

Bilateral prophylactic mastectomy has been shown to reduce the risk of breast cancer by at least 95 percent in women who have a deleterious (disease-causing) mutation in the *BRCA1* gene or the *BRCA2* gene and by up to 90 percent in women who have a strong family history of breast cancer.

Bilateral prophylactic salpingo-oophorectomy has been shown to reduce the risk of ovarian cancer by approximately 90 percent and the risk of breast cancer by approximately 50 percent in women at very high risk of developing these diseases.

Which Women Might Consider Having Surgery to Reduce Their Risk of Breast Cancer?

Women who inherit a deleterious mutation in the *BRCA1* gene or the *BRCA2* gene or mutations in certain other genes that greatly increase the risk of developing breast cancer may consider having bilateral prophylactic mastectomy and/or bilateral prophylactic salpingo-oophorectomy to reduce this risk.

In two studies, the estimated risks of developing breast cancer by age 70 years were 55 to 65 percent for women who carry a deleterious mutation in the *BRCA1* gene and 45 to 47 percent for women who carry a deleterious mutation in the *BRCA2* gene. Estimates of the lifetime risk of breast cancer for women with Cowden syndrome, which is caused by certain mutations in the *PTEN* gene, ranging from 25 to 50 percent or higher, and for women with Li-Fraumeni syndrome, which is caused by certain mutations in the *TP53* gene, from 49 to 60 percent. (By contrast, the lifetime risk of breast cancer for the average American woman is about 12%.)

Other women who are at very high risk of breast cancer may also consider bilateral prophylactic mastectomy, including:

- Those with a strong family history of breast cancer (such as having a mother, sister, and/or daughter who was diagnosed with bilateral breast cancer or with breast cancer before age 50 years or having multiple family members with breast or ovarian cancer)

- Those with lobular carcinoma *in situ* (LCIS) plus a family history of breast cancer (LCIS is a condition in which abnormal cells are found in the lobules of the breast. It is not cancer, but women with LCIS have an increased risk of developing invasive breast cancer in either breast. Many breast surgeons consider prophylactic mastectomy to be an overly aggressive approach for women with LCIS who do not have a strong family history or other risk factors.)

- Those who have had radiation therapy to the chest (including the breasts) before the age of 30 years—for example, if they were treated with radiation therapy for Hodgkin lymphoma. (Such women are at high risk of developing breast cancer throughout their lives.)

Can a Woman Have Risk-Reducing Surgery If She Has Already Been Diagnosed with Breast Cancer?

Yes. Some women who have been diagnosed with cancer in one breast, particularly those who are known to be at very high risk, may consider having the other breast (called the "contralateral breast") removed as well, even if there is no sign of cancer in that breast. Prophylactic surgery to remove a contralateral breast during breast-cancer surgery (known as "contralateral prophylactic mastectomy") reduces the risk of breast cancer in that breast, although it is not yet known whether this risk reduction translates into longer survival for the patient.

However, doctors often discourage contralateral prophylactic mastectomy for women with cancer in one breast who do not meet the criteria of being at very high risk of developing a contralateral breast cancer. For such women, the risk of developing another breast cancer, either in the same or the contralateral breast, is very small, especially if they receive adjuvant chemotherapy or hormone therapy as part of their cancer treatment.

Given that most women with breast cancer have a low risk of developing the disease in their contralateral breast, women who are not known to be at very high risk but who remain concerned about cancer development in their other breast may want to consider options other than surgery to further reduce their risk of a contralateral breast cancer.

What Are the Potential Harms of Risk-Reducing Surgeries?

As with any other major surgery, bilateral prophylactic mastectomy and bilateral prophylactic salpingo-oophorectomy have potential complications or harms, such as bleeding or infection. Also, both surgeries are irreversible.

Bilateral prophylactic mastectomy can also affect a woman's psychological well-being due to a change in body image and the loss of normal breast functions. Although most women who choose to have this surgery are satisfied with their decision, they can still experience anxiety and concerns about body image. The most common psychological side effects include difficulties with body appearance, with feelings of femininity, and with sexual relationships. Women who undergo total mastectomies lose nipple sensation, which may hinder sexual arousal.

Bilateral prophylactic salpingo-oophorectomy causes a sudden drop in estrogen production, which will induce early menopause in a premenopausal woman (this is also called "surgical menopause"). Surgical menopause can cause an abrupt onset of menopausal symptoms, including hot flashes, insomnia, anxiety, and depression, and some of these symptoms can be severe. The long-term effects of surgical menopause include decreased sex drive, vaginal dryness, and decreased bone density.

Women who have severe menopausal symptoms after undergoing bilateral prophylactic salpingo-oophorectomy may consider using short-term menopausal hormone therapy after surgery to alleviate these symptoms. (The increase in breast-cancer risk associated with certain types of menopausal hormone therapy is much less than the decrease in breast-cancer risk associated with bilateral prophylactic salpingo-oophorectomy.)

What Are the Cancer Risk Reduction Options for Women Who Are at Increased Risk of Breast Cancer but Not at the Highest Risk?

Risk-reducing surgery is not considered an appropriate cancer prevention option for women who are not at the highest risk of breast cancer (that is, for those who do not carry a high-penetrance gene mutation that is associated with breast cancer or who do not have a clinical or medical history that puts them at very high risk). However, some women who are not at very high risk of breast cancer but are, nonetheless, considered as being at increased risk of the disease may choose to use drugs to reduce their risk.

Healthcare providers use several types of tools, called "risk assessment models," to estimate the risk of breast cancer for women who do not have a deleterious mutation in *BRCA1*, *BRCA2*, or another gene associated with breast-cancer risk. One widely used tool is the Breast Cancer Risk Assessment Tool (BCRAT) (www.bcrisktool.cancer.gov), a computer model that takes a number of factors into account in estimating the risks of breast cancer over the next 5 years and up to age 90 years (lifetime risk). Women who have an estimated 5-year risk of 1.67 percent or higher are classified as "high-risk," which means that they have a higher than average risk of developing breast cancer. This high-risk cut-off (that is, an estimated 5-year risk of 1.67 percent or higher) is widely used in research studies and in clinical counseling.

Two drugs, tamoxifen, and raloxifene, are approved by the U.S. Food and Drug Administration (FDA) to reduce the risk of breast cancer in women who have a 5-year risk of developing breast cancer of 1.67 percent or more. Tamoxifen is approved for risk reduction in both premenopausal and postmenopausal women, and raloxifene is approved for risk reduction in postmenopausal women only. In large randomized clinical trials, tamoxifen, taken for 5 years, reduced the risk of invasive breast cancer by about 50 percent in high-risk postmenopausal women; raloxifene, taken for 5 years, reduced breast-cancer risk by about 38 percent in high-risk postmenopausal women. Both drugs block the activity of estrogen, thereby inhibiting the growth of some breast cancers. The U.S. Preventive Services Task Force (USPSTF) recommends that women at increased risk of breast cancer talk with their healthcare professional about the potential benefits and harms of taking tamoxifen or raloxifene to reduce their risk.

Another drug, exemestane, has shown to reduce the incidence of breast cancer in postmenopausal women who are at increased risk of the disease by 65 percent. Exemestane belongs to a class of drugs called "aromatase inhibitors," which block the production of estrogen by the body. It is not known, however, whether any of these drugs reduces the very high risk of breast cancer for women who carry a known mutation that is strongly associated with an increased risk of breast cancer, such as deleterious mutations in *BRCA1* and *BRCA2*.

Some women who have undergone breast-cancer surgery, regardless of their risk of recurrence, may be given drugs to reduce the likelihood that their breast cancer will recur. (This additional treatment is called "adjuvant therapy.") Such treatment also reduces the already low risks of contralateral and second-primary breast cancers. Drugs that are used as adjuvant therapy to reduce the risk of breast cancer after breast-cancer surgery include tamoxifen, aromatase inhibitors, traditional chemotherapy agents, and trastuzumab.

What Can Women at Very High Risk Do If They Do Not Want to Undergo Risk-Reducing Surgery?

Some women who are at very high risk of breast cancer (or of contralateral breast cancer) may undergo more frequent breast-cancer screening (also called "enhanced screening"). For example, they may have yearly mammograms and yearly magnetic resonance imaging (MRI) screening—with these tests staggered so that the breasts are imaged every six months—as well as clinical breast examinations performed regularly by a healthcare professional. Enhanced screening may increase the chance of detecting breast cancer at an early stage, when it may have a better chance of being treated successfully.

Women who carry mutations in some genes that increase their risk of breast cancer may be more likely to develop radiation-associated breast cancer than the general population because those genes are involved in the repair of deoxyribonucleic acid (DNA) breaks, which can be caused by exposure to radiation. Women who are at high risk of breast cancer should ask their healthcare provider about the risks of diagnostic tests that involve radiation (mammograms or X-rays). Ongoing clinical trials are examining various aspects of enhanced screening for women who are at high risk of breast cancer.

Chemoprevention (the use of drugs or other agents to reduce cancer risk or delay its development) may be an option for some women who wish to avoid surgery. Tamoxifen and raloxifene both have been approved by the FDA to reduce the risk of breast cancer in women at increased risk. Whether these drugs can be used to prevent breast cancer in women at much higher risk, such as women with harmful mutations in *BRCA1* or *BRCA2* or other breast-cancer susceptibility genes, is not yet clear, although tamoxifen may be able to help lower the risk of contralateral breast cancer among *BRCA1* and *BRCA2* mutation carriers previously diagnosed with breast cancer.

Does Health Insurance Cover the Cost of Risk-Reducing Surgeries?

Many health-insurance companies have official policies about whether and under what conditions they will pay for prophylactic mastectomy (bilateral or contralateral) and bilateral prophylactic salpingo-oophorectomy for breast and ovarian cancer risk reduction. However, the criteria used for considering these procedures as medically necessary may vary among insurance companies. Some insurance companies may require a second opinion or a letter of medical necessity from the healthcare provider before they will approve coverage of any surgical procedure. A woman who is considering prophylactic surgery to reduce her risk of breast and/or ovarian cancer should discuss insurance coverage issues with her doctor and insurance company before choosing to have the surgery.

The Women's Health and Cancer Rights Act (WHCRA), enacted in 1999, requires most health plans that offer mastectomy coverage to also pay for breast reconstruction surgery after mastectomy. More information about WHCRA can be found through the U.S. Department of Labor (DOL).

Who Should a Woman Talk to When Considering Surgery to Reduce Her Risk of Breast Cancer?

The decision to have any surgery to reduce the risk of breast cancer is a major one. A woman who is at high risk of breast cancer may wish to get a second opinion on risk-reducing surgery as well as on alternatives to surgery.

A woman who is considering prophylactic mastectomy may also want to talk with a surgeon who specializes in breast reconstruction. Other healthcare professionals, including a breast health specialist, medical social worker, or cancer clinical psychologist or psychiatrist, can also help a woman consider her options for reducing her risk of breast cancer.

Many factors beyond the risk of disease itself may influence a woman's decision about whether to undergo risk-reducing surgery. For example, for women who have been diagnosed with cancer in one breast, these factors can include distress about the possibility of having to go through cancer treatment a second time and the worry and inconvenience associated with long-term breast surveillance. For this reason, women who are considering risk-reducing surgery may want to talk with other women who have considered or had the procedure. Support groups can help connect women with others who have had similar cancer experiences. The searchable NCI database National Organizations That Offer Cancer-Related Services (www.supportorgs.cancer.gov/home.aspx?js=1) has listings for many support groups.

Finally, if a woman has a strong family history of breast cancer, ovarian cancer, or both, she and other members of her family may want to obtain genetic counseling services. A genetic counselor or other healthcare provider trained in genetics can review the family's risks of disease and help family members obtain genetic testing for mutations in cancer-predisposing genes, if appropriate.

Part Four

Screening, Diagnosis, and Stages of Breast Cancer

Chapter 29

Breast-Cancer Screening and Exams

Chapter Contents

Section 29.1

Overview of Breast-Cancer Screening

This section includes text excerpted from "Breast
Cancer Screening (PDQ®)—Patient Version,"
National Cancer Institute (NCI), October 26, 2018.

What Is Screening?

Screening is looking for signs of disease, such as breast cancer
before a person has symptoms. The goal of screening tests is to find
cancer at an early stage when it can be treated and may be cured.
Sometimes a screening test finds cancer that is very small or very slow
growing. These cancers are unlikely to cause death or illness during
the person's lifetime.

Scientists are trying to better understand which people are more
likely to get certain types of cancer. For example, they look at the
person's age, their family history, and certain exposures during their
lifetime. This information helps doctors recommend who should be
screened for cancer, which screening tests should be used, and how
often the tests should be done.

It is important to remember that your doctor does not necessarily
think you have cancer if he or she suggests a screening test. Screening
tests are done when you have no cancer symptoms. Women who have
a strong family history or a personal history of cancer or other risk
factors may also be offered genetic testing.

If a screening test result is abnormal, you may need to have more
tests done to find out if you have cancer. These are called "diagnostic
tests," rather than screening tests.

What Does Breast-Cancer Screening Involve?

Breast-cancer screening involves the following:

- Tests are used to screen for different types of cancer when a
  person does not have symptoms.

- Mammography is the most common screening test for breast cancer.

- Magnetic resonance imaging (MRI) may be used to screen
  women who have a high risk of breast cancer.

Whether a woman should be screened for breast cancer and the
screening test to use depends on certain factors.

- Other screening tests have been or are being studied in clinical trials.

- Breast exam

- Thermography

- Tissue sampling

Screening tests for breast cancer are being studied in clinical trials.

Tests Are Used to Screen for Different Types of Cancer When a Person Does Not Have Symptoms

Scientists study screening tests to find those with the fewest harms and most benefits. Cancer screening trials also are meant to show whether early detection (finding cancer before it causes symptoms) helps a person live longer or decreases a person's chance of dying from the disease. For some types of cancer, the chance of recovery is better if the disease is found and treated at an early stage.

Mammography Is the Most Common Screening Test for Breast Cancer

A mammogram is an X-ray picture of the breast. Mammography may find tumors that are too small to feel. It may also find ductal carcinoma *in situ* (DCIS). In DCIS, abnormal cells line the breast duct, and in some women may become invasive cancer.

Mammography is less likely to find breast tumors in women with dense breast tissue. Because both tumors and dense breast tissue appear white on a mammogram, it can be harder to find a tumor when there is dense breast tissue. Younger women are more likely to have dense breast tissue.

Many factors affect whether mammography is able to detect (find) breast cancer:

- The age and weight of the patient

- The size and type of tumor

- Where the tumor has formed in the breast

- How sensitive the breast tissue is to hormones

- How dense the breast tissue is

- The timing of the mammography within the woman's menstrual cycle

- The quality of the mammogram pictures

- The skill of the radiologist in reading the mammogram

Women aged 50 to 69 years who have screening mammograms have a lower chance of dying from breast cancer than women who do not have screening mammograms.

Fewer women are dying of breast cancer in the United States, but it is not known whether the lower risk of dying is because the cancer was found early by screening or whether the treatments were better.

Magnetic Resonance Imaging May Be Used to Screen Women Who Have a High Risk of Breast Cancer

MRI is a procedure that uses a magnet, radio waves, and a computer to make a series of detailed pictures of areas inside the body. This procedure is also called "nuclear magnetic resonance imaging (NMRI)." MRI does not use any X-rays and the woman is not exposed to radiation.

MRI may be used as a screening test for women who have a high risk of breast cancer. Factors that put women at high risk include the following:

- Certain gene changes, such as changes in the *BRCA1* or *BRCA2* genes

- A family history (first degree relative, such as a mother, daughter or sister) with breast cancer

- Certain genetic syndromes, such as Li-Fraumeni (LFS) or Cowden syndrome (CS)

An MRI is more likely than mammography to find a breast mass that is not cancer.

Whether a Woman Should Be Screened for Breast Cancer and the Screening Test to Use Depends on Certain Factors

Women with risk factors for breast cancer, such as certain changes in the *BRCA1* or *BRCA2* gene or certain genetic syndromes may be screened at a younger age and more often.

Women who have had radiation treatment to the chest, especially at a young age, may start routine breast-cancer screening at an earlier age. The benefits and risks of mammograms and MRIs for these women have not been studied.

Breast-cancer screening has not been shown to benefit the following women:

- Elderly women who, if diagnosed with breast cancer through screening, will usually die of other causes

- In women with an average risk of developing breast cancer, screening mammography before age 40 has not shown any benefit

- In women who are not expected to live for a long time and have other diseases or conditions, finding and treating early-stage breast cancer may reduce their quality of life (QOL) without helping them live longer

Other Screening Tests Have Been or Are Being Studied in Clinical Trials

Studies have been done to find out if the following breast-cancer screening tests are useful in finding breast cancer or helping women with breast cancer live longer.

Breast Exam

A clinical breast exam (CBE) is an exam of the breast by a doctor or other health professional. She or he will carefully feel the breasts and under the arms for lumps or anything else that seems unusual. It is not known if having CBEs decreases the chance of dying from breast cancer.

Breast self-exams may be done by women or men to check their breasts for lumps or other changes. If you feel any lumps or notice any other changes in your breasts, talk to your doctor. Doing regular breast self-exams has not been shown to decrease the chance of dying from breast cancer.

Thermography

Thermography is a procedure in which a special camera that senses heat is used to record the temperature of the skin that covers the breasts. Tumors can cause temperature changes that may show up on the thermogram.

There have been no randomized clinical trials of thermography to find out how well it detects breast cancer or the harms of the procedure.

Tissue Sampling

Breast-tissue sampling is taking cells from breast tissue to check under a microscope. Breast-tissue sampling as a screening test has not been shown to decrease the risk of dying from breast cancer.

Screening Tests for Breast Cancer Are Being Studied in Clinical Trials

Information about clinical trials supported by National Cancer Institute (NCI) can be found on NCI clinical trials webpage. Clinical trials supported by other organizations can be found on the Clinical-Trials.gov website.

Section 29.2

Breast Self-Exam

"Breast Self-Exam," © 2016 Omnigraphics. Reviewed February 2019.

Breast self-examination is a technique people can use to visually and manually check their own breast tissue for lumps or other changes. Many healthcare practitioners and cancer-prevention organizations recommend performing monthly breast self-examinations beginning at age 18 as a method of early detection for breast cancer. People who conduct regular self-exams become familiar with the normal appearance and feel of their breast tissue, which enables them to recognize changes and discover lumps that may require medical attention. Some of the changes that should be checked by a doctor include:

- New lumps or areas of thickness, which may or may not be painful
- Discharge of fluid from the nipples
- Dimpling, puckering, rashes, or other changes to the skin
- Changes to the size or shape of the breast

Finding lumps or noticing changes should not be a cause for alarm, however. An estimated 80 percent of lumps found in self-examinations are not cancerous, and most breast problems are caused by something other than cancer. In fact, some experts do not recommend self-examinations by people over 40 with no increased risk of breast cancer. They argue that the potential benefits of early detection are outweighed by the risks of undergoing tests and treatments that are unnecessary. Instead, they recommend regular checkups at a doctor's office as well as annual mammograms.

Self-Examination Procedures

Ideally, breast self-examinations should be performed on a monthly basis. For women who are menstruating, the best time is usually toward the end of the monthly period, when the breasts are less likely to be tender. For those who no longer have periods, experts recommend choosing a certain day of the month. Performing self-examinations on a regular schedule make it easier to compare the results and recognize changes in breast tissue.

Visual Examination

The first part of the process involves a visual examination of the breasts. This examination should be conducted while standing in front of a mirror in three different positions: with your arms hanging naturally at your sides; with your arms raised above your head; and with your hands on your hips and your upper body leaning forward from the waist. Be sure to look from the right and left sides as well as from the front. Check carefully for any changes to the following:

Size and Shape

Make sure your breasts appear to be their usual size and shape, and that no sudden changes have occurred. Although one breast may normally be larger than the other, you should not see any visible swelling or bulging.

Skin and Veins

Check the skin on your breasts for anything that appears unusual, such as puckering, dimpling, or distortion. Also look for areas of redness, soreness, rashes, or texture changes. Make sure that the veins beneath the skin appear as they usually do. You should not see a noticeable increase in the size or number of veins in one breast as compared to the other breast.

Nipples

Check for any physical changes to the appearance or position of the nipples, such as a sudden inversion. Also check the skin for redness, itching, scaliness, or swelling. Look for any fluid discharge, which may appear watery, milky, sticky, or bloody.

Manual Examination

The second part of the process involves a manual examination of each breast using the fingers of the opposite hand. It should cover the entire surface area of each breast, from the collarbone down to the abdomen, and from the armpit across to the cleavage. This examination should be conducted while lying down, and then again while standing up. The main steps are as follows:

1. Lie down on your back and place a pillow beneath your right shoulder.

2. Place your right arm on top of your head.

3. Use the pads of the three middle fingers on your left hand to examine your right breast.

4. Move your fingers in small circles, about the size of a quarter.

5. Vary the amount of pressure you apply in order to feel all levels of your breast tissue. Use light pressure to feel just beneath the skin, and firm pressure to feel the deep tissue against the ribcage.

6. Begin under the armpit and work from top to bottom along the outer part of your breast.

7. After completing one vertical strip, move over one finger width and begin a new strip, working from bottom to top. Do not lift the fingers between rows.

8. Check the entire breast area in an up-and-down pattern, as if mowing a lawn.

9. Repeat the process by using the left hand to examine the right breast.

10. Examine both breasts again while standing. Many women find it convenient to perform this part of the self-examination in the shower, while the skin is wet and soapy.

If you discover a lump in one breast, check to see if the same kind of lump exists in the other breast. If so, the lumps are probably normal. Many women have fibrocystic lumps that occur throughout both breasts, which may make self-examination difficult. By performing regular self-examinations, women can become familiar with the normal appearance of their breast tissue and consult with medical professionals if they notice any changes.

References

1. "Breast Self-Examination," Healthwise, February 20, 2015.
2. "The Five Steps of a Breast Self-Exam," Breastcancer.org, 2016.
3. "How to Do a Breast Self-Exam," Maurer Foundation, March 26, 2016.

Section 29.3

Harms of Breast-Cancer Screening

This section includes text excerpted from "Breast Cancer Screening (PDQ®)—Patient Version," National Cancer Institute (NCI), October 26, 2018.

Screening Tests Can Have Harms

Not all breast cancers will cause death or illness in a woman's lifetime, so they may not need to be found or treated.

Decisions about screening tests can be difficult. Not all screening tests are helpful and most have harms. Before having any screening test, you may want to discuss the test with your doctor. It is important to know the harms of the test and whether it has been proven to reduce the risk of dying from cancer.

The harms of mammography are discussed below:

False-Positive Test Results Can Occur

Screening test results may appear to be abnormal even though no cancer is present. A false-positive test result (one that shows there is cancer when there really isn't) is usually followed by more tests (such as biopsy), which also have risks.

When a breast biopsy result is abnormal, getting a second opinion from a different pathologist may confirm a correct breast-cancer diagnosis.

Most abnormal test results turn out not to be cancer. False-positive results are more common in the following:

- Younger women (under age 50)

- Women who have had previous breast biopsies

- Women with a family history of breast cancer

- Women who take hormones for menopause

False-positive results are more likely the first time screening mammography is done than with later screenings. For every ten women who have a single mammogram, one will have a false-positive result. The chance of having a false-positive result goes up the more mammograms a woman has. Comparing a current mammogram with a past mammogram lowers the risk of a false-positive result.

The skill of the radiologist also can affect the chance of a false-positive result.

False-Positive Results Can Lead to Extra Testing and Cause Anxiety

If a mammogram is abnormal, more tests may be done to diagnose cancer. Women can become anxious during diagnostic testing. Even if it is a false-positive test and cancer is not diagnosed, the result can lead to anxiety anywhere from a few days to years later.

Several studies show that women who feel anxiety after false-positive test results are more likely to schedule regular breast-screening exams in the future.

False-Negative Test Results Can Delay Diagnosis and Treatment

Screening test results may appear to be normal even though breast cancer is present. This is called a false-negative test result. A woman who has a false-negative test result may delay seeking medical care even if she has symptoms. About one in five cancers are missed by mammography.

The chance of a false-negative test result is more common in women who:

- Are younger

- Have dense breast tissue

- Have cancer that is not dependent on hormones (estrogen (ER) and progesterone (PR))

- Have cancer that is fast growing

Finding Breast Cancer May Lead to Breast-Cancer Treatment and Side Effects, but It May Not Improve a Woman's Health or Help Her Live Longer

Some breast cancers found by screening mammography may never cause health problems or become life-threatening. Finding these cancers is called "overdiagnosis." When these cancers are found, having treatment may cause serious side effects and may not lead to a longer, healthier life.

Mammography Exposes the Breast to Low Doses of Radiation

Being exposed to high radiation doses is a risk factor for breast cancer. The radiation dose with a mammogram is very low. Women who start getting mammograms after age 50 have very little risk that the overall exposure to radiation from mammograms throughout their lives will cause harm. Women with large breasts or with breast implants may be exposed to slightly higher radiation doses during screening mammography.

There May Be Pain or Discomfort during a Mammogram

During a mammogram, the breast is placed between two plates that are pressed together. Pressing the breast helps to get a better X-ray of the breast. Some women have pain or discomfort during a mammogram. The amount of pain may also depend on the following:

- The phase of the woman's menstrual cycle

- The woman's anxiety level

- How much pain the woman expected

Talk to Your Doctor about Your Risk of Breast Cancer and Your Need for Screening Tests

Talk to your doctor or other healthcare providers about your risk of breast cancer, whether a screening test is right for you, and the benefits and harms of the screening test. You should take part in the decision about whether you want to have a screening test, based on what is best for you.

Section 29.4

Breast-Cancer Screening for Women with Silicone Gel-Filled Breast Implants

This section contains text excerpted from the following sources: Text in this section begins with excerpts from "Silicone Gel-Filled Breast Implants," U.S. Food and Drug Agency (FDA), August 28, 2018. Text under the heading "Breast Cancer" is excerpted from "FDA Update on the Safety of Silicone Gel-Filled Breast Implants," U.S. Food and Drug Administration (FDA), June 2011. Reviewed February 2019.

Breast implants are not lifetime devices. The longer a woman has implants, the more likely it is that she will need to have surgery to remove or replace them.

The most frequent complications and adverse outcomes experienced by breast implant patients include capsular contracture, reoperation, and implant removal (with or without replacement). Other common complications include implant rupture, wrinkling, asymmetry, scarring, pain, and infection. In addition, women with breast implants may have a very low but increased likelihood of being diagnosed with anaplastic large cell lymphoma (ALCL).

MRI continues to be an effective method of detecting silent rupture of silicone gel-filled breast implants. If you have silicone gel-filled breast implants, the Food and Drug Agency (FDA) recommends that you receive MRI screening for silent rupture three years after receiving your implant and every two years after that.

There is no apparent association between silicone gel-filled breast implants and connective tissue disease, breast cancer, or reproductive problems. However, in order to definitively rule out these and other complications, studies would need to be much larger and longer than those conducted so far.

The FDA issued an Update on the Safety of Silicone Gel-Filled Breast Implants. This update included preliminary results of the studies required by the manufacturers at the time of approval as well as a review of other available scientific data.

The Summary of Safety and Effectiveness for each of the five approved silicone gel-filled breast implants details safety information known at the time of FDA approval. As the FDA learns of new safety information, it requires companies to update their product labeling. The most current safety information about silicone gel-filled breast implants can be found in the labeling.

Breast Cancer

Women who receive silicone gel-filled breast implants for augmentation do not appear to be at increased risk of developing breast cancer. In fact, studies suggest they may be at average or even lower risk— with some estimating a risk reduction of 10 to 50 percent.

Survival rates for women with breast cancer who receive silicone gel-filled breast implants as part of breast reconstruction appear to be unaffected by the presence of an implant.

Some reports have observed an increase in cancer risk for patients with cosmetic breast implants (not specifically silicone gel-filled breast implants), including brain, cervical, vulvar, lung, and nonmelanoma skin cancer. However, these observations appear unrelated to the effects of the implants themselves. Post-approval studies have not identified an increased cancer risk among silicone gel-filled breast implant recipients.

One possible exception is the rare development of anaplastic large cell lymphoma (ALCL) in women with breast implants. Reports in the scientific community have suggested a possible association between anaplastic lymphoma kinase (ALK)-negative ALCL and silicone gel-filled and saline-filled breast implants. In a thorough review of scientific literature published from January 1997 through May 2010, the FDA identified 34 unique cases of ALCL in women with breast implants throughout the world. The FDA's adverse event reporting systems also contain 17 reports of ALCL in women with breast implants. Additional cases have been identified through the FDA's contact with

181

other regulatory authorities, scientific experts, and breast implant manufacturers. In total, the FDA is aware of approximately 60 case reports of ALCL in women with breast implants worldwide.

Other than ALCL, the available epidemiologic evidence does not support a clinical association of silicone gel-filled breast implants with increased cancer risk in humans. Results from several published large scale cohort studies with long-term follow-up provide no evidence of an association between breast implants and cancer.

Screening for Breast Cancer

Screening mammograms are X-ray images of the breast used to look for changes in the breast tissue that are too small to cause noticeable symptoms; in some cases, these represent breast cancers. Breast implants may make it difficult to see breast tissue on standard mammograms; additional X-ray images, called implant displacement views, can be obtained at the time of a mammogram and should be used to examine the breast tissue more completely in breast implant patients.

The National Cancer Institute advises women with breast implants to receive screening mammography, at experienced centers, at intervals based on their age and risk factors. Women should be sure to notify the mammography facility and the technologist conducting the exam that they have breast implants.

Section 29.5

3D Technologies Changing Breast-Cancer Diagnosis

This section includes text excerpted from "3D Technologies Poised to Change How Doctors Diagnose Cancers," U.S. Food and Drug Administration (FDA), September 30, 2014. Reviewed February 2019.

Scientists at the Food and Drug Administration are studying the next generation of screening and diagnostic devices, some of which borrow from the world of entertainment. Soon, three-dimensional (3D) images in actual 3D might help your doctor find hidden tumors and better diagnose cancers, thanks to the regulatory work being done by a team at FDA's Division of Imaging, Diagnostics, and Software Reliability.

The team is led by Division Director Kyle Myers, a physicist with a Ph.D. in optical sciences. It includes Aldo Badano, Ph.D., a world-renowned expert in display evaluation technology, and Brian Garra, M.D., a diagnostic radiologist doing research in regulatory science at FDA.

They are studying how clinicians receive visual information and analyze it to diagnose a disease. At the center of their research are breast-cancer screening devices, which are making the leap from traditional two-dimensional (2D) screening such as mammography to 3D breast tomosynthesis, 3D ultrasound and breast computerized tomography (CT). This technology is very exploratory and years away from becoming standard in your doctor's office.

New Era in Breast-Cancer Detection

There are many new technologies being developed for breast-cancer screening, especially 3D alternatives that may eventually replace today's 2D mammography. FDA has already approved two of these state-of-the-art devices: The Selenia Dimensions 3D System, which provides 3D breast tomosynthesis images of the breast for breast-cancer diagnosis; and the GE Healthcare's SenoClaire, which uses a combination of 2D mammogram images and 3D breast tomosynthesis images.

The technologies under development include 3D breast tomosynthesis, which artificially creates 3D images of the breast from a limited set of 2D images. Tomosynthesis reveals sections of the breast that can be hidden by overlapping tissue in a standard mammogram.

"The problem of overlapping shadows has confounded breast-cancer screening because mammograms don't show cancers that are hidden by overlapping tissue," Myers says. And compounding the problem is overlapping tissue that can look like cancer but isn't. "The new technologies we're studying overcome these barriers," she adds.

Another benefit of 3D breast tomosynthesis: It's more accurate than mammography in pinpointing the size and location of cancer tumors in dense breast tissue, Myers says. With 3D breast tomosynthesis, doctors can detect abnormalities earlier and better see small tumors because the images are clearer and have greater contrast.

"Clinical studies have shown that 3D breast tomosynthesis can increase the cancer detection rate, reduce the number of women sent for biopsy who don't have cancer, or achieve some balance of these two goals of this new screening technology," she adds.

There's also a lot of research and development in 3D ultrasound, which automatically scans the breast and generates 3D data that can be sliced and examined from any direction. Garra, who is a leader in this field, says 3D ultrasound improves breast-cancer detection in women with dense breast tissue.

"Both 3D breast tomosynthesis and 3D ultrasound detect breast cancer. But for radiologists and other doctors, there are many more images to examine, and that can reduce the speed at which studies can be interpreted," he says.

Another promising technology—the dedicated breast CT system— creates a full 3D representation of the breast. The scan is taken while the patient lies face down on a bed with her breast suspended through a cup and the X-ray machine rotates around it. For patients, the procedure is more comfortable than regular mammography because the breast isn't compressed. Also, there's less radiation exposure than during a CT exam of the entire chest because only the breast is exposed to X-rays.

Health care practitioners using this technology have to learn how to read and interpret hundreds of high-resolution images produced by the scanner. But what makes the task easier is that the images have less distortion than mammography, and the system is optimized to differentiate between the breast's soft tissue and cancer tissue.

"These images will be very different from 2D mammograms. They're truly 3D images of the breast from any orientation. You can scroll through the slices—up and down, left and right—and get a unique view of the breast like never before," Myers says. "It gives doctors tremendous freedom in how they look at the interior of the breast and evaluate its structures. It's almost like seeing the anatomy itself."

New Era in How We See

How can radiologists look at these images and convert them into three dimensions? That's where Badano's work comes in. His research lab is exploring various display device technologies to improve how radiologists review 3D images. The studied technologies include devices supported by mobile technologies and special-purpose 3D displays developed specifically for 3D imaging systems.

"These are no longer conventional images, so you need to examine them in the 3D space," he says. "Using a 2D display might no longer be ideal." Device manufacturers are building on technologies developed primarily for other markets, including the gaming industry, to show 3D images in actual 3D. But the work is painstaking and far from ready for medical use.

"As people have experienced in movie theaters and when playing video games, 3D displays have problems, including the image resolution and added noise. When wearing 3D glasses, our brain needs to separate the images from the left eye and the right eye and reconstruct a 3D object," Badano says. "In the lab, we're doing experiments to see how different technologies handle these tradeoffs."

One of the challenges is that 3D displays for medical imaging require better resolution. For medical use, the specifications are high—" and so are the stakes," he adds.

Chapter 30

HER2 Breast-Cancer Testing

What Is HER2 Breast-Cancer Testing?

HER2 stands for human epidermal growth factor receptor 2. It is a gene that makes a protein found on the surface of all breast cells. It is involved in normal cell growth.

Genes are the basic units of heredity, passed down from your mother and father. In certain cancers, especially breast cancer, the *HER2* gene mutates (changes) and makes extra copies of the gene. When this happens, the *HER2* gene makes too much HER2 protein, causing cells to divide and grow too fast.

Cancers with high levels of the HER2 protein are known as HER2-positive. Cancers with low levels of the protein are known as HER2-negative. About 20 percent of breast cancers are HER2-positive.

HER2 testing looks at a sample of tumor tissue. The most common ways to test tumor tissue are:

- **Immunohistochemistry (IHC) testing** measures the HER2 protein on the surface of the cells

- **Fluorescence *in situ* hybridization (FISH) testing** looks for extra copies of the *HER2* gene

Both types of tests can tell whether you have HER2-positive cancer. Treatments that specifically target HER2-positive breast cancer can be very effective.

This chapter includes text excerpted from "HER2 (Breast Cancer) Testing," MedlinePlus, National Institutes of Health (NIH), November 2, 2018.

187

Other names: Human epidermal growth factor receptor 2, ERBB2 amplification, HER2 overexpression, HER2/neu tests

What Is HER2 Breast-Cancer Testing Used For?

HER2 testing is mostly used to find out whether cancer is HER2-positive. It is also sometimes used to see if cancer is responding to treatment or if cancer has returned after treatment.

Why Do You Need HER2 Breast-Cancer Testing?

If you've been diagnosed with breast cancer, you may need this test to find out if your cancer is HER2-positive or HER2-negative. If you are already being treated for HER2-positive breast cancer, you may need this test to:

- Find out if your treatment is working. Normal levels of HER2 may mean you are responding to treatment. High levels may mean the treatment is not working.

- Find out if cancer has come back after treatment

What Happens during a HER2 Breast-Cancer Test

Most HER2 testing involves taking a sample of tumor tissue in a procedure called a "biopsy." There are three main types of biopsy procedures:

- **Fine needle aspiration biopsy**, which uses a very thin needle to remove a sample of breast cells or fluid

- **Core needle biopsy**, which uses a larger needle to remove a sample

- **Surgical biopsy**, which removes a sample in a minor, outpatient procedure

Fine needle aspiration and core needle biopsies usually include the following steps:

- You will lay on your side or sit on an exam table.

- A healthcare provider will clean the biopsy site and inject it with an anesthetic so you won't feel any pain during the procedure.

188

- Once the area is numb, the provider will insert either a fine aspiration needle or core biopsy needle into the biopsy site and remove a sample of tissue or fluid.

- You may feel a little pressure when the sample is withdrawn.

- Pressure will be applied to the biopsy site until the bleeding stops.

- Your provider will apply a sterile bandage at the biopsy site.

In a surgical biopsy, a surgeon will make a small cut in your skin to remove all or part of a breast lump. A surgical biopsy is sometimes done if the lump can't be reached with a needle biopsy. Surgical biopsies usually include the following steps.

- You will lie on an operating table. An IV (intravenous line) may be placed in your arm or hand.

- You may be given medicine, called a "sedative," to help you relax.

- You will be given local or general anesthesia so you won't feel pain during the procedure.

- For local anesthesia, a healthcare provider will inject the biopsy site with medicine to numb the area.

- For general anesthesia, a specialist called an "anesthesiologist" will give you medicine so you will be unconscious during the procedure.

- Once the biopsy area is numb or you are unconscious, the surgeon will make a small cut into the breast and remove part or all of a lump. Some tissue around the lump may also be removed.

- The cut in your skin will be closed with stitches or adhesive strips.

The type of biopsy you have will depend on different factors, including the size and location of the tumor. HER2 can also be measured in a blood test, but blood testing for HER2 has not been proven to be useful for most patients. So, it is not usually recommended.

After your tissue sample has been taken, it will be tested in one of two ways:

- HER2 protein levels will be measured.

- The sample will be looked at for extra copies of the *HER2* gene.

189

Will You Need to Do Anything to Prepare for the HER2 Breast-Cancer Test?

You won't need any special preparations if you are getting local anesthesia (numbing of the biopsy site). If you are getting general anesthesia, you will probably need to fast (not eat or drink) for several hours before surgery. Your surgeon will give you more specific instructions. Also, if you are getting a sedative or general anesthesia, be sure to arrange for someone to drive you home. You may be groggy and confused after you wake up from the procedure.

Are There Any Risks Associated with the HER2 Breast-Cancer Test?

You may have a little bruising or bleeding at the biopsy site. Sometimes the site gets infected. If that happens, you will be treated with antibiotics. A surgical biopsy may cause some additional pain and discomfort. Your healthcare provider may recommend or prescribe medicine to help you feel better.

There is very little risk to having a blood test. You may have slight pain or bruising at the spot where the needle was put in, but most symptoms go away quickly.

What Do the Results of HER2 Breast-Cancer Test Mean?

If HER2 protein levels are higher than normal or extra copies of the *HER2* gene are found, it probably means you have HER2-positive cancer. If your results show normal amounts of HER2 protein or the normal number *HER2* genes, you probably have HER2-negative cancer.

If your results were not clearly positive or negative, you will probably get retested, either using a different tumor sample or using a different testing method. Most often, IHC (testing for the HER2 protein) is done first, followed by FISH (testing for extra copies of the gene). IHC testing is less expensive and provides faster results than FISH. But most breast specialists think FISH testing is more accurate.

Treatments for HER2-positive breast cancer can substantially shrink cancerous tumors, with very few side effects. These treatments are not effective in HER2-negative cancers.

If you are being treated for HER2-positive cancer, normal results may mean you are responding to treatment. Results that show higher than normal amounts may mean your treatment is not working, or that cancer has come back after treatment.

Is There Anything Else That You Need to Know about HER2 Breast-Cancer Testing?

While it's much more common in women, breast cancer, including HER2-positive breast cancer, can also affect men. If a man has been diagnosed with breast cancer, HER2 testing may be recommended.

In addition, both men and women may need HER2 testing if they have been diagnosed with certain cancers of the stomach and esophagus. These cancers sometimes have high levels of the HER2 protein and may respond well to HER2-positive cancer treatments.

Chapter 31

PDL1 (Immunotherapy) Tests

What Is a PDL1 Test?

This test measures the amount of PDL1 on cancer cells. PDL1 is a protein that helps keep immune cells from attacking nonharmful cells in the body. Normally, the immune system fights foreign substances like viruses and bacteria, and not your own healthy cells. Some cancer cells have high amounts of PDL1. This allows the cancer cells to "trick" the immune system, and avoid being attacked as foreign, harmful substances.

If your cancer cells have a high amount of PDL1, you may benefit from a treatment called immunotherapy. Immunotherapy is a therapy that boosts your immune system to help it recognize and fight cancer cells. Immunotherapy has been shown to be very effective in treating certain types of cancers. It also tends to have fewer side effects than other cancer therapies.

Other names: Programmed death-ligand 1, PD-LI, PDL-1 by immunohistochemistry (IHC)

What Is PDL1 Test Used For?

PDL1 testing is used to find out if you have cancer that may benefit from immunotherapy.

This chapter includes text excerpted from "PDL1 (Immunotherapy) Tests," MedlinePlus, National Institutes of Health (NIH), November 5, 2018.

Why Do You Need a PDL1 Test?

You may need PDL1 testing if you've been diagnosed with one of the following cancers:

- Breast cancer
- Nonsmall cell lung cancer
- Melanoma
- Hodgkin lymphoma
- Bladder cancer
- Kidney cancer

High levels of PDL1 are often found in these, as well as some other types of cancer. Cancers that have high levels of PDL1 can often be treated effectively with immunotherapy.

What Happens during a PDL1 Test

Most PDL1 tests are done in a procedure called a "biopsy." There are three main types of biopsy procedures:

- **Fine needle aspiration biopsy**, which uses a very thin needle to remove a sample of breast cells or fluid
- **Core needle biopsy**, which uses a larger needle to remove a sample
- **Surgical biopsy**, which removes a sample in a minor, outpatient procedure

Fine needle aspiration and core needle biopsies usually include the following steps:

- You will lay on your side or sit on an exam table.
- A healthcare provider will clean the biopsy site and inject it with an anesthetic so you won't feel any pain during the procedure.
- Once the area is numb, the provider will insert either a fine aspiration needle or core biopsy needle into the biopsy site and remove a sample of tissue or fluid.
- You may feel a little pressure when the sample is withdrawn.
- Pressure will be applied to the biopsy site until the bleeding stops.

- Your provider will apply a sterile bandage at the biopsy site.

In a surgical biopsy, a surgeon will make a small cut in your skin to remove all or part of a breast lump. A surgical biopsy is sometimes done if the lump can't be reached with a needle biopsy. Surgical biopsies usually include the following steps.

- You will lie on an operating table. An IV (intravenous line) may be placed in your arm or hand.

- You may be given medicine, called a "sedative," to help you relax.

- You will be given local or general anesthesia so you won't feel pain during the procedure.

- For **local anesthesia**, a healthcare provider will inject the biopsy site with medicine to numb the area.

- For **general anesthesia**, a specialist called an "anesthesiologist" will give you medicine so you will be unconscious during the procedure.

- Once the biopsy area is numb or you are unconscious, the surgeon will make a small cut into the breast and remove part or all of a lump. Some tissue around the lump may also be removed.

- The cut in your skin will be closed with stitches or adhesive strips.

There are different types of biopsies. The type of biopsy you get will depend on the location and size of your tumor.

Will You Need to Do Anything to Prepare for PDL1 Test?

You won't need any special preparations if you are getting local anesthesia (numbing of the biopsy site). If you are getting general anesthesia, you will probably need to fast (not eat or drink) for several hours before surgery. Your surgeon will give you more specific instructions. Also, if you are getting a sedative or general anesthesia, be sure to arrange for someone to drive you home. You may be groggy and confused after you wake up from the procedure.

What Are the Risks Associated with the PDL1 Test?

You may have a little bruising or bleeding at the biopsy site. Sometimes the site gets infected. If that happens, you will be treated with antibiotics. A surgical biopsy may cause some additional pain and discomfort. Your healthcare provider may recommend or prescribe medicine to help you feel better.

What Do the PDL1 Test Results Mean?

If your results show your tumor cells have high levels of PDL1, you may be started on immunotherapy. If your results do not show high levels of PDL1, immunotherapy may not be effective for you. But you may benefit from another type of cancer treatment. If you have questions about your results, talk to your healthcare provider.

Is There Anything Else You Need to know about a PDL1 Test?

Immunotherapy does not work for everyone, even if you have tumors with high levels of PDL1. Cancer cells are complex and often unpredictable. Healthcare providers and researchers are still learning about immunotherapy and how to predict who will benefit the most from this treatment.

Chapter 32

Mammograms

Chapter Contents

Section 32.1

Questions and Answers about Mammograms

This section includes text excerpted from "Mammograms,"
Office on Women's Health (OWH), U.S. Department of
Health and Human Services (HHS), November 22, 2018.

What Is a Mammogram?

A mammogram is a low-dose X-ray exam of the breasts to look for
changes that are not normal. The results are recorded on X-ray film or
directly into a computer for a doctor called a "radiologist" to examine.

A mammogram allows the doctor to have a closer look for changes
in breast tissue that cannot be felt during a breast exam. It is used for
women who have no breast complaints and for women who have breast
symptoms, such as a change in the shape or size of a breast, a lump,
nipple discharge, or pain. Breast changes occur in almost all women.
In fact, most of these changes are not cancer and are called "benign,"
but only a doctor can know for sure. Breast changes can also happen
monthly, due to your menstrual period.

What Is the Best Method of Detecting Breast Cancer as Early as Possible?

A high-quality mammogram plus a clinical breast exam (CBE), an
exam done by your doctor, is the most effective way to detect breast
cancer early. Finding breast cancer early greatly improves a woman's
chances for successful treatment.

Like any test, mammograms have both benefits and limitations.
For example, some cancers can't be found by a mammogram, but they
may be found in a CBE.

Checking your own breasts for lumps or other changes is called a
"breast self-exam (BSE)." Studies so far have not shown that BSE alone
helps reduce the number of deaths from breast cancer. BSE should not
take the place of routine CBEs and mammograms.

If you choose to do BSE, remember that breast changes can occur
because of pregnancy, aging, menopause, menstrual cycles, or from
taking birth control pills or other hormones. It is normal for breasts
to feel a little lumpy and uneven. Also, it is common for breasts to be
swollen and tender right before or during a menstrual period. If you
notice any unusual changes in your breasts, contact your doctor.

How Is a Mammogram Done?

You stand in front of a special X-ray machine. The person who takes the X-rays, called a "radiologic technician," places your breasts, one at a time, between an X-ray plate and a plastic plate. These plates are attached to the X-ray machine and compress the breasts to flatten them. This spreads the breast tissue out to obtain a clearer picture. You will feel pressure on your breast for a few seconds. It may cause you some discomfort; you might feel squeezed or pinched. This feeling only lasts for a few seconds, and the flatter your breast, the better the picture. Most often, two pictures are taken of each breast—one from the side and one from above. A screening mammogram takes about 20 minutes from start to finish.

Are There Different Types of Mammograms?

Mammograms are of different types.

- **Screening mammograms** are done for women who have no symptoms of breast cancer. It usually involves two X-rays of each breast. Screening mammograms can detect lumps or tumors that cannot be felt. They can also find microcalcifications or tiny deposits of calcium in the breast, which sometimes mean that breast cancer is present.

- **Diagnostic mammograms** are used to check for breast cancer after a lump or other symptom or sign of breast cancer has been found. Signs of breast cancer may include pain, thickened skin on the breast, nipple discharge, or a change in breast size or shape. This type of mammogram also can be used to find out more about breast changes found on a screening mammogram or to view breast tissue that is hard to see on a screening mammogram. A diagnostic mammogram takes longer than a screening mammogram because it involves more X-rays in order to obtain views of the breast from several angles. The technician can magnify a problem area to make a more detailed picture, which helps the doctor make a correct diagnosis.

A digital mammogram also uses X-rays to produce an image of the breast, but instead of storing the image directly on film, the image is stored directly on a computer. This allows the recorded image to be magnified for the doctor to take a closer look. Current research has not shown that digital images are better at showing cancer than X-ray film images in general. But, women with dense breasts who are pre or perimenopausal, or who are younger than age 50, may benefit from having a digital rather than a film mammogram. Digital mammography may offer these benefits:

- Long-distance consultations with other doctors may be easier because the images can be shared by computer

- Slight differences between normal and abnormal tissues may be more easily noted

- The number of follow-up tests needed may be fewer

- Fewer repeat images may be needed, reducing exposure to radiation

How Often Should You Get a Mammogram?

The U.S. Preventive Services Task Force (USPSTF) recommends:

- Women ages 50 to 74 years should get a mammogram every 2 years

- Women younger than age 50 should talk to a doctor about when to start and how often to have a mammogram

What Can Mammograms Show?

The radiologist will look at your X-rays for breast changes that do not look normal and for differences in each breast. She or he will compare your past mammograms with your most recent one to check for changes. The doctor will also look for lumps and calcifications.

- **Lump or mass.** The size, shape, and edges of a lump sometimes can give doctors information about whether or not it may be cancer. On a mammogram, a growth that is benign often looks smooth and round with a clear, defined edge. Breast cancer often has a jagged outline and an irregular shape.

- **Calcification.** Calcification is a deposit of the mineral calcium in the breast tissue. Calcifications appear as small white spots on a mammogram. There are two types:

  - **Macrocalcifications** are large calcium deposits often caused by aging. These usually are not a sign of cancer.

  - **Microcalcifications** are tiny specks of calcium that may be found in an area of rapidly dividing cells.

If calcifications are grouped together in a certain way, it may be a sign of cancer. Depending on how many calcium specks you have, how big they are, and what they look like, your doctor may suggest that you have other tests. Calcium in the diet does not create calcium deposits, or calcifications, in the breast.

What If Your Screening Mammogram Shows a Problem?

If you have a screening-test result that suggests cancer, your doctor must find out whether it is due to cancer or to some other cause. Your doctor may ask about your personal and family medical history. You may have a physical exam. Your doctor also may order some of these tests:

- **Diagnostic mammogram,** to focus on a specific area of the breast

- **Ultrasound,** an imaging test that uses sound waves to create a picture of your breast. The pictures may show whether a lump is solid or filled with fluid. A cyst is a fluid-filled sac. Cysts are not cancer. But a solid mass may be cancer. After the test, your doctor can store the pictures on video or print them out. This exam may be used along with a mammogram.

- **Magnetic resonance imaging (MRI),** which uses a powerful magnet linked to a computer. MRI makes detailed pictures of breast tissue. Your doctor can view these pictures on a monitor or print them on film. MRI may be used along with a mammogram.

- **Biopsy,** a test in which fluid or tissue is removed from your breast to help find out if there is cancer. Your doctor may refer you to a surgeon or to a doctor who is an expert in breast disease for a biopsy.

Where Can You Get a High-Quality Mammogram?

Women can get high-quality mammograms in breast clinics, hospital radiology departments, mobile vans, private radiology offices, and doctors' offices. The U.S. Food and Drug Administration (FDA) certifies mammography facilities that meet strict quality standards for their X-ray machines and staff and are inspected every year. You can ask your doctor or the staff at the mammography center about FDA certification before making your appointment. A list of FDA-certified facilities can be found on the Internet.

Your doctor, local medical clinic, or local or state health department can tell you where to get no-cost or low-cost mammograms. You can also call the National Cancer Institute's (NCI) Cancer Information Service (CIS) toll-free at 800-422-6237.

What If You Have Breast Implants?

Women with breast implants should also have mammograms. A woman who had an implant after breast-cancer surgery in which the entire breast was removed (mastectomy) should ask her doctor whether she needs a mammogram of the reconstructed breast.

If you have breast implants, be sure to tell your mammography facility that you have them when you make your appointment. The technician and radiologist must be experienced in X-raying patients with breast implants. Implants can hide some breast tissue, making it harder for the radiologist to see a problem when looking at your mammogram. To see as much breast tissue as possible, the X-ray technician will gently lift the breast tissue slightly away from the implant and take extra pictures of the breasts.

How Do You Get Ready for Your Mammogram?

First, check with the place you are having the mammogram for any special instructions you may need to follow before you go. Here are some general guidelines to follow:

- If you are still having menstrual periods, try to avoid making your mammogram appointment during the week before your period. Your breasts will be less tender and swollen. The mammogram will hurt less and the picture will be better.

- If you have breast implants, be sure to tell your mammography facility that you have them when you make your appointment.

- Wear a shirt with shorts, pants, or a skirt. This way, you can undress from the waist up and leave your shorts, pants, or skirt on when you get your mammogram.

- Don't wear any deodorant, perfume, lotion, or powder under your arms or on your breasts on the day of your mammogram appointment. These things can make shadows show up on your mammogram.

- If you have had mammograms at another facility, have those X-ray films sent to the new facility so that they can be compared to the new films.

Are There Any Problems with Mammograms?

Although they are not perfect, mammograms are the best method to find breast changes that cannot be felt. If your mammogram shows a breast change, sometimes other tests are needed to better understand it. Even if the doctor sees something on the mammogram, it does not mean it is cancer.

As with any medical test, mammograms have limits. These limits include:

- **They are only part of a complete breast exam.** Your doctor also should do a clinical breast exam. If your mammogram finds something abnormal, your doctor will order other tests.

- **Finding cancer does not always mean saving lives.** Even though mammography can detect tumors that cannot be felt, finding a small tumor does not always mean that a woman's life will be saved. Mammography may not help a woman with fast-growing cancer that has already spread to other parts of her body before being found.

- **False negatives can happen.** This means everything may look normal, but cancer is actually present. False negatives don't happen often. Younger women are more likely to have a false negative mammogram than are older women. The dense breasts of younger women make breast cancers harder to find in mammograms.

- **False positives can happen.** This is when the mammogram results look like cancer is present, even though it is not. False positives are more common in younger women, women who have had breast biopsies, women with a family history of breast cancer, and women who are taking estrogen, such as menopausal hormone therapy (MHT).

- **Mammograms (as well as dental X-rays and other routine X-rays) use very small doses of radiation.** The risk of any harm is very slight, but repeated X-rays could cause cancer. The benefits nearly always outweigh the risk. Talk to your doctor about the need for each X-ray. Ask about shielding to protect parts of the body that are not in the picture. You should always let your doctor and the technician know if there is any chance that you are pregnant.

Section 32.2

Digital Mammography

This section includes text excerpted from "Frequently Asked Questions about Digital Mammography," U.S. Food and Drug Administration (FDA), November 14, 2017.

What Is Digital Mammography?

Full field digital mammography (FFDM, also known simply as "digital mammography") is a mammography system where the X-ray film used in screen-film mammography (SFM) is replaced by solid-state detectors (SSD), similar to those found in digital cameras, which convert X-rays into electrical signals. The electrical signals are used to produce images of the breast that can be seen on a computer screen or printed on special films to look like screen-film mammograms. Types of digital mammography include direct radiography (the most common type, which captures the image directly onto a flat-panel detector (FPD)), computed radiography (CR) (which involves the use of a cassette that contains an imaging plate), or digital breast tomosynthesis (DBT).

What Is Digital Breast Tomosynthesis?

DBT is a relatively new technology. In DBT, the X-ray tube moves in an arc around the breast and takes multiple images from different angles. Similar to computed tomography (CT) scan, these images are then reconstructed into parallel "slices" through the breast. This allows interpreting physicians to see through layers of overlapping tissue.

How Can Women Find a FDA-Certified Digital Mammography Facility?

Digital mammography has been in use since 2001. Ninety-six percent of all certified mammography facilities in the United States. use digital units of some type. You can find a list of certified facilities, searchable by state or ZIP Code, at www.fda.gov/findmammography.

Do Private Insurance Companies, Medicare, and Medicaid Pay for Digital Mammography Exams, Such as Digital Breast Tomosynthesis?

You should contact your insurance provider before the procedure to determine what procedures are covered by your insurance plan. The telephone number for questions about Medicare reimbursement is 800-633-4227. To find the number for MEDICAID, look in your local directory.

Section 32.3

Nipple Aspirate Test Is No Substitute for Mammogram

This section includes text excerpted from "Nipple Aspirate Test Is No Substitute for Mammogram," U.S. Food and Drug Administration (FDA), October 27, 2017.

A mammogram is a low-dose X-ray picture of the breast—and it's still the best way for healthcare providers to screen women for breast cancer. (Breast-cancer screening lets healthcare providers check for cancer before there are signs and symptoms of the disease.)

Unfortunately, in the past, other tests have been falsely described as alternatives to mammograms. One such test is the nipple aspirate, which involves drawing fluid from a woman's breast with a special pump and testing it for abnormal cells. Companies have marketed this test as a way to screen for abnormal cells (instead of a mammogram), but the U.S. Food and Drug Administration (FDA) is reminding you that this kind of test cannot be used alone to screen for or diagnose breast cancer. In fact, if women were to skip a mammogram in favor of an unproven test, it could result in serious health consequences if breast cancer goes undetected.

Furthermore, the FDA is unaware of any valid scientific data to show that a nipple aspirate test, when used on its own, is an effective screening tool for any medical condition, including the detection of breast cancer or other breast diseases. And after the FDA initiated regulatory action against a company promoting such a test, the company voluntarily removed it from the market.

While the FDA believes that there are no nipple aspirate devices currently on the market, the agency urges healthcare providers and patients who may come in contact with the device to consider reporting it to MedWatch, the FDA's Safety Information and Adverse Event (AE) Reporting Program.

About U.S. Food and Drug Administration Actions and False Claims for Nipple Aspirate Tests

The FDA can take action when companies sell medical devices that make false medical claims. For instance, in February 2013, the FDA issued a warning letter to Atossa Genetics (ATOS), Inc., a company that was selling a nipple aspirate test with false or misleading labeling touting the test as FDA-cleared. The FDA asked the firm to take prompt action to correct the violations addressed in the warning letter. In October 2013, Atossa initiated a voluntary recall to remove the ForeCYTE Breast Health Test from the market.

In addition to stating that the test can help women 18 years and older determine their risk level for breast cancer, Atossa had claimed that its test was "literally a Pap smear for breast cancer." (A Pap smear is a screening test for cervical cancer.) But this claim was unsubstantiated, according to FDA medical officer Michael Cummings, M.D., who reviews obstetrical and gynecological devices for the agency.

"The cervical Pap smear has a known clinical benefit supported by extensive clinical studies over many years," Cummings says. "Its scientific ability to screen for cervical cancer is unquestioned." The nipple aspirate test had no such evidence supporting it, he says.

A healthcare provider can follow up on an abnormal Pap smear with a procedure that will allow appropriately targeted biopsies. (A biopsy is a procedure that removes cells or tissue from your body to check for damage or disease.) However, an abnormal nipple aspirate report does not allow a targeted biopsy to confirm the presence of diseases.

In addition, the nipple aspirate test may produce results that are falsely positive or falsely negative. (Aspirate fluid containing few cells, or no cells at all, may miss cancers and give women dangerously false reassurance.)

More Information about Mammograms

The FDA is responsible for implementing a system for certifying facilities that perform mammography—and for reviewing new mammography devices to determine whether they may be marketed—to protect the public health.

If you're worried about how a mammogram feels, talk to your healthcare provider about what you can expect. A mammogram can be uncomfortable for the woman being screened because it briefly presses down on the breast to flatten out the breast tissue and increase the clarity of the X-ray image.

Also talk with your healthcare provider if you have specific questions about mammography (including when or how frequently you should be screened), or if you have other questions about breast-cancer screening.

The bottom line: Mammography is still the best test for breast-cancer screening.

Section 32.4

Thermogram No Substitute for Mammogram

This section includes text excerpted from "Breast Cancer Screening: Thermogram No Substitute for Mammogram," U.S. Food and Drug Administration (FDA), October 27, 2017.

The U.S. Food and Drug Administration (FDA) is reminding you that mammography—a low-dose X-ray image of the breast—is still the most effective breast-cancer screening test. Proper breast-cancer screening lets healthcare providers check for cancer even before there may be signs and symptoms of the disease.

Unfortunately, the FDA has received reports from healthcare providers and patients that some health centers are providing information that can mislead patients into believing that thermography—a type of test that shows patterns of heat and blood flow on or near the surface of the body—is a proven alternative to mammography. But the FDA is not aware of any scientific evidence to support these claims.

Indeed, thermography has not been shown to be effective as a standalone test for either breast-cancer screening or diagnosis in detecting early-stage breast cancer.

"Plenty of evidence shows that mammography is still the most effective screening method for detecting breast cancer in its early, most treatable stages," reiterates Helen J. Barr, M.D., director of the Division of Mammography Quality Standards (DMQS) in the FDA Center for Devices and Radiological Health (CDRH). "You should not rely solely on thermography for the screening or diagnosis of breast cancer."

More about Misleading Thermography Claims—and U.S. Food and Drug Administration Actions to Protect the Public

The FDA regulates the medical devices used for breast-cancer screening.

About one in eight women will be diagnosed with breast cancer sometime in their lives, reports the National Cancer Institute (NCI), part of the National Institutes of Health (NIH). Rarely, men also can have breast cancer. But there has been a decline in breast-cancer deaths in recent years, and one reason is that cancers have been detected earlier through mammography, according to the American Cancer Society (ACS).

In fact, the greatest danger from thermography is that those who opt for this method instead of mammography may miss the chance to detect cancer at its earliest stage.

Thermography has only been cleared by the FDA as an "adjunctive" tool—meaning for use alongside a primary test like mammography. Patients who undergo a thermography test alone should not be reassured of the findings because the device was not cleared to be used other than with another testing method like mammography.

Moreover, some websites claim that thermography can find breast cancer years before it would be detected through other methods and have unproven claims about improved detection of cancer in dense breasts. The FDA is aware of no evidence that supports these claims.

The FDA has taken regulatory action (including issuing warning letters) against healthcare providers and thermography manufacturers who try to mislead patients into believing that the thermography can take the place of mammography. To protect the public health, the FDA's regulatory action can include scheduling a regulatory meeting, sending a warning letter or other correspondence, an establishment inspection, and judicial actions.

The FDA continues to monitor this situation.

Advice for Patients Getting Breast-Cancer Screening

Some women have sought out thermography because it is painless and doesn't require exposure to radiation.

If you're worried about how a mammogram feels, talk to your healthcare provider about what you can expect. A mammogram can be uncomfortable for the person being screened because it briefly presses down on the breast to flatten out the breast tissue and increase the clarity of the X-ray image.

Also talk to your healthcare provider if you have specific questions about mammography, including questions about when and how frequently you should be screened. As a rule, you should also call your healthcare provider if you notice any change in either of your breasts such as a lump, thickening or nipple leakage, or changes in how the nipple looks.

Section 32.5

Mammogram Myths

This section includes text excerpted from "4 Mammography Myths,"
U.S. Food and Drug Administration (FDA), January 19, 2018.

Knowing the truth about mammograms could help save your life or the life of someone you love. Over 60 percent of breast-cancer cases are diagnosed before they spread. Nearly 90 percent of women who find and treat their breast cancer is cancer-free at five years. Mammograms can help reduce the number of deaths from breast cancer among women ages 40 to 70.

Myth: Mammograms don't help.

Fact: Regular mammograms are the best tests doctors have to find breast cancer early, sometimes up to three years before it can be felt.

Myth: Mammograms cause cancer.

Fact: Mammograms utilize very small doses of radiation—it's like getting an X-ray.

The risk of harm is extremely low. Thanks to technology, radiation doses in mammography have consistently decreased with time while consistently increasing inaccuracy. The benefits of detecting and treating something that is life-threatening far outweigh the extremely small potential of harm from radiation exposure.

Myth: Mammograms are inaccurate.

Fact: Although they are not perfect, mammograms are the best tool we have in early detection. Overall, when cancer is present, mammograms are about 80 percent effective in identifying it. It is possible to get a false-negative result (when a mammogram misses cancer that is present). Although this happens about 20 percent of the time, repeated and regular screenings reduce this percentage. It is also possible to get a false-positive result (when a mammogram indicates the presence of cancer where there is none present). These results usually require follow-up with additional testing and most women called back for this additional testing do not have cancer.

Myth: Mammograms are painful.

Fact: Everyone's pain threshold is different, but the compression involved in a mammogram is more often described as temporary discomfort. It's necessary to ensure that everything can be seen clearly on a mammogram. It could be unpleasant for a few moments, but it's a small tradeoff for living cancer-free, or catching breast cancer early and fighting it successfully. It may also help to know that your breasts may be more sensitive if you are about to get or have your period—so you may want to schedule your routine mammogram in the middle of your cycle.

Know before you go.

- Knowing how to prepare for your mammogram can help ease your mind and speed the process.

- Don't wear deodorant, perfume, lotion, or powder under your arms or on your breasts on the day of your exam. Foreign particles could show up in an X-ray.

- Only get a mammogram at facilities certified by the FDA or one of its state counterparts. This ensures the staff is trained and you'll receive quality treatment. There were 8,675 Mammography Quality Standards Act (MQSA)-certified facilities as of April 2013, and 38,619,078 mammograms have been performed at these sites. You can find a site by visiting www.fda.gov/findmammography.

- Let technologists and staff know if you have breast implants. They may need to take more pictures than a regular mammogram.

- You have the right to a written report of the results within 30 days of receiving a mammogram, as well as the original mammogram X-ray pictures. Call if you don't get your results, rather than assuming that everything is normal.

- Bring prior mammograms or have them sent to the center if possible.

- Tell the clinic if you have physical disabilities that may make it hard for you to sit up, lift your arms, or hold your breath.

Section 32.6

Direct-to-Patient Mammogram Results: It's the Law

This section includes text excerpted from "Direct-to-Patient Mammogram Results: It's the Law," U.S. Food and Drug Administration (FDA), February 15, 2018.

It is a world of lightning-fast technology. In the radiology world, advances in teleradiology (the transmission of radiological images from one location to another for the purposes of interpretation or comparison) and the availability of workstations where physicians can review and manipulate digital images means that mammogram results and follow up may be available to women and their healthcare providers more quickly nowadays than in the past. In some cases, patients who require additional imaging or workup can go from a screening mammogram to a needle biopsy the same day.

Everyone involved in mammography, from the U.S. Food and Drug Administration (FDA) to mammography facilities and their dedicated mammography technologists, interpreting physicians, and administrative staff, recognizes the importance of and shares a role in ensuring that an effective mechanism exists for communicating mammography results. While healthcare providers routinely receive their patients' test results, the Mammography Quality Standards Act (MQSA) regulations have a unique provision that requires mammography facilities to send each patient a written summary of the mammography report in lay terms. While there are different approaches to achieving this goal, the regulations require that facilities maintain a system to ensure timely communication of mammography results to patients.

The content and format of the lay summary letters are left to the discretion of the facility; however, the regulations are clear about how and when patients must receive their results; the written summary must be sent within 30 days of the mammogram. If a patient's mammogram is interpreted as "Suspicious" or "Highly Suggestive of Malignancy," the MQSA requires the facility to make reasonable attempts to communicate those results to the patient and her referring healthcare provider as soon as possible.

For patients who are self-referred, the written mammography report, as well as the written lay summary, must be provided to the patient herself. Furthermore, the regulations also require that facilities that accept patients for mammography who do not have a healthcare provider must maintain a system for referring such patients to a healthcare provider when clinically indicated.

Many facilities choose to provide verbal results to patients to expedite healthcare and alleviate the anxiety of waiting for results. Just as verbal results to a healthcare provider must be followed up by a written medical report, any verbal communication of mammogram results to a patient must be supplemented with written communication. The intent of the regulation is that the patient herself has a written record of her results in easy to understand language, separate from the medical report delivered to her referring healthcare provider.

One common situation where verbal results might be conveyed is when a mammography exam results in an "incomplete: need additional imaging evaluation" assessment. In addition, the facility must also provide, within 30 days of the examination, a written lay summary indicating that additional imaging is needed. If the results of the follow-up diagnostic mammographic images are available within 30 days of the screening mammogram, the facility has the option of combining the results into one lay summary letter addressing both the screening and the diagnostic workup. If one combined lay summary is provided, the FDA suggests that it state specifically that it refers to both the screening and the diagnostic mammograms. If there are results from other types of follow-up imaging, for example, ultrasound, available within the 30-day timeframe, these may also be included in such a combined report.

Whether it's mailed, sent electronically, or handed to the patient, every patient that receives a mammographic exam must receive the results of that mammogram in written form. Although not required by the MQSA, facilities that have non-English reading populations may want to consider providing lay summary letters in another language to accommodate the needs of their patient population. Not only is effective communication of mammography results to women themselves a good check and balance system to ensure that results are communicated, but it also gives women direct knowledge about of their own breast health and empowers their involvement in further action, whether that be continuing routine screening or engaging in recommended further evaluation.

Chapter 33

Breast Magnetic Resonance Imaging

What Is a Breast Magnetic Resonance Imaging?

Magnetic resonance imaging (MRI) is a noninvasive diagnostic test that generates a series of detailed images of internal organs and body structures using a magnetic field and radio waves. These images are combined by a computer and examined by a radiologist to aid in the detection of cancer and other abnormalities. MRI of the breast is often performed following a diagnosis of breast cancer to gather additional information about the extent of the disease. Breast MRI is also used as a screening tool along with mammograms in women at high risk for developing breast cancer.

The Breast Magnetic Resonance Imaging Procedure

While undergoing a breast MRI, the patient typically lies face down on a table with her breasts positioned through special openings. In most cases, a contrast dye is injected into a vein in her arm either before or during the procedure. The dye helps create clearer images to make any abnormalities easier to detect. The table then slides into a large, cylindrical machine that looks like a tunnel.

"Breast Magnetic Resonance Imaging (MRI)," © 2016 Omnigraphics. Reviewed February 2019.

With a technician operating the MRI machine from a separate room, it creates a strong magnetic field around the patient and then sends pulses of radio waves from a scanner. Although this process is completely painless, the magnetic field and radio waves change the alignment of hydrogen atoms in the patient's body. The activity of the hydrogen atoms is analyzed by a computer, which converts the information into a detailed image of the breast. This image appears on a viewing monitor.

Advantages of Breast Magnetic Resonance Imaging

Breast MRI offers a number of advantages in screening and diagnosis of breast cancer and other breast abnormalities. Since MRIs do not use radiation, they are less dangerous for younger women or for women at high risk for breast cancer who must undergo multiple screenings per year. In addition, research has shown that breast MRI is capable of finding some small breast legions that might be missed by mammography or other screening methods. Because it is highly sensitive, breast MRI can also help detect breast cancer in women with dense breast tissue or breast implants.

Breast MRI is often used as a screening tool to find early breast cancers in women at high risk, including those with a strong family history of the disease, a BRCA gene mutation, precancerous breast changes such as lobular carcinoma *in situ* (LCIS), or a history of receiving radiation to the chest area. Breast MRI also may be used to further evaluate abnormalities or assess the extent of breast cancer detected through other means. Some of the common uses of breast MRI include:

- Detecting small lesions or abnormalities not visible using mammography or ultrasound

- Evaluating the size and location of breast cancer that may have spread to more than one area of the breast

- Determining whether breast cancer may have spread into the chest wall

- Evaluating the opposite breast for changes in women who have been recently diagnosed with cancer in one breast

- Determining the best surgical treatment options for removing breast cancer

- Checking for recurrence of breast cancer in women with lumpectomy scars that may produce inaccurate mammogram results

- Assessing whether a silicone gel breast implant may have leaked or ruptured

Risks of Breast Magnetic Resonance Imaging

Although it offers many advantages, breast MRI also has some limitations. Since it can miss some breast cancers that will usually be detected by mammography, it should not be considered a substitute or replacement for mammograms. In addition, a breast MRI may produce false-positive results by identifying areas as suspicious that turn out to be benign. This may lead to unwarranted anxiety and unnecessary testing for the patient.

While breast MRI is generally considered safe and painless, it does involve a few potential risks, such as:

- Allergic reaction to the contrast dye, which can also cause complications for patients with kidney problems

- Danger related to exposure to a strong magnet for patients with implanted medical devices, such as pacemakers or cochlear implants, or internal metal objects, such as plates, screws, clips, or wire mesh

- Anxiety attacks for patients with severe claustrophobia

- Potential harm to a fetus during the first trimester, which may make MRI testing inadvisable for women who are pregnant

References

1. "Breast Magnetic Resonance Imaging (MRI)," Johns Hopkins Medical, n.d.

2. "Breast MRI for the Early Detection of Breast Cancer," Cancer. net, March 2014.

3. "Tests and Procedures: Breast MRI," Mayo Clinic, August 22, 2013.

Chapter 34

Breast Biopsy

Chapter Contents

Section 34.1

Indroduction to Breast Biopsy

This section includes text excerpted from "Breast Biopsy,"
MedlinePlus, National Institutes of Health (NIH), November 7, 2018.

What Is a Breast Biopsy?

A breast biopsy is a procedure that removes a small sample of breast tissue for testing. The tissue is looked at under a microscope to check for breast cancer. There are different ways to do a breast biopsy procedure. One method uses a special needle to remove tissue. Another method removes tissue in minor, outpatient surgery.

A breast biopsy can determine whether you have breast cancer. But most women who have a breast biopsy do not have cancer.

Other names: core needle biopsy; core biopsy, breast; fine-needle aspiration; open surgery biopsy.

What Is Breast Biopsy Used For?

A breast biopsy is used to confirm or rule out breast cancer. It is done after other breast tests, such as a mammogram, or a physical breast exam, show there might be a chance of breast cancer.

Why Do You Need a Breast Biopsy?

You may need a breast biopsy if:

- You or your healthcare provider felt a lump in your breast

- Your mammogram, magnetic resonance imaging (MRI), or ultrasound tests show a lump, shadow, or other areas of concern

- You have changes in your nipple, such as bloody discharge

If your healthcare provider has ordered a breast biopsy, it does not necessarily mean you have breast cancer. The majority of breast lumps that are tested are benign, which means noncancerous.

What Happens during a Breast Biopsy

There are three main types of breast-biopsy procedures:

- **Fine needle aspiration (FNA) biopsy**, which uses a very thin needle to remove a sample of breast cells or fluid

- **Core needle biopsy**, which uses a larger needle to remove a sample

- **Surgical biopsy,** which removes a sample in a minor, outpatient procedure

Fine needle aspiration and **core needle biopsies** usually include the following steps:

- You will lay on your side or sit on an exam table.

- A healthcare provider will clean the biopsy site and inject it with an anesthetic, so you won't feel any pain during the procedure.

- Once the area is numb, the provider will insert either a fine aspiration needle or core biopsy needle into the biopsy site and remove a sample of tissue or fluid.

- You may feel a little pressure when the sample is withdrawn.

- Pressure will be applied to the biopsy site until the bleeding stops.

- Your provider will apply a sterile bandage at the biopsy site.

In a **surgical biopsy**, a surgeon will make a small cut in your skin to remove all or part of a breast lump. A surgical biopsy is sometimes done if the lump can't be reached with a needle biopsy. Surgical biopsies usually include the following steps:

- You will lie on an operating table. An IV (intravenous) line may be placed in your arm or hand.

- You may be given medicine, called a "sedative," to help you relax.

- You will be given local or general anesthesia, so you won't feel pain during the procedure.

- For local anesthesia, a healthcare provider will inject the biopsy site with medicine to numb the area.

- For general anesthesia, a specialist called an anesthesiologist will give you medicine, so you will be unconscious during the procedure.

- The biopsy area is numb or you are unconscious, the surgeon will make a small cut into the breast and remove part or all of a lump. Some tissue around the lump may also be removed.

- The cut in your skin will be closed with stitches or adhesive strips.

The type of biopsy you have will depend on different factors, including the size of the lump and what the lump or area of concern looks like on a breast test.

Will You Need to Do Anything to Prepare for the Breast Biopsy?

You won't need any special preparations if you are getting local anesthesia (numbing of the biopsy site). If you are getting general anesthesia, you will probably need to fast (not eat or drink) for several hours before surgery. Your surgeon will give you more specific instructions. Also, if you are getting a sedative or general anesthesia, be sure to arrange for someone to drive you home. You may be groggy and confused after you wake up from the procedure.

Are There Any Risks due to the Breast Biopsy?

You may have a little bruising or bleeding at the biopsy site. Sometimes the site gets infected. If that happens, you will be treated with antibiotics. A surgical biopsy may cause some additional pain and discomfort. Your healthcare provider may recommend or prescribe medicine to help you feel better.

What Do the Results Mean?

It may take several days to a week to get your results. Typical results may show:

- **Normal.** No cancer or abnormal cells were found.

- **Abnormal, but benign**. These show breast changes that are not cancer. These include calcium deposits and cysts. Sometimes more testing and/or follow-up treatment may be needed.

- **Cancer cells found.** Your results will include information about cancer to help you and your healthcare provider develop a treatment plan that best meets your needs. You will probably be referred to a provider who specializes in breast-cancer treatment.

Is There Anything Else You Need to Know about a Breast Biopsy?

In the United States, tens of thousands of women and hundreds of men die of breast cancer every year. A breast biopsy, when appropriate, can help find breast cancer at an early stage when it's most treatable. If breast cancer is found early, when it is confined to the breast only, the 5-year survival rate is 99 percent. This means, on average, that 99 out of 100 people with breast cancer that was detected early are still alive 5 years after being diagnosed. If you have questions about breast cancer screening, such as mammograms or a breast biopsy, talk to your healthcare provider.

Section 34.2

Sentinel Lymph Node Biopsy

This section includes text excerpted from "Sentinel Lymph Node Biopsy," National Cancer Institute (NCI), August 11, 2011. Reviewed February 2019.

What Are Lymph Nodes?

Lymph nodes are small round organs that are part of the body's lymphatic system. They are found widely throughout the body and are connected to one another by lymph vessels. Groups of lymph nodes are located in the neck, underarms, chest, abdomen, and groin. A clear fluid called "lymph" flows through lymph vessels and lymph nodes.

Lymph originates from a fluid, known as "interstitial fluid," that has diffused, or "leaked," out of small blood vessels called "capillaries." This fluid contains many substances, including blood plasma, proteins, glucose, and oxygen. It bathes most of the body's cells, providing them with the oxygen and nutrients they need for growth and survival. Interstitial fluid also picks up waste products from cells as well as other materials, such as bacteria and viruses, to help remove them from the body's tissues. Interstitial fluid eventually collects in lymph vessels, where it becomes known as "lymph." Lymph flows through the body's lymph vessels to reach two large ducts at the base of the neck, where it is emptied into the bloodstream.

Lymph nodes are important parts of the body's immune system. They contain B lymphocytes, T lymphocytes, and other types of immune system cells. These cells monitor lymph for the presence of foreign substances, such as bacteria and viruses. If a foreign substance is detected, some of the cells will become activated and immune response will be triggered.

Lymph nodes are also important in helping to determine whether cancer cells have developed the ability to spread to other parts of the body. Many types of cancer spread through the lymphatic system, and one of the earliest sites of spread for these cancers is nearby lymph nodes.

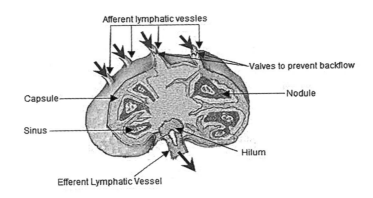

Figure 34.1. *Lymph Node Structure* (Source: "Lymph Nodes," National Cancer Institute (NCI).)

What Is a Sentinel Lymph Node?

A sentinel lymph node is defined as the "first lymph node to which cancer cells are most likely to spread from a primary tumor." Sometimes, there can be more than one sentinel lymph node.

What Is a Sentinel Lymph Node Biopsy?

A sentinel lymph node biopsy (SLNB) is a procedure in which the sentinel lymph node is identified, removed, and examined to determine whether cancer cells are present.

A negative SLNB result suggests that cancer has not developed the ability to spread to nearby lymph nodes or other organs. A positive SLNB result indicates that cancer is present in the sentinel lymph node and may be present in other nearby lymph nodes (called "regional lymph nodes") and, possibly, other organs. This information can help a doctor determine the stage of cancer (extent of the disease within the body) and develop an appropriate treatment plan.

What Happens during a Sentinel Lymph Node Biopsy

A surgeon injects a radioactive substance, a blue dye, or both near the tumor to locate the position of the sentinel lymph node. The surgeon then uses a device that detects radioactivity to find the sentinel node or looks for lymph nodes that are stained with the blue dye. Once the sentinel lymph node is located, the surgeon makes a small incision (about 1/2 inch) in the overlying skin and removes the node.

The sentinel node is then checked for the presence of cancer cells by a pathologist. If cancer is found, the surgeon may remove additional lymph nodes, either during the same biopsy procedure or during a follow-up surgical procedure. SLNBs may be done on an outpatient basis or may require a short stay in the hospital.

SLNB is usually done at the same time the primary tumor is removed. However, the procedure can also be done either before or after removal of the tumor.

What Are the Benefits of Sentinel Lymph Node Biopsy?

In addition to helping doctors stage cancers and estimate the risk that tumor cells have developed the ability to spread to other parts of the body, SLNB may help some patients avoid more extensive lymph node surgery. Removing additional nearby lymph nodes to look for cancer cells may not be necessary if the sentinel node is negative for cancer.

What Are the Adverse Effects of Lymph Node Surgery?

All lymph node surgery can have adverse effects, and some of these effects may be reduced or avoided if fewer lymph nodes are removed. The potential adverse effects of lymph node surgery include the following:

- **Lymphedema, or tissue swelling.** During SLNB or more extensive lymph node surgery, lymph vessels leading to and from the sentinel node or group of nodes are cut, thereby disrupting the normal flow of lymph through the affected area. This disruption may lead to an abnormal buildup of lymph fluid. In addition to swelling, patients with lymphedema may experience pain or discomfort in the affected area, and the overlying skin may become thickened or hard. In the case of extensive lymph node surgery in an armpit or groin, the swelling may affect an entire arm or leg. In addition, there is an increased risk of infection in the affected area or limb. Very rarely, chronic lymphedema due to extensive lymph node removal may cause cancer of the lymphatic vessels called "lymphangiosarcoma."

- **Seroma**, or the buildup of lymph fluid at the site of the surgery

- **Numbness, tingling,** or **pain** at the site of the surgery

- **Difficulty in moving** the affected body part

Is Sentinel Lymph Node Biopsy Associated with Other Harms?

SLNB, like other surgical procedures, can cause short-term pain, swelling, and bruising at the surgical site and increase the risk of infection. In addition, some patients may have skin or allergic reactions to the blue dye used in SLNB. Another potential harm is a false-negative biopsy result—that is, cancer cells are not seen in the sentinel lymph node although they are present and may have already spread to other regional lymph nodes or other parts of the body. A false-negative biopsy result gives the patient and the doctor a false sense of security about the extent of cancer in the patient's body.

Is Sentinel Lymph Node Biopsy Used to Help Stage All Types of Cancer?

No. SLNB is most commonly used to help stage breast cancer and melanoma. However, it is being studied with other cancer types, including colorectal cancer (CRC), gastric cancer, esophageal cancer, head and neck cancer, thyroid cancer, and nonsmall cell lung cancer.

What Has Research Shown about the Use of Sentinel Lymph Node Biopsy in Breast Cancer?

Breast cancer cells are most likely to spread first to lymph nodes located in the axilla, or armpit area, next to the affected breast. However, in breast cancers close to the center of the chest (near the breastbone), cancer cells may spread first to lymph nodes inside the chest (under the breastbone) before they can be detected in the axilla.

The number of lymph nodes in the axilla varies from person to person but usually ranges from 20 to 40. Historically, removal of these lymph nodes (in an operation called "axillary lymph node dissection," or ALND) was done for two reasons: to help stage breast cancer and to help prevent a regional recurrence of the disease. (Regional recurrence of breast cancer occurs when breast cancer cells that have migrated to nearby lymph nodes give rise to a new tumor.)

Because removing multiple lymph nodes at the same time has been associated with adverse effects, the possibility that SLNB alone might be sufficient for staging breast cancer in women who have no clinical signs of axillary lymph node metastasis, such as swollen or "matted" (clumped or stuck together) nodes, was investigated.

In a phase III trial involving 5,611 women with breast cancer and no clinical signs of axillary metastasis, researchers from the National Surgical Adjuvant Breast and Bowel Project (NSABP), which is a National Cancer Institute (NCI) clinical trials cooperative group, randomly assigned participants to receive SLNB alone or SLNB plus ALND. The women in the two groups whose sentinel lymph node(s) were negative for cancer (a total of 3,989 women) were then followed for an average of eight years. Most of the women (87.5%) had a lumpectomy, and the rest had a mastectomy. Nearly 88 percent of the women also received adjuvant systemic therapy (AST) (chemotherapy, hormonal therapy, or both), and 82 percent had external-beam radiation therapy (EBRT) to the affected breast.

The researchers found no differences in overall survival and disease-free survival between the two groups of women. Based on these results, it was concluded that ALND might not be necessary for women with clinically negative axillary lymph nodes and a negative SLNB whose breast cancer is treated with surgery, adjuvant systemic therapy, and external-beam radiation therapy.

Subsequently, the American College of Surgeons Oncology Group (ACOSOG), which is another NCI clinical trials cooperative group, reported findings from an additional phase III clinical trial, this one testing whether women with a positive sentinel lymph node but no

227

clinical evidence of axillary lymph node metastasis could be safely treated with tumor removal and no further lymph node surgery other than the SLNB. In this trial, 891 women were randomly assigned to SLNB only, or ALND after SLNB. All of the women were treated with lumpectomy. More than 95 percent of them also received adjuvant systemic therapy (chemotherapy, hormone therapy (HT), or both), and about 90 percent received external-beam radiation therapy to the affected breast.

When the results of this trial were reported, the patients had been followed for a median of 6.3 years. The two groups of women had a similar 5-year overall survival (92.5% in the SLNB-only group versus 91.8 percent in the SLNB plus ALND group) and 5-year disease-free survival (83.9% in the SLNB-only group and 82.2 percent in the SLNB plus ALND group). The researchers concluded that SLNB alone is safe and does not affect the survival of women who have sentinel lymph node metastasis but no clinical signs of other lymph node involvement and whose breast cancer is treated with surgery, systemic therapy, and external-beam radiation therapy. The excellent outcome in this trial for women treated with SLNB without ALND is likely due, at least in part, to the ability of local radiation therapy and modern systemic treatments to effectively treat breast cancer cells that may have spread to other axillary lymph nodes besides the sentinel node or to other parts of the body.

Chapter 35

Testing New Approaches to Breast-Cancer Screening

A goal of precision medicine for cancer is to match patients with the most appropriate treatments based on information about the genetic and molecular changes in their tumors. This approach can also help patients avoid treatments that would be unlikely to help and could cause harm.

In the field of cancer screening, individualized approaches could help doctors identify individuals at risk of cancer who need to be screened with tests and testing intervals that are appropriate for each person's level of risk. Those who are not at risk could avoid the potential harms of screening, such as false-positive test results and overdiagnosis.

Interest in bringing precision to cancer screening has increased in recent years, particularly in the area of breast cancer. In 2016, for example, researchers in California launched a clinical trial to test a new approach to breast-cancer screening. The Women Informed to Screen Depending on Measures of Risk (WISDOM) clinical trial is using several measures, such as safety, to compare annual mammography with a more individualized approach called "risk-based screening."

For participants in the risk-based group, researchers will recommend the age to start (and stop) screening and the screening interval

---

This chapter includes text excerpted from "In an Era of Precision Medicine, Testing New Approaches to Breast Cancer Screening," National Cancer Institute (NCI), May 9, 2017.

based on each woman's risk score, which is determined by analyzing factors such as certain genetic alterations, family medical history, and breast density.

"We are trying to bring precision medicine into the arena of screening," said Laura Esserman, M.D., who directs the Carol Franc Buck Breast Care Center at the University of California, San Francisco, and is co-leading the WISDOM trial. "The idea is to learn how we can do a better job of screening for breast cancer."

Moving toward Precision Cancer Prevention

The trial aims to recruit 100,000 women. Women in the study are encouraged to be randomly assigned to receive annual mammograms or risk-based screening. Recognizing that some participants would join only if they could choose annual mammograms or choose risk-based screening, the researchers give all participants the option of joining the group they prefer.

Women who are assigned to the risk-based screening arm will receive a risk assessment that includes the sequencing of 9 genes strongly associated with breast cancer and the evaluation of more than 80 other genetic markers of breast-cancer risk. For those with the highest risk scores, such as women who have harmful mutations in the *BRCA* genes, the researchers will recommend annual mammography and annual magnetic resonance imaging (MRI) beginning at age 40.

"By design, everyone in the trial is at least 40 years old, so we would start screening the women at highest risk immediately," said Jeffrey Tice, M.D., of the Division of General Internal Medicine at University of California, San Francisco, and one of the leaders of the study. Under the ideal scheduling of mammography and breast MRI, these women would have one of the imaging tests every 6 months, he added.

For women in the risk-based screening arm with the lowest risk scores, the researchers would recommend screening with mammography every 2 years beginning at age 50.

"Many of us involved in this trial feel that the one-size-fits-all approach to breast-cancer screening is not optimal for patients, and it's not an optimal use of resources," said Dr. Tice. "But we need to test the risk-based approach in a clinical trial so that we can evaluate the evidence."

The goal of the WISDOM trial is to determine whether risk-based screening is as safe as annual screening (that is, no increase in advanced-stage breast cancers compared with the annual screening group) and less morbid (that is, involves fewer mammograms and biopsies).

Another question is whether risk-based screening helps to reduce false-positive results and the detection of indolent or slow-growing tumors that would not have caused harm in the woman's lifetime, a phenomenon known as "overdiagnosis." The researchers will also determine which approach is preferred by women based on feedback about satisfaction and anxiety.

The study could also yield insights into questions about the psycho-social effects of clinical deoxyribonucleic acid (DNA) testing. Currently, the trial is sequencing 9 genes and using data on about 80 genetic markers associated with breast-cancer risk to help in calculating the participants' risk level, but in the coming months that number should exceed 100, according to Dr. Tice.

Focusing on High-Risk Individuals

As the WISDOM trial was getting underway, a working group of the Cancer Moonshot[SM] Blue Ribbon Panel recommended that National Cancer Institute (NCI) launch two demonstration projects in cancer screening that focus on inherited syndromes that put individuals at high risk of developing cancer: Lynch syndrome and hereditary breast and ovarian cancer syndrome (HBOC).

By screening individuals who may have one of these syndromes—all patients with colorectal cancer, in the case of Lynch syndrome, and breast and ovarian cancer patients whose family histories suggest a hereditary syndrome, in the case of HBOC—for genetic alterations known to cause them, doctors could identify candidates, including family members, for increased surveillance. These individuals could then be monitored closely for early signs of cancer, according to the report.

Targeting individuals at high risk for cancer, whether or not they have an inherited predisposition, is "a major component of precision cancer prevention," noted the authors of a recent commentary on cancer prevention in the era of precision medicine.

Eva Szabo, M.D., of NCI's Division of Cancer Prevention and Nina Brahme, Ph.D., of the U.S. Food and Drug Administration (FDA), wrote that more information about the early molecular changes associated with the development of cancer is needed to realize the promise of individualized approaches to cancer prevention and early detection.

"To make progress in precision prevention, we really need a better understanding of the early phases of cancer development," Dr. Szabo said in an interview. This will require multidisciplinary studies involving experts in fields such as genomics, epigenetics, immunology, and the microbiome, she added.

A proposed project called the "Pre-Cancer Genome Atlas" could potentially help, Dr. Szabo noted. This collaborative effort would involve profiling the genomes of premalignant lesions and associated changes in nearby tissues over time; these results would be analyzed along with clinical data.

"We have a golden opportunity," Dr. Szabo said. "The technology for conducting these kinds of studies has improved dramatically, and we know so much more about how to do these kinds of analyses than we did a decade ago."

Investigating Risk Factors

Tools that can reliably assess an individual's risk of developing cancer are essential for the success of risk-based screening strategies. "Healthcare providers need accurate risk-prediction models so they can identify individuals who are at risk for the disease," said Karla Kerlikowske, M.D., of the University of California, San Francisco's Helen Diller Family Comprehensive Cancer Center.

In the case of breast cancer, most women with the disease have at least one known risk factor (such as dense breasts or high body mass index) that is easily assessed at the time of diagnosis, according to a recent study led by Dr. Kerlikowske. In the study, more than 90 percent of women had at least one risk factor when diagnosed with breast cancer.

This information could potentially be used to inform risk-based screening in the future, noted Dr. Kerlikowske. "In our study, the most prevalent and strongest risk factor among women developing breast cancer was breast density," said Natalie Engmann, a Ph.D. candidate at UCSF and the study's first author.

The study authors concluded that to individualize breast-cancer prevention, risk models need to include breast density. The Breast Cancer Surveillance Consortium Risk Calculator (www.tools.bcsc-scc.org/BC5yearRisk/intro.htm) is the only risk prediction model that incorporates a clinical measure of breast density.

Improving Screening Methods

For Dr. Esserman, the falling costs of sequencing DNA have created an opportunity to explore new approaches to screening that incorporate genetic information.

"There's no reason we can't improve on the model we have today," she said, noting that the seminal clinical trials that led to the current guidelines were conducted decades ago, long before the introduction of current tools such as tests for estrogen, progesterone, and HER2 receptors. "Women should demand and expect changes in how we screen for this disease."

As the tools and methods for screening improve, Dr. Esserman predicted, doctors can start to do less screening for people who are at lower risk. "This is the way the field is going to evolve—toward putting resources to the people who need them the most," she added.

Chapter 36

Understanding Your Laboratory Test and Breast Pathology Reports

What Are Laboratory Tests?

A laboratory test is a procedure in which a sample of blood, urine, other bodily fluid, or tissue is examined to get information about a person's health. Some laboratory tests provide precise and reliable information about specific health problems. Other tests provide more general information that helps doctors identify or rule out possible health problems. Doctors often use other types of tests, such as imaging tests, in addition to laboratory tests to learn more about a person's health.

How Are Laboratory Tests Used in Cancer Medicine?

Laboratory tests are used in cancer medicine in many ways:

- To screen for cancer or precancerous conditions before a person has any symptoms of the disease

This chapter contains text excerpted from the following sources: Text under the heading "What Are Laboratory Tests?" is excerpted from "Understanding Laboratory Tests," National Cancer Institute (NCI), December 11, 2013. Reviewed February 2019; Text under the heading "What Is a Pathology Report?" is excerpted from "Pathology Reports," National Cancer Institute (NCI), September 23, 2010. Reviewed February 2019.

- To help diagnose cancer

- To provide information about the stage of cancer (that is, its severity); for malignant tumors, this includes the size and/or extent (reach) of the original (primary) tumor and whether or not the tumor has spread (metastasized) to other parts of the body

- To plan treatment

- To monitor a patient's general health during treatment and to check for potential side effects of the treatment

- To determine whether a cancer is responding to treatment

- To find out whether cancer has recurred (come back)

Which Laboratory Tests Are Used in Cancer Medicine?

Categories of some common laboratory tests used in cancer medicine are listed below in alphabetical order.

Blood Chemistry Test

What it measures. The amounts of certain substances that are released into the blood by the organs and tissues of the body, such as metabolites, electrolytes, fats, and proteins, including enzymes. Blood chemistry tests usually include tests for blood urea nitrogen (BUN) and creatinine.

How it is used. Diagnosis and monitoring of patients during and after treatment. High or low levels of some substances can be signs of disease or side effects of treatment.

Cancer Gene Mutation Testing

What it measures. The presence or absence of specific inherited mutations in genes that are known to play a role in cancer development. Examples include tests to look for *BRCA1* and *BRCA2* gene mutations, which play a role in the development of breast, ovarian, and other cancers.

How it is used. Assessment of cancer risk

Complete Blood Count (CBC)

What it measures. Numbers of the different types of blood cells, including red blood cells (RBCs), white blood cells (WBCs), and platelets, in a sample of blood. This test also measures the amount of hemoglobin (the protein that carries oxygen) in the blood, the percentage of the total blood volume that is taken up by red blood cells (hematocrit), the size of the RBCs, and the amount of hemoglobin in RBCs.

How it is used. Diagnosis, particularly in leukemias, and monitoring during and after treatment

Cytogenetic Analysis

What it measures. Changes in the number and/or structure of chromosomes in a patient's WBCs or bone marrow cells

How it is used. Diagnosis, deciding on appropriate treatment

Immunophenotyping

What it measures. Identifies cells based on the types of antigens present on the cell surface

How it is used. Diagnosis, staging, and monitoring of cancers of the blood system and other hematologic disorders, including leukemias, lymphomas, myelodysplastic syndromes (MCS), and myeloproliferative disorders (MPD). It is most often done on blood or bone marrow samples, but it may also be done on other bodily fluids or biopsy tissue samples.

Sputum Cytology (Sputum Culture)

What it measures. The presence of abnormal cells in sputum (mucus and other matter brought up from the lungs by coughing)

How it is used. Diagnosis of lung cancer

Tumor Marker Tests

What they measure. Some measure the presence, levels, or activity of specific proteins or genes in a tissue, blood, or other bodily fluids that may be signs of cancer or certain benign (noncancerous) conditions. A tumor that has a greater than normal level of a tumor marker may respond to treatment with a drug that targets that marker. For example, cancer cells that have high levels of the human epidermal growth factor receptor 2 (*HER2*)/*neu* gene or protein may respond to treatment with a drug that targets the HER2/neu protein.

Some tumor marker tests analyze deoxyribonucleic acid (DNA) to look for specific gene mutations that may be present in cancers but not normal tissues. Examples include *EGFR* gene mutation analysis to help determine treatment and assess prognosis in nonsmall cell lung cancer and *BRAF* gene mutation analysis to predict response to targeted therapies in melanoma and colorectal cancer (CRC).

Still, other tumor marker tests, called "multigene tests (or multi-parameter gene expression tests)," analyze the expression of a specific group of genes in tumor samples. These tests are used for prognosis and treatment planning. For example, the 21-gene signature can help patients with lymph node-negative, estrogen receptor-positive breast cancer decide if there may be a benefit to treating with chemotherapy in addition to hormone therapy, or not.

How they are used. Diagnosis, deciding on appropriate treatment, assessing response to treatment, and monitoring for cancer recurrence

Urinalysis

What it measures. The color of urine and its contents, such as sugar, protein, RBCs, and WBCs.

How it is used. Detection and diagnosis of kidney cancer and urothelial cancers

Urine Cytology

What it measures. The presence of abnormal cells shed from the urinary tract into urine to detect disease.

How it is used. Detection and diagnosis of bladder cancer and other urothelial cancers, monitoring patients for cancer recurrence.

How to Interpret Your Test Results

With some laboratory tests, the results obtained for healthy people can vary somewhat from person to person. Factors that can cause person-to-person variation in laboratory test results include a person's age, sex, race, medical history, and general health. In fact, the results obtained from a single person given the same test on different days can also vary. For these tests, therefore, the results are considered normal if they fall between certain lower and upper limits or values. This range of normal values is known as the "normal range," the "reference range," and the "reference interval." When healthy people take such tests, it is expected that their results will fall within the normal range 95 percent of the time. (5% of the time, the results from healthy people will fall outside the normal range and will be marked as "abnormal.") Reference ranges are based on test results from large numbers of people who have been tested in the past.

Some test results can be affected by certain foods and medications. For this reason, people may be asked to not eat or drink for several hours before a laboratory test or to delay taking medications until after the test.

For many tests, it is possible for someone with cancer to have results that fall within the normal range. Likewise, it is possible for someone who doesn't have cancer to have test results that fall outside the normal range. This is one reason that many laboratory tests alone cannot provide a definitive diagnosis of cancer or other diseases.

In general, laboratory test results must be interpreted in the context of the overall health of the patient and are considered along with the results of other examinations, tests, and procedures. A doctor who is familiar with a patient's medical history and the current situation is the best person to explain test results and what they mean.

What If a Laboratory Test Result Is Unclear or Inconclusive?

If a test result is unclear or inconclusive, the doctor will likely repeat the test to be certain of the result and may order additional tests. The doctor may also compare the latest test result to previous results, if available, to get a better idea of what is normal for that person.

What Are Some Questions to Ask the Doctor about Laboratory Tests?

It can be helpful to take a list of questions to the doctor's office. Questions about a laboratory test might include:

• What will this test measure?

• Why is this test being ordered?

• Does this test have any risks or side effects?

• How should I prepare for the test?

• When will the test results be available?

- How will the results be given (a letter, a phone call, online)?
- Will this test need to be done more than once?

How Reliable Are Laboratory Tests and Their Results?

The results of laboratory tests affect many of the decisions a doctor makes about a person's healthcare, including whether additional tests are necessary, developing a treatment plan, or monitoring a person's response to treatment. It is very important, therefore, that the laboratory tests themselves are trustworthy and that the laboratory that performs the tests meets rigorous state and federal regulatory standards.

The U.S. Food and Drug Administration (FDA) regulates the development and marketing of all laboratory tests that use test kits and equipment that are commercially manufactured in the United States. After the FDA approves a laboratory test, other federal and state agencies make sure that the test materials and equipment meet strict standards while they are being manufactured and then used in a medical or clinical laboratory.

All laboratory testing that is performed on humans in the United States (except testing done in clinical trials and other types of human research) is regulated through the Clinical Laboratory Improvement Amendments (CLIA), which were passed by Congress in 1988. The CLIA laboratory certification program is administered by the Centers for Medicare & Medicaid Services (CMS) in conjunction with the FDA and the Centers for Disease Control and Prevention (CDC). CLIA ensures that laboratory staff is appropriately trained and supervised and that testing laboratories have quality control programs in place so that test results are accurate and reliable.

To enroll in the CLIA program, laboratories must complete a certification process that is based on the level of complexity of tests that the laboratory will perform. The more complicated the test, the more demanding the requirements for certification. Laboratories must demonstrate that they can perform tests as accurately and as precisely as the manufacturer did to gain FDA approval of the test. Laboratories must also evaluate the tests regularly to make sure that they continue to meet the manufacturer's specifications. Laboratories undergo regular unannounced on-site inspections to ensure they are following the requirements outlined in CLIA to receive and maintain certification.

Some states have additional requirements that are equal to or more stringent than those outlined in CLIA. CMS has determined that Washington and New York have state licensure programs that are exempt from CLIA program requirements. Therefore, licensing authorities in Washington and New York have primary responsibility for oversight of their state's laboratory practices.

What Is a Pathology Report?

A pathology report is a document that contains the diagnosis determined by examining cells and tissues under a microscope. The report may also contain information about the size, shape, and appearance of a specimen as it looks to the naked eye. This information is known as the "gross description."

A pathologist is a doctor who does this examination and writes the pathology report. Pathology reports play an important role in cancer diagnosis and staging (describing the extent of cancer within the body, especially whether it has spread), which helps determine treatment options.

How Is Tissue Obtained for Examination by the Pathologist?

In most cases, a doctor needs to do a biopsy or surgery to remove cells or tissues for examination under a microscope.

Some common ways a biopsy can be done are as follows:

- A needle is used to withdraw tissue or fluid.

- An endoscope (a thin, lighted tube) is used to look at areas inside the body and remove cells or tissues.

- Surgery is used to remove part of the tumor or the entire tumor. If the entire tumor is removed, typically some normal tissue around the tumor is also removed.

Tissue removed during a biopsy is sent to a pathology laboratory, where it is sliced into thin sections for viewing under a microscope. This is known as "histologic (tissue) examination" and is usually the best way to tell if cancer is present. The pathologist may also examine cytologic (cell) material. Cytologic material is present in urine, cerebrospinal fluid (CSF) (the fluid around the brain and spinal cord), sputum (mucus from the lungs), peritoneal (abdominal cavity) fluid, pleural (chest cavity) fluid, cervical/vaginal smears, and in fluid removed during a biopsy.

How Is Tissue Processed after a Biopsy or Surgery? What Is a Frozen Section?

The tissue removed during a biopsy or surgery must be cut into thin sections, placed on slides, and stained with dyes before it can be examined under a microscope. Two methods are used to make the tissue firm enough to cut into thin sections: frozen sections and paraffin-embedded (permanent) sections. All tissue samples are prepared as permanent sections, but sometimes frozen sections are also prepared.

Permanent sections are prepared by placing the tissue in fixative (usually formalin) to preserve the tissue, processing it through additional solutions, and then placing it in paraffin wax. After the wax has hardened, the tissue is cut into very thin slices, which are placed on slides and stained. The process normally takes several days. A permanent section provides the best quality for examination by the pathologist and produces more accurate results than a frozen section.

Frozen sections are prepared by freezing and slicing the tissue sample. They can be done in about 15 to 20 minutes while the patient is in the operating room. Frozen sections are done when an immediate answer is needed; for example, to determine whether the tissue is cancerous so as to guide the surgeon during the course of an operation.

How Long after the Tissue Sample Is Taken Will the Pathology Report Be Ready?

The pathologist sends a pathology report to the doctor within 10 days after the biopsy or surgery is performed. Pathology reports are written in the technical medical language. Patients may want to ask their doctors to give them a copy of the pathology report and to explain the report to them. Patients also may wish to keep a copy of their pathology report in their own records.

What Information Does a Pathology Report Usually Include?

The pathology report may include the following information:

- **Patient information.** Name, birth date, biopsy date

- **Gross description.** Color, weight, and size of tissue as seen by the naked eye

- **Microscopic description.** How the sample looks under the microscope and how it compares with normal cells

- **Diagnosis.** Type of tumor/cancer and grade (how abnormal the cells look under the microscope and how quickly the tumor is likely to grow and spread)

- **Tumor size.** Measured in centimeters

- **Tumor margins.** There are three possible findings when the biopsy sample is the entire tumor:

  - Positive margins mean that cancer cells are found at the edge of the material removed

  - Negative, not involved, clear, or free margins mean that no cancer cells are found at the outer edge

  - Close margins are neither negative nor positive

- **Other information.** Usually, notes about samples that have been sent for other tests or a second opinion

- **Details of a pathologist.** Pathologist's signature and name and address of the laboratory

What Might the Pathology Report Say about the Physical and Chemical Characteristics of the Tissue?

After identifying the tissue as cancerous, the pathologist may perform additional tests to get more information about the tumor that cannot be determined by looking at the tissue with routine stains, such as hematoxylin (H) and eosin (E), under a microscope. The pathology report will include the results of these tests. For example, the pathology report may include information obtained from immunochemical stains (IHC). IHC uses antibodies to identify specific antigens on the surface of cancer cells. IHC can be used to:

- Determine where cancer started

- Distinguish among different cancer types, such as carcinoma, melanoma, and lymphoma

- Help diagnose and classify leukemias and lymphomas

The pathology report may also include the results of flow cytometry. Flow cytometry is a method of measuring properties of cells in a sample, including the number of cells, percentage of live cells, cell size and shape, and presence of tumor markers on the cell surface. Tumor markers are substances produced by tumor cells or by other cells in the body in response to cancer or certain noncancerous conditions.) Flow

243

cytometry can be used in the diagnosis, classification, and management of cancers such as acute leukemia, chronic lymphoproliferative disorders (LPD), and non-Hodgkin lymphoma.

Finally, the pathology report may include the results of molecular diagnostic and cytogenetic studies. Such studies investigate the presence or absence of malignant cells and genetic or molecular abnormalities in specimens.

What Information about the Genetics of the Cells Might Be Included in the Pathology Report?

Cytogenetics uses tissue culture and specialized techniques to provide genetic information about cells, particularly genetic alterations. Some genetic alterations are markers or indicators of specific cancer. For example, the Philadelphia chromosome (Ph) is associated with chronic myelogenous leukemia (CML). Some alterations can provide information about prognosis, which helps the doctor make treatment recommendations. Some tests that might be performed on a tissue sample include:

- **Fluorescence in situ hybridization (FISH).** Determines the positions of particular genes. It can be used to identify chromosomal abnormalities and to map genes.

- **Polymerase chain reaction (PCR).** A method of making many copies of particular DNA sequences of relevance to the diagnosis.

- **Real-time PCR or quantitative PCR.** A method of measuring how many copies of a particular DNA sequence are present.

- **Reverse-transcriptase polymerase chain reaction (RT-PCR).** A method of making many copies of a specific ribonucleic acid (RNA) sequence.

- **Southern blot hybridization.** Detects specific DNA fragments.

- **Western blot hybridization.** Identifies and analyzes proteins or peptides.

Can Individuals Get a Second Opinion about Their Pathology Results?

Although most cancers can be easily diagnosed, sometimes patients or their doctors may want to get a second opinion about the pathology results. Patients interested in getting a second opinion should talk with their doctor. They will need to obtain the slides and/or paraffin block from the pathologist who examined the sample or from the hospital where the biopsy or surgery was done.

Many institutions provide second opinions on pathology specimens. The National Cancer Institute (NCI)-designated cancer centers or academic institutions are reasonable places to consider. Patients should contact the facility in advance to determine if this service is available, the cost, and shipping instructions.

Chapter 37

Breast-Cancer Diagnosis: Questions to Ask

You may want to ask your doctor some of the following questions before you decide on your cancer treatment.

Questions about Cancer Treatment

Some of the questions that you can ask related to your breast-cancer treatment are listed below.

- What are the ways to treat my type and stage of cancer?
- What are the benefits and risks of each of these treatments?
- What treatment do you recommend? Why do you think it is best for me?
- When will I need to start treatment?
- Will I need to be in the hospital for treatment? If so, for how long?
- What is my chance of recovery with this treatment?
- How will we know if the treatment is working?
- Would a clinical trial (research study) be right for me?

This chapter includes text excerpted from "Questions to Ask Your Doctor about Your Treatment," National Cancer Institute (NCI), August 9, 2018.

- How do I find out about studies for my type and stage of cancer?
- Where will I go for treatment?
- How is the treatment given?
- How long will each treatment session take?
- How many treatment sessions will I have?
- Should a family member or friend come with me to my treatment sessions?

Questions about Finding a Specialist and Getting a Second Opinion

Some of the questions related to your search for a specialist or to whom you should go for getting a second opinion regarding breast-cancer treatment are listed below.

- Will I need a specialist(s) for my cancer treatment?
- Will you help me find a doctor to give me another opinion on the best treatment plan for me?

Questions about Side Effects

The breast-cancer treatment that you may be taking up, might have side effects. Consult with your healthcare provider regarding the side effects by asking the following questions:

- What are the possible side effects of the treatment?
- What side effects may happen during or between my treatment sessions?
- Are there any side effects that I should call you about right away?
- Are there any lasting effects of the treatment?
- Will this treatment affect my ability to have children?
- How can I prevent or treat side effects?

Questions about Medicines and Other Products You Might Be Taking

You may be put under medication during or after your treatment. You can ask your healthcare provider regarding the medicines and other products that you may have to take:

- Do I need to tell you about the medicines I am taking now?

- Should I tell you about dietary supplements (such as vitamins, minerals, herbs, or fish oil) that I am taking?

- Could any drugs or supplements change the way that cancer treatment works?

Chapter 38

Breast-Cancer Staging

What Is Breast-Cancer Staging?

After breast cancer has been diagnosed, tests are done to find out if cancer cells have spread within the breast or to other parts of the body. The process used to find out whether cancer has spread within the breast or to other parts of the body is called "staging." The information gathered from the staging process determines the stage of the disease. It is important to know the stage in order to plan treatment. The results of some of the tests used to diagnose breast cancer are also used to stage the disease.

The following tests and procedures also may be used in the staging process:

- **Sentinel lymph node biopsy (SLNB)**—the removal of the sentinel lymph node during surgery. The sentinel lymph node is the first lymph node in a group of lymph nodes to receive lymphatic drainage from the primary tumor. It is the first lymph node the cancer is likely to spread to from the primary tumor. A radioactive substance and/or blue dye is injected near the tumor. The substance or dye flows through the lymph ducts to the lymph nodes. The first lymph node to receive the

This chapter includes text excerpted from "Breast Cancer Treatment (PDQ®)—Patient Version," National Cancer Institute (NCI), December 28, 2018.

substance or dye is removed. A pathologist views the tissue under a microscope to look for cancer cells. If cancer cells are not found, it may not be necessary to remove more lymph nodes. Sometimes, a sentinel lymph node is found in more than one group of nodes.

- **Chest X-ray**—an X-ray of the organs and bones inside the chest. An X-ray is a type of energy beam that can go through the body and onto film, making a picture of areas inside the body.

- **Computerized tomography (CT)/computerized axial tomography (CAT) scan**—a procedure that makes a series of detailed pictures of areas inside the body, taken from different angles. The pictures are made by a computer linked to an X-ray machine. A dye may be injected into a vein or swallowed to help the organs or tissues show up more clearly. This procedure is also called "computed tomography," "computerized tomography," or "computerized axial tomography (CAT)."

- **Bone scan**—a procedure to check if there are rapidly dividing cells, such as cancer cells, in the bone. A very small amount of radioactive material is injected into a vein and travels through the bloodstream. The radioactive material collects in the bones with cancer and is detected by a scanner.

- **Positron emission tomography (PET) scan**—a procedure to find malignant tumor cells in the body. A small amount of radioactive glucose (sugar) is injected into a vein. The PET scanner rotates around the body and makes a picture of where glucose is being used in the body. Malignant tumor cells show up brighter in the picture because they are more active and take up more glucose than normal cells do.

How Cancer Spreads

There are three ways that cancer spreads in the body. Cancer can spread through tissue, the lymph system, and the blood:

- **Tissue.** Cancer spreads from where it began by growing into nearby areas.

- **Lymph system.** Cancer spreads from where it began by getting into the lymph system. The cancer travels through the lymph vessels to other parts of the body.

- **Blood.** Cancer spreads from where it began by getting into the blood. The cancer travels through the blood vessels to other parts of the body.

When cancer spreads to another part of the body, it is called 'metastasis.' Cancer cells break away from where they began (the primary tumor) and travel through the lymph system or blood.

- **Lymph system.** Cancer gets into the lymph system, travels through the lymph vessels, and forms a tumor (metastatic tumor) in another part of the body.

- **Blood.** Cancer gets into the blood, travels through the blood vessels, and forms a tumor (metastatic tumor) in another part of the body.

The metastatic tumor is the same type of cancer as the primary tumor. For example, if breast cancer spreads to the bone, the cancer cells in the bone are actually breast-cancer cells. The disease is metastatic-breast cancer, not bone cancer.

How Staging Is Done for Breast Cancer

To plan the best treatment and understand your prognosis, it is important to know the breast-cancer stage. There are three types of breast-cancer stage groups:

- **Clinical prognostic stage** is used first to assign a stage for all patients based on health history, physical exam, imaging tests (if done), and biopsies. The clinical prognostic stage is described by the TNM system, tumor grade, and biomarker status (Estrogen receptors (ER) and Progesterone receptors (PR), human epidermal growth factor receptor 2 (HER2)). In clinical staging, mammography or ultrasound is used to check the lymph nodes for signs of cancer.

- **Pathological prognostic stage (PPS)** is then used for patients who have surgery as their first treatment. The PPS is based on all clinical information, biomarker status, and laboratory test results from breast tissue and lymph nodes removed during surgery.

- **Anatomic stage (AS)** is based on the size and the spread of cancer as described by the TNM system. The Anatomic Stage is used in parts of the world where biomarker testing is not available. It is not used in the United States.

TNM System for Breast Cancer

The TNM system is used to describe the size of the primary tumor and the spread of cancer to nearby lymph nodes or other parts of the body. For breast cancer, the TNM system describes the tumor as follows:

Tumor (T). The size and location of the tumor.

- TX: Primary tumor cannot be assessed.

- T0: No sign of a primary tumor in the breast.

- Tis: Carcinoma *in situ* (CIS). There are two types of breast carcinoma in situ:

  - Tis (DCIS). Ductal carcinoma *in situ* (DCIS) is a condition in which abnormal cells are found in the lining of a breast duct. The abnormal cells have not spread outside the duct to other tissues in the breast. In some cases, DCIS may become invasive breast cancer that is able to spread to other tissues. At this time, there is no way to know which lesions can become invasive.

  - Tis (Paget disease). Paget disease (PD) of the nipple is a condition in which abnormal cells are found only in the skin cells of the nipple. It is not staged according to the TNM system. If Paget disease and invasive breast cancer are present, the TNM system is used to stage the invasive breast cancer.

- T1: The tumor is 20 millimeters or smaller. There are four subtypes of a T1 tumor depending on the size of the tumor:

  - T1mi: the tumor is 1 millimeter or smaller.

  - T1a: the tumor is larger than 1 millimeter but not larger than 5 millimeters.

  - T1b: the tumor is larger than 5 millimeters but not larger than 10 millimeters.

  - T1c: the tumor is larger than 10 millimeters but not larger than 20 millimeters.

- T2: The tumor is larger than 20 millimeters but not larger than 50 millimeters.

- T3: The tumor is larger than 50 millimeters.

  - T4: The tumor is described as one of the following:

- T4a: the tumor has grown into the chest wall.

- T4b: the tumor has grown into the skin—an ulcer has formed on the surface of the skin on the breast, small tumor nodules have formed in the same breast as the primary tumor, and/or there is swelling of the skin on the breast.

- T4c: the tumor has grown into the chest wall and the skin.

- T4d: inflammatory breast cancer (IBC)—one-third or more of the skin on the breast is red and swollen (also called peau d'orange).

Lymph node (N). When the lymph nodes are removed by surgery and studied under a microscope by a pathologist, pathologic staging is used to describe the lymph nodes. The pathologic staging of lymph nodes is described below.

- NX: The lymph nodes cannot be assessed.

- N0: No sign of cancer in the lymph nodes, or tiny clusters of cancer cells not larger than 0.2 millimeters in the lymph nodes.

- N1: Cancer is described as one of the following:

  - N1mi: cancer has spread to the axillary (armpit area) lymph nodes and is larger than 0.2 millimeters but not larger than two millimeters.

  - N1a: cancer has spread to one to three axillary lymph nodes (ALN) and cancer in at least one of the lymph nodes is larger than two millimeters.

  - N1b: cancer has spread to lymph nodes near the breastbone on the same side of the body as the primary tumor, and the cancer is larger than 0.2 millimeters and is found by sentinel lymph node biopsy. Cancer is not found in the axillary lymph nodes.

  - N1c: cancer has spread to one to three axillary lymph nodes and cancer in at least one of the lymph nodes is larger than two millimeters. Cancer is also found by sentinel lymph node biopsy in the lymph nodes near the breastbone on the same side of the body as the primary tumor.

- N2: Cancer is described as one of the following:

  - N2a: cancer has spread to four to nine axillary lymph nodes and cancer in at least one of the lymph nodes is larger than two millimeters.

- N2b: cancer has spread to lymph nodes near the breastbone and the cancer is found by imaging tests. Cancer is not found in the axillary lymph nodes by sentinel lymph node biopsy or lymph node dissection.

- N3: Cancer is described as one of the following:

- N3a: cancer has spread to 10 or more axillary lymph nodes and cancer in at least one of the lymph nodes is larger than 2 millimeters, or cancer has spread to lymph nodes below the collarbone.

- N3b: cancer has spread to one to nine axillary lymph nodes and cancer in at least one of the lymph nodes is larger than two millimeters. Cancer has also spread to lymph nodes near the breastbone and the cancer is found by imaging tests, or cancer has spread to four to nine axillary lymph nodes and cancer in at least one of the lymph nodes is larger than two millimeters. Cancer has also spread to lymph nodes near the breastbone on the same side of the body as the primary tumor, and the cancer is larger than 0.2 millimeters and is found by sentinel lymph node biopsy.

- N3c: cancer has spread to lymph nodes above the collarbone on the same side of the body as the primary tumor.

When the lymph nodes are checked using mammography or ultrasound, it is called clinical staging. The clinical staging of lymph nodes is not described here.

Metastasis (M)—the spread of cancer to other parts of the body.

- M0: There is no sign that cancer has spread to other parts of the body.

- M1: Cancer has spread to other parts of the body, most often the bones, lungs, liver, or brain. If cancer has spread to distant lymph nodes, cancer in the lymph nodes is larger than 0.2 millimeters.

The Grading System

The grading system describes a tumor based on how abnormal the cancer cells and tissue look under a microscope and how quickly the cancer cells are likely to grow and spread. Low-grade cancer cells look more like normal cells and tend to grow and spread more slowly than high-grade cancer cells. To describe how abnormal the cancer cells and tissue are, the pathologist will assess the following three features:

- How much of the tumor tissue has normal breast ducts?

- The size and shape of the nuclei in the tumor cells.

- How many dividing cells are present, which is a measure of how fast the tumor cells are growing and dividing.

For each feature, the pathologist assigns a score of one to three; a score of "one" means the cells and tumor tissue look the most like normal cells and tissue, and a score of "three" means the cells and tissue look the most abnormal. The scores for each feature are added together to get a total score between three and nine.

Three grades are possible:

- Total score of three to five: G1 (Low grade or well differentiated).

- Total score of six to seven: G2 (Intermediate grade or moderately differentiated).

- Total score of eight to nine: G3 (High grade or poorly differentiated).

Biomarker Testing

Healthy breast cells, and some breast cancer cells, have receptors (biomarkers) that attach to the hormones estrogen and progesterone. These hormones are needed for healthy cells, and some breast cancer cells, to grow and divide. To check for these biomarkers, samples of tissue containing breast cancer cells are removed during a biopsy or surgery. The samples are tested in a laboratory to see whether the breast cancer cells have estrogen or progesterone receptors.

Another type of receptor (biomarker) that is found on the surface of all breast-cancer cells is called "HER2." HER2 receptors are needed for the breast-cancer cells to grow and divide.

For breast cancer, biomarker testing includes the following:

- **Estrogen receptor (ER).** If the breast cancer cells have estrogen receptors, the cancer cells are called ER-positive (ER+). If the breast cancer cells do not have estrogen receptors, the cancer cells are called ER-negative (ER-).

- **Progesterone receptor (PR).** If the breast cancer cells have progesterone receptors, the cancer cells are called PR positive

(PR+). If the breast cancer cells do not have progesterone receptors, the cancer cells are called PR negative (PR-).

- **Human epidermal growth factor type 2 receptor (HER2/ neu or HER2).** If the breast cancer cells have larger than normal amounts of HER2 receptors on their surface, the cancer cells are called HER2 positive (HER2+). If the breast cancers cells have a normal amount of HER2 on their surface, the cancer cells are called HER2 negative (HER2-). HER2+ breast cancer is more likely to grow and divide faster than HER2- breast cancer.

Sometimes the breast cancer cells will be described as triple negative or triple positive.

- **Triple negative.** If the breast cancer cells do not have estrogen receptors, progesterone receptors, or a larger than normal amount of HER2 receptors, the cancer cells are called triple negative.

- **Triple positive**. If the breast cancer cells do have estrogen receptors, progesterone receptors, and a larger than normal amount of HER2 receptors, the cancer cells are called triple positive.

It is important to know the estrogen receptor, progesterone receptor, and HER2 receptor status to choose the best treatment. There are drugs that can stop the receptors from attaching to the hormones estrogen and progesterone and stop the cancer from growing. Other drugs may be used to block the HER2 receptors on the surface of the breast cancer cells and stop the cancer from growing.

The TNM System, the grading system, and biomarker status are combined to find out the breast cancer stage. Here are three examples that combine the TNM system, the grading system, and the biomarker status to find out the Pathological Prognostic breast cancer stage for a woman whose first treatment was surgery:

- If the tumor size is 30 millimeters (T2), has not spread to nearby lymph nodes (N0), has not spread to distant parts of the body (M0), and is:

  - Grade 1
  - HER2+
  - ER-
  - PR-

The cancer is stage IIA.

- If the tumor size is 53 millimeters (T3), has spread to 4 to 9 axillary lymph nodes (N2), has not spread to other parts of the body (M0), and is:

  - Grade 2
  - HER2+
  - ER+
  - PR-

The tumor is stage IIIA.

- If the tumor size is 65 millimeters (T3), has spread to 3 axillary lymph nodes (N1a), has spread to the lungs (M1), and is:

  - Grade 1
  - HER2+
  - ER-
  - PR-

The cancer is stage IV.

Talk to Your Doctor

Talk to your doctor to find out what your breast cancer stage is and how it is used to plan the best treatment for you. After surgery, your doctor will receive a pathology report that describes the size and location of the primary tumor, the spread of cancer to nearby lymph nodes, tumor grade, and whether certain biomarkers are present. The pathology report and other test results are used to determine your breast cancer stage.

You are likely to have many questions. Ask your doctor to explain how staging is used to decide the best options to treat your cancer and whether there are clinical trials that might be right for you.

The treatment of breast cancer depends partly on the stage of the disease.

Part Five

Breast-Cancer Treatments

Chapter 39

Breast-Cancer Treatment—An Overview

Different types of treatments are available for patients with breast cancer. Some treatments are standard (the currently used treatment), and some are being tested in clinical trials. A treatment clinical trial is a research study meant to help improve current treatments or obtain information on new treatments for patients with cancer. When clinical trials show that a new treatment is better than the standard treatment, the new treatment may become the standard treatment. Patients may want to think about taking part in a clinical trial. Some clinical trials are open only to patients who have not started treatment.

Standard Treatments for Breast Cancer

The five types of standard treatment that are used to treat breast cancer are described below.

Surgery

Most patients with breast cancer have surgery to remove cancer.

Sentinel lymph node biopsy (SLNB) is the removal of the sentinel lymph node during surgery. The sentinel lymph node is the first lymph node in a group of lymph nodes to receive lymphatic drainage from

This chapter includes text excerpted from "Breast Cancer Treatment (PDQ®)— Patient Version," National Cancer Institute (NCI), December 28, 2018.

the primary tumor. It is the first lymph node the cancer is likely to spread to from the primary tumor. A radioactive substance and/or blue dye is injected near the tumor. The substance or dye flows through the lymph ducts to the lymph nodes. The first lymph node to receive the substance or dye is removed. A pathologist views the tissue under a microscope to look for cancer cells. If cancer cells are not found, it may not be necessary to remove more lymph nodes. Sometimes, a sentinel lymph node is found in more than one group of nodes. After the sentinel lymph node biopsy, the surgeon removes the tumor using breast-conserving surgery or mastectomy. If cancer cells were found, more lymph nodes will be removed through a separate incision. This is called a "lymph node dissection."

Types of surgery include the following:

- **Breast-conserving surgery**—operation to remove cancer and some normal tissue around it, but not the breast itself. Part of the chest wall lining may also be removed if the cancer is near it. This type of surgery may also be called lumpectomy, partial mastectomy, segmental mastectomy, quadrantectomy, or breast-sparing surgery.

- **Total mastectomy**—surgery to remove the whole breast that has cancer. This procedure is also called a simple mastectomy. Some of the lymph nodes under the arm may be removed and checked for cancer. This may be done at the same time as the breast surgery or after. This is done through a separate incision.

- **Modified radical mastectomy (MRM)**—surgery that is performed to remove the whole breast that has cancer, many of the lymph nodes under the arm, the lining over the chest muscles, and sometimes, part of the chest wall muscles.

Chemotherapy may be given before surgery to remove the tumor. When given before surgery, chemotherapy will shrink the tumor and reduce the amount of tissue that needs to be removed during surgery. Treatment is given before surgery is called preoperative therapy or neoadjuvant therapy.

After the doctor removes all cancer that can be seen at the time of the surgery, some patients may be given radiation therapy, chemotherapy, targeted therapy, or hormone therapy after surgery, to kill any cancer cells that are left. Treatment given after the surgery, to lower the risk that cancer will come back, is called "postoperative therapy" or adjuvant therapy.

If a patient is going to have a mastectomy, breast reconstruction (surgery to rebuild the shape of the breast after a mastectomy) may be considered. Breast reconstruction may be done at the time of the mastectomy or at some time after. The reconstructed breast may be made with the patient's own (nonbreast) tissue or by using implants filled with saline or silicone gel. Before the decision to get an implant is made, patients can call the U.S. Food and Drug Administration's (FDA) Center for Devices and Radiological Health (CDRH) at 888-463-6332.

Radiation Therapy

Radiation therapy is a cancer treatment that uses high-energy X-rays or other types of radiation to kill cancer cells or keep them from growing. There are two types of radiation therapy:

- **External radiation therapy** uses a machine outside the body to send radiation toward cancer.

- **Internal radiation therapy** uses a radioactive substance sealed in needles, seeds, wires, or catheters that are placed directly into or near cancer.

The way the radiation therapy is given depends on the type and stage of the cancer being treated. External radiation therapy is used to treat breast cancer. Internal radiation therapy with strontium-89 (a radionuclide) is used to relieve bone pain caused by breast cancer that has spread to the bones. Strontium-89 is injected into a vein and travels to the surface of the bones. Radiation is released and kills cancer cells in the bones.

Chemotherapy

Chemotherapy is a cancer treatment that uses drugs to stop the growth of cancer cells, either by killing the cells or by stopping them from dividing. When chemotherapy is taken by mouth or injected into a vein or muscle, the drugs enter the bloodstream and can reach cancer cells throughout the body (systemic chemotherapy). When chemotherapy is placed directly into the cerebrospinal fluid (CSF), an organ or a body cavity such as the abdomen, the drugs mainly affect cancer cells in those areas (regional chemotherapy).

The way the chemotherapy is given depends on the type and stage of the cancer being treated. Systemic chemotherapy is used in the treatment of breast cancer.

Hormone Therapy

Hormone therapy is a cancer treatment that removes hormones or blocks their action and stops cancer cells from growing. Hormones are substances made by glands in the body and circulated in the bloodstream. Some hormones can cause certain cancers to grow. If tests show that the cancer cells have places where hormones can attach (receptors), drugs, surgery, or radiation therapy is used to reduce the production of hormones or block them from working. The hormone estrogen, which makes some breast cancers grow, is made mainly by the ovaries. Treatment to stop the ovaries from making estrogen is called ovarian ablation.

Hormone therapy with tamoxifen is often given to patients with early localized breast cancer that can be removed by surgery and those with metastatic breast cancer (cancer that has spread to other parts of the body). Hormone therapy with tamoxifen or estrogens can act on cells all over the body and may increase the chance of developing endometrial cancer. Women taking tamoxifen should have a pelvic exam every year to look for any signs of cancer. Any vaginal bleeding, other than menstrual bleeding, should be reported to a doctor as soon as possible.

Hormone therapy with a luteinizing hormone-releasing hormone (LHRH) agonist is given to some premenopausal women who have just been diagnosed with hormone receptor-positive breast cancer. LHRH agonists decrease the body's estrogen and progesterone.

Hormone therapy with an aromatase inhibitor is given to some postmenopausal women who have hormone receptor-positive breast cancer. Aromatase inhibitors (AI) decrease the body's estrogen by blocking an enzyme called aromatase from turning androgen into estrogen. Anastrozole, letrozole, and exemestane are types of aromatase inhibitors.

For the treatment of early localized breast cancer that can be removed by surgery, certain aromatase inhibitors may be used as adjuvant therapy instead of tamoxifen or after two to three years of tamoxifen use. For the treatment of metastatic breast cancer, aromatase inhibitors are being tested in clinical trials to compare them to hormone therapy with tamoxifen.

In women with hormone receptor-positive breast cancer, at least five years of adjuvant hormone therapy reduces the risk that cancer will recur (come back).

Other types of hormone therapy include megestrol acetate (MGA) or antiestrogen therapy such as fulvestrant.

Targeted Therapy

Targeted therapy is a type of treatment that uses drugs or other substances to identify and attack specific cancer cells without harming normal cells. Monoclonal antibodies (MOAB), tyrosine kinase inhibitors (TKI), cyclin-dependent kinase (CDK) inhibitors, mammalian target of rapamycin (mTOR) inhibitors, and pharmacological inhibitors (PARP) are types of targeted therapies used in the treatment of breast cancer.

Monoclonal antibody (MAB) therapy is a cancer treatment that uses antibodies made in the laboratory, from a single type of immune system cell. These antibodies can identify substances on cancer cells or normal substances that may help cancer cells grow. The antibodies attach to the substances and kill the cancer cells, block their growth, or keep them from spreading. Monoclonal antibodies are given by infusion. They may be used alone or to carry drugs, toxins, or radioactive material directly to cancer cells. Monoclonal antibodies may be used in combination with chemotherapy as adjuvant therapy.

Types of monoclonal antibody therapy include the following:

- **Trastuzumab** is a monoclonal antibody that blocks the effects of the growth factor protein human epidermal growth factor receptor 2 (HER2), which sends growth signals to breast-cancer cells. It may be used with other therapies to treat HER2 positive breast cancer.

- **Pertuzumab** is a monoclonal antibody that may be combined with trastuzumab and chemotherapy to treat breast cancer. It may be used to treat certain patients with HER2 positive breast cancer that has metastasized (spread to other parts of the body). It may also be used as neoadjuvant therapy or adjuvant therapy in certain patients with early-stage HER2 positive breast cancer.

- **Ado-trastuzumab** emtansine is a monoclonal antibody linked to an anticancer drug. This is called an antibody-drug conjugate (ADC). It is used to treat HER2 positive breast cancer that has spread to other parts of the body or recurred (come back).

Tyrosine kinase inhibitors are targeted therapy drugs that block signals needed for tumors to grow. Tyrosine kinase inhibitors may be used with other anticancer drugs as adjuvant therapy. Tyrosine kinase inhibitors include the following:

- **Lapatinib** is a tyrosine kinase inhibitor that blocks the effects of the HER2 protein and other proteins inside tumor cells. It may be used with other drugs to treat patients with HER2 positive breast cancer that has progressed after treatment with trastuzumab.

- **Neratinib** is a tyrosine kinase inhibitor that blocks the effects of the HER2 protein and other proteins inside tumor cells. It may be used to treat patients with early-stage HER2 positive breast cancer after treatment with trastuzumab.

Cyclin-dependent kinase inhibitors are targeted therapy drugs that block proteins called cyclin-dependent kinases, which cause the growth of cancer cells. Cyclin-dependent kinase inhibitors include the following:

- **Palbociclib** is a cyclin-dependent kinase inhibitor used with the drug letrozole to treat breast cancer that is estrogen receptor positive and HER2 negative and has spread to other parts of the body. It is used in postmenopausal women whose cancer has not been treated with hormone therapy. Palbociclib may also be used with fulvestrant in women whose disease has gotten worse after treatment with hormone therapy.

- **Ribociclib** is a cyclin-dependent kinase inhibitor used with letrozole to treat breast cancer that is hormone receptor positive and HER2 negative and has come back or spread to other parts of the body. It is used in postmenopausal women whose cancer has not been treated with hormone therapy.

- **Abemaciclib** is a cyclin-dependent kinase inhibitor used to treat hormone receptor positive and HER2 negative breast cancer that is advanced or has spread to other parts of the body. It may be used alone or with other drugs to treat breast cancer that has gotten worse after other treatment.

Mammalian target of rapamycin (mTOR) inhibitors blocks a protein called mTOR, which may keep cancer cells from growing and prevent the growth of new blood vessels that tumors need to grow. mTOR inhibitors include the following:

- **Everolimus** is an mTOR inhibitor used in postmenopausal women with advanced hormone receptor-positive breast cancer that is also HER2 negative and has not gotten better with other treatment.

PARP inhibitors are a type of targeted therapy that blocks deoxyribonucleic acid (DNA) repair and may cause cancer cells to die.

Olaparib is a PARP inhibitor used to treat patients with mutations in the *BRCA1* or *BRCA2* genes and HER2 negative breast cancer that has spread to other parts of the body. PARP inhibitor therapy is being studied for the treatment of patients with triple-negative breast cancer (TNBC).

Side Effects due to Some Treatments

Some treatments for breast cancer may cause side effects that continue or appear months or years after treatment has ended. These are called "late effects."

Late effects of radiation therapy are not common, but may include:

- **Inflammation of the lung** after radiation therapy to the breast, especially when chemotherapy is **given at the same time.**

- **Arm lymphedema**, especially when radiation therapy is given after lymph node dissection.

- In women younger than 45 years who receive radiation therapy to the chest wall after mastectomy, there may be a higher risk of developing breast cancer in the other breast.

Late effects of chemotherapy depend on the drugs used, but may include:

- Heart failure

- Blood clots

- Premature menopause (PMM)

- Second cancer, such as leukemia

Late effects of targeted therapy with trastuzumab, lapatinib, or pertuzumab may include heart problems such as heart failure.

Chapter 40

How to Find a Doctor If You Have Cancer

If you have been diagnosed with cancer, finding a doctor and a treatment facility for your cancer care is an important step to getting the best treatment possible.

You will have many things to consider when choosing a doctor. It's important for you to feel comfortable with the specialist that you choose because you will be working closely with that person to make decisions about your cancer treatment.

Choosing a Doctor

When choosing a doctor for your cancer care, it may be helpful to know some of the terms used to describe a doctor's training and credentials. Most physicians who treat people with cancer are medical doctors (they have an M.D. degree) or osteopathic doctors (they have a D.O. degree). Standard training includes four years of study at a college or university, four years of medical school, and three to seven years of postgraduate medical education (PGME) through internships and residencies. Doctors must pass an exam to become licensed to practice medicine in their state.

Specialists are doctors who have done their residency training in a specific field such as internal medicine. Independent specialty boards

This chapter includes text excerpted from "Finding Healthcare Services," National Cancer Institute (NCI), August 25, 2017.

certify physicians after they have met needed requirements, including meeting certain education and training standards, being licensed to practice medicine, and passing an examination given by their specialty board. Once they have met these requirements, physicians are said to be "board certified."

Some specialists who treat cancer are:

- **Medical oncologist** specializes in treating cancer

- **Hematologist** focuses on diseases of the blood and related tissues, including the bone marrow, spleen, and lymph nodes

- **Radiation oncologist** uses X-rays and other forms of radiation to diagnose and treat disease

- **Surgeon** performs operations on almost any area of the body and may specialize in a certain type of surgery

Finding a Doctor Who Specializes in Cancer Care

To find a doctor who specializes in cancer care, ask your primary care doctor to suggest someone. Or you may know of a specialist through the experience of a friend or family member. Also, your local hospital should be able to provide you with a list of specialists who practice there.

Another option for finding a doctor is your nearest National Cancer Institute (NCI)-designated cancer center. The Find a Cancer Center page www.cancer.gov provides contact information to help healthcare providers and cancer patients with referrals to all NCI-designated cancer centers in the United States.

The online directories listed below may also help you find a cancer care specialist.

- **The American Board of Medical Specialists (ABMS)**, which creates and implements the standards for certifying and evaluating doctors, has a list of doctors that have met specific requirements and passed specialty exams.

- **The American Medical Association (AMA)** Doctor provides information on licensed doctors in the United States.

- **The American Society of Clinical Oncology (ASCO)** member database has the names and affiliations of nearly 30,000 oncologists worldwide.

- **The American College of Surgeons** (ACoS) lists member surgeons by region and specialty in their Find a Surgeon database. The ACoS can also be reached at 800-621-4111.

- **The American Osteopathic Association (AOA)** Find a Doctor database provides an online list of practicing osteopathic physicians who are AOA members. The AOA can also be reached at 800-621-1773.

Local medical societies may also maintain lists of doctors in each specialty for you to check. Public and medical libraries may have print directories of doctors' names listed geographically by specialty.

Depending on your health insurance plan, your choice may be limited to doctors who participate in your plan. Your insurance company can give you a list of doctors who take part in your plan. It's important to contact the office of the doctor you're considering to be sure that he or she is accepting new patients through your plan. It's also important to do this if you're using a federal or state health insurance program such as Medicare or Medicaid.

If you can change health insurance plans, you may want to decide which doctor you would like to use first and then choose the plan that includes your chosen physician. You also have the option of seeing a doctor outside your plan and paying more of the costs yourself.

To help make your decision when you're considering what doctor to choose, think about if the doctor:

- Has the education and training needed to meet your needs

- Has someone who covers for them if they are unavailable and who would have access to your medical records

- Has a helpful support staff

- Explains things clearly, listens to you, and treats you with respect

- Encourages you to ask questions

- Has office hours that meet your needs

- Is easy to get an appointment with

If you are choosing a surgeon, you will want to ask:

- Are they board certified?

- How often do they perform the type of surgery you need?

- How many of these procedures have they performed?

- At what hospital(s) do they practice?

It's important for you to feel good about the doctor you choose. You will be working with this person closely as you make decisions about your cancer treatment.

Chapter 41

Getting a Second Opinion after a Breast-Cancer Diagnosis

If you have been diagnosed with cancer, finding a doctor and a treatment facility for your cancer care is an important step to getting the best treatment possible. You will have many things to consider when choosing a doctor. It's important for you to feel comfortable with the specialist that you choose because you will be working closely with that person to make decisions about your cancer treatment.

Need for Second Opinion

After you talk to a doctor about the diagnosis and treatment plan for your cancer, you may want to get another doctor's opinion before you begin treatment. This is known as getting a "second opinion."

How to Get a Second Opinion

You can do this by asking another specialist to review all the materials related to your case. The doctor who gives the second opinion may agree with the treatment plan proposed by your first doctor, or

---

This chapter includes text excerpted from "Finding Healthcare Services," National Cancer Institute (NCI), August 25, 2017.

they may suggest changes or another approach. Either way, getting a second opinion may:

- Give you more information

- Answer any questions you may have

- Give you a greater sense of control

- Help you feel more confident, knowing you have explored all your options

Nothing Wrong in Getting a Second Opinion

Getting a second opinion is very common. Yet some patients worry that their doctor will be offended if they ask for a second opinion. Usually, the opposite is true. Most doctors welcome a second opinion. And many health insurance companies pay for a second opinion or even require them, particularly if a doctor recommends surgery.

What You Should Do While Getting a Second Opinion

When talking with your doctor about getting a second opinion, it may be helpful to express that you're satisfied with your care but want to be certain you're as informed as possible about your treatment options. It's best to involve your doctor in the process of getting a second opinion, because he or she will need to make your medical records (such as your test results and X-rays) available to the doctor giving the second opinion. You may wish to bring a family member along for support when asking for a second opinion.

Resources You Can Try

If your doctor can't suggest another specialist for a second opinion, many of the resources listed above for finding a doctor can help you find a specialist for a second opinion. You can also call National Cancer Institute's (NCI) Contact Center at 800-422-6237 for guidance.

Chapter 42

Choosing a Treatment Facility

As with choosing a doctor, your choice of facilities may be limited to those that take part in your health insurance plan. If you have already found a doctor for your cancer treatment, you may need to choose a treatment facility based on where your doctor practices. Or your doctor may be able to recommend a facility that provides quality care to meet your needs.

Questions to Consider before Choosing a Treatment Facility

Some questions to ask when considering a treatment facility are:

- Does it have experience and success in treating my condition?

- Has it been rated by state, consumer, or other groups for its quality of care?

- How does it check on and work to improve its quality of care?

This chapter includes text excerpted from "Finding Healthcare Services," National Cancer Institute (NCI), August 25, 2017.

- Has it been approved by a nationally recognized accrediting body, such as the American Chemical Society (ACS) Commission on Cancer (COC) and/or The Joint Commission?

- Does it explain patients' rights and responsibilities? Are copies of this information available to patients?

- Does it offer support services, such as social workers and resources, to help me find financial assistance if I need it?

- Is it conveniently located?

Check with Your Health-Insurance Provider

If you belong to a health-insurance plan, ask your insurance company if the facility you are choosing is approved by your plan. If you decide to pay for treatment yourself because you choose to go outside of your network or don't have insurance, discuss the possible costs with your doctor beforehand. You will want to talk to the hospital billing department as well. Nurses and social workers may also be able to give you more information about coverage, eligibility, and insurance issues.

Resources That May Help You in Finding a Hospital or Treatment Facility

The following resources may help you find a hospital or treatment facility for your care:

- **National Cancer Institute (NCI)**, To find a cancer center, www.cancer.gov page provides contact information for NCI-designated cancer centers located throughout the country.

- **The American College of Surgeon's (ACoS) Commission on Cancer (CoC)**. The ACoS website www.facs.org has a searchable database of cancer care programs they have accredited. They can also be reached at 312-202-5085 or by e-mail at CoC@facs.org.

- **The Joint Commission** evaluates and accredits healthcare organizations and programs in the United States. It also provides guidance about choosing a treatment facility and offers an online Quality Check® service that patients can use to check whether a specific facility has been accredited by the Joint Commission and to view its performance reports. They also can be reached at 630-792-5000.

Chapter 43

Adjuvant and Neoadjuvant Therapy for Breast Cancer

What Is Adjuvant Therapy for Breast Cancer?

Adjuvant therapy for breast cancer is any treatment given after primary therapy to increase the chance of long-term, disease-free survival. Primary therapy is the main treatment used to reduce or eliminate the cancer. Primary therapy for breast cancer usually includes surgery—a mastectomy (removal of the breast) or a lumpectomy (surgery to remove the tumor and a small amount of normal tissue around it; a type of breast-conserving surgery). During either type of surgery, one or more nearby lymph nodes are also removed to see if cancer cells have spread to the lymphatic system. When a woman has breast-conserving surgery, primary therapy almost always includes radiation therapy.

Even in early-stage breast cancer, cells may break away from the primary tumor and spread to other parts of the body (metastasize). Therefore, doctors give adjuvant therapy to kill any cancer cells that may have spread, even if they cannot be detected by imaging or laboratory tests. Studies have shown that adjuvant therapy for breast cancer may increase the chance of long-term survival by preventing a recurrence.

This chapter includes text excerpted from "Adjuvant and Neoadjuvant Therapy for Breast Cancer," National Cancer Institute (NCI), June 16, 2009. Reviewed February 2019.

What Types of Adjuvant Therapies Are Used for Breast Cancer?

Most adjuvant therapies are systemic: they use substances that travel through the bloodstream, reaching and affecting cancer cells all over the body. Adjuvant therapy for breast cancer can include chemotherapy, hormonal therapy, the targeted drug trastuzumab (Herceptin), radiation therapy, or a combination of treatments.

Adjuvant chemotherapy uses drugs to kill cancer cells. Research has shown that adjuvant chemotherapy for early-stage breast cancer helps to prevent cancer from returning. Usually, more than one drug is given during adjuvant chemotherapy (called combination chemotherapy).

Hormonal therapy deprives breast-cancer cells of the hormone estrogen, which many breast tumors need to grow. A commonly used hormonal treatment is the drug tamoxifen, which blocks estrogen's activity in the body. Studies have shown that tamoxifen helps prevent original cancer from returning and also helps to prevent the development of new cancers in the other breast; however, many women develop resistance to the drug over time. Tamoxifen can be given to both premenopausal and postmenopausal women.

Postmenopausal women may also receive hormonal therapy with a newer type of drug called an aromatase inhibitor (AI), either after tamoxifen therapy or instead of tamoxifen therapy. Rather than blocking estrogen's activity, as tamoxifen does, AIs prevent the body from making estrogen. Clinical trials suggest that AIs may be more effective than tamoxifen in preventing breast cancer recurrence in some women. Using AIs to block estrogen production in premenopausal women is not very effective, in part because the ovary is stimulated to make more estrogen when blood levels of estrogen fall below normal. This does not occur in postmenopausal women, whose ovaries have stopped making estrogen.

Some premenopausal women may undergo ovarian ablation or suppression, which greatly reduces the amount of estrogen produced by the body, either permanently or temporarily. Premenopausal women who have *BRCA1* or *BRCA2* gene mutations are at very high risk of breast cancer recurrence as well as of ovarian cancer and may decide to have their ovaries surgically removed as part of adjuvant therapy. The surgical removal of the ovaries also decreases the risk of ovarian cancer. Other premenopausal women who have a lower risk of recurrence may be prescribed drugs that temporarily suppress the function of the ovaries, in addition to tamoxifen.

Trastuzumab is a monoclonal antibody that targets cancer cells that make too much of, or overexpress, a protein called HER2. When cancer cells overexpress HER2 protein, they are said to be HER2 positive. Approximately 20 percent of all breast cancers are HER2 positive. Clinical trials have shown that targeted therapy with trastuzumab in addition to chemotherapy decreases the risk of relapse for women with HER2-positive tumors.

Radiation therapy is usually given after breast-conserving surgery and may be given after a mastectomy. (When doctors give radiation therapy after breast-conserving surgery, it is usually considered part of primary therapy.) For women at high risk of recurrence, doctors may use radiation therapy after mastectomy to kill cancer cells that may be left in tissues next to the breast, such as the chest wall or nearby lymph nodes. Radiation therapy is a type of local therapy, not systemic therapy.

How Is Adjuvant Therapy Given, and for How Long?

Adjuvant chemotherapy is given orally (by mouth) or by injection into a blood vessel. It is given in cycles, consisting of a treatment period followed by a recovery period. The number of cycles depends on the types of drugs used. Most patients do not have to stay in the hospital for chemotherapy—they can be treated as an outpatient or at the doctor's office. Adjuvant chemotherapy usually does not last for much more than six months.

Hormonal therapy is usually given orally, as a pill.

- Most women who undergo hormonal therapy take tamoxifen every day for five years.

- Some women may take an aromatase inhibitor every day for five years instead of tamoxifen.

- Some women may receive additional treatment with an aromatase inhibitor after five years of tamoxifen.

- Finally, some women may switch to taking an aromatase inhibitor after two or three years of tamoxifen, for a total of five or more years of hormonal therapy.

- Trastuzumab is given by infusion into a blood vessel every one to three weeks for a year.

Radiation therapy given after mastectomy is divided into small doses given once a day over the course of several weeks. Radiation therapy may not be given at the same time as some types of chemo-therapy or hormonal therapy.

How Do Doctors Decide Who Needs Adjuvant Therapy?

Not all women with breast cancer need adjuvant therapy. Patients at higher risk of cancer recurrence are more likely to need adjuvant therapy. Doctors look at both prognostic and predictive factors to decide which patients might benefit from adjuvant treatments. Prognostic factors help doctors estimate how likely a tumor is to recur. Predictive factors help doctors estimate how likely cancer cells are to respond to a particular treatment.

In addition to a woman's age and menopausal status, several other prognostic factors are used to determine the risk of recurrence.

- **Stage of cancer.** Cancer stage refers to the size of the tumor and whether it is in the breast only or has spread to nearby lymph nodes or other places in the body. Larger tumors (especially those that are more than five centimeters—about two inches—in diameter) are more likely to recur than small tumors. Breast cancer often first spreads to the lymph nodes under the arm (axillary lymph nodes). During surgery, doctors usually remove some of these underarm lymph nodes to determine whether they contain cancer cells. Cancer that has spread to these lymph nodes is more likely to recur.

- **Tumor grade.** This term refers to how closely the tumor cells resemble normal breast cells when viewed under a microscope. Tumors with cells that bear little or no resemblance to normal breast cells (called "poorly differentiated tumors") are more likely to recur. Women with tumor cells that look like normal breast cells (called "well-differentiated tumors") tend to have a better prognosis.

- **Proliferative capacity of the tumor.** Proliferative capacity refers to how fast the tumor cells divide or multiply, to form more cells. Women who have tumor cells that have low proliferative capacity (that is, the cells divide less often and grow more slowly) tend to have a better prognosis.

- **Hormone receptor status.** The cells of many breast tumors express receptors for the hormones estrogen and progesterone. Tumors with cells that do not express hormone receptors are more likely to recur. Doctors can determine whether a tumor expresses hormone receptors with laboratory tests.

- **HER2 status.** Tumors that produce too much of a protein called HER2 are more likely to recur. Doctors can determine whether a tumor produces too much HER2 with a laboratory test.

Two major predictive factors are currently used to determine whether cancer cells might respond to particular treatments:

- **Hormone receptor status.** As mentioned above, the cells of many breast tumors express receptors for the hormones estrogen and progesterone. These hormones bind to the receptors and help the cancer cells grow. Blocking the activity of these hormones with hormonal therapy stops the growth of the cancer cells. Hormonal therapy will not help patients whose tumors do not express hormone receptors.

- **HER2 status.** Tumors that produce too much of the protein HER2 can be treated with trastuzumab, which can cut the risk of recurrence by up to about half. Women whose tumors do not produce too much HER2 do not benefit from treatment with trastuzumab.

Clinical trials are underway to see if genetic information collected from tumors can help predict which women will benefit from adjuvant chemotherapy.

Prognostic and predictive factors cannot determine exactly which patients may benefit from adjuvant therapy and which patients may benefit from primary therapy alone. Decisions about adjuvant therapy must be made on an individual basis. This complicated decision-making process is best carried out by consulting an oncologist, a doctor who specializes in cancer treatment. In addition to the factors described above, doctors will take into account a woman's general health and her personal treatment preferences.

What Is Neoadjuvant Therapy?

Neoadjuvant therapy is treatment given before primary therapy. A woman may receive neoadjuvant chemotherapy for breast cancer to shrink a tumor that is inoperable in its current state, so it can be surgically removed. A woman whose tumor can be removed by mastectomy may instead receive neoadjuvant therapy to shrink the tumor enough to allow breast-conserving surgery.

Neoadjuvant chemotherapy is given in the same manner as adjuvant chemotherapy. If a tumor does not respond (shrink) or continues to grow during neoadjuvant chemotherapy, the doctor may stop treatment and try another type of chemotherapy or perform surgery instead, depending on the stage of cancer.

Clinical trials are examining whether hormonal therapy or trastuzumab is effective when given before surgery.

What Are the Side Effects of Adjuvant and Neoadjuvant Therapy?

Chemotherapy: The side effects of chemotherapy depend mainly on the drugs a woman receives. As with other types of treatment, side effects vary from person to person. In general, anticancer drugs affect rapidly dividing cells. These include blood cells, which fight infection, cause the blood to clot, and carry oxygen to all parts of the body. When blood cells are affected by anticancer drugs, patients are more likely to get infections and bruise or bleed easily and may have less energy during treatment and for some time afterward. Cells in hair follicles and cells that line the digestive tract also divide rapidly. As a result of chemotherapy, patients may lose their hair and may have other side effects, such as loss of appetite, nausea, vomiting, diarrhea, or mouth sores.

Doctors can prescribe medications to help control nausea and vomiting caused by chemotherapy. They also monitor patients for any signs of other problems and may adjust the dose or schedule of treatment if problems arise. In addition, doctors advise women who have a lowered resistance to infection because of low blood cell counts to avoid crowds and people who are sick or have colds. The side effects of chemotherapy are generally short-term. They gradually go away during the recovery part of the chemotherapy cycle or after the treatment is over. However, some chemotherapy drugs, called anthracyclines, can increase the risk of heart problems. Women who receive an anthracycline as part of their treatment should be monitored closely by their doctors for heart problems for the rest of their lives.

Hormonal therapy: In general, the side effects of tamoxifen are similar to some of the symptoms of menopause. The most common side effects are hot flashes, vaginal discharge, and nausea. Tamoxifen also increases the risk of cataract development. Not all women who take tamoxifen have these symptoms. Most of these side effects do not require medical attention.

Doctors carefully monitor women taking tamoxifen for any signs of more serious side effects. Among women who have not had a hysterectomy (surgery to remove the uterus), the risk of developing uterine cancer is increased for those taking tamoxifen. Women who take tamoxifen should talk with their doctor about having regular pelvic exams and should be examined promptly if they have pelvic pain or any abnormal vaginal bleeding. Women taking tamoxifen, particularly those who are receiving chemotherapy along with tamoxifen, have a greater risk of developing a blood clot.

Aromatase inhibitors also cause hot flashes, vaginal dryness, and other symptoms of menopause. Women taking an aromatase inhibitor may also experience joint pain (arthralgia) or muscle pain (myalgia) during treatment.

Women taking aromatase inhibitors may have a higher risk of heart problems than those taking tamoxifen. Aromatase inhibitors also reduce bone density and increase the risk of bone fractures. Doctors should carefully monitor women taking aromatase inhibitors for any signs of heart damage or changes in bone density. A type of drug called a bisphosphonate can help reduce bone loss caused by aromatase inhibitors for patients at high risk of fractures.

Trastuzumab: Side effects from trastuzumab can include nausea, vomiting, hot flashes, and joint pain. Trastuzumab can also increase the risk of heart problems. Women receiving trastuzumab should be monitored closely by their doctors for any reduction in the heart's ability to pump blood, both during and after treatment.

Radiation therapy: Skin in the area treated by radiation may become red, dry, tender, and itchy, and the breast may feel heavy and tight. These problems usually go away over time. Women receiving radiation therapy may become very tired, especially in the later weeks of treatment.

Careful studies have shown that the risks of adjuvant therapy for breast cancer are outweighed by the benefit of treatment— that is, increasing the chance of long-term survival. However, it is important for women to share any concerns they may have about their treatment or side effects with their doctor or other healthcare provider.

What Are Doctors and Scientists Doing to Learn More about Adjuvant and Neoadjuvant Therapy for Breast Cancer?

Doctors and scientists are conducting research studies called clinical trials to learn how to treat breast cancer more effectively. In these studies, researchers compare two or more groups of patients who receive different treatments. Clinical trials allow researchers to examine the effectiveness of new treatments in comparison with standard ones, as well as to compare the side effects of the treatments.

Researchers are also investigating whether molecular information obtained from a woman's tumor can be used to decide if the woman would benefit from adjuvant therapy. Two large clinical trials sponsored by NCI, a part of the National Institutes of Health, are currently underway in this area of research.

The Trial Assigning Individualized Options for Treatment (TAILORx) is examining whether molecular markers that are frequently associated with risk of recurrence among women who have early-stage breast cancer can be used to assign patients to the most appropriate and effective treatment. TAILORx is using a test called Oncotype DX™, which calculates the risk of recurrence based on the levels of expression of 21 genes in breast tumors, in over 10,000 women recruited at 900 sites in the United States and Canada. Based on their risk of recurrence, women will be assigned to one of three different treatment groups: women with a high risk of recurrence will receive chemotherapy plus hormonal therapy; women with a low risk of recurrence will receive hormonal therapy alone; and women with an intermediate risk of recurrence will be randomly assigned to receive adjuvant hormonal therapy, with or without chemotherapy. Because the degree of benefit of chemotherapy for women with an intermediate risk of recurrence is unknown, TAILORx seeks to determine whether the Oncotype DX test will be helpful in future treatment planning for this group.

In the Microarray In Node-negative Disease may Avoid Chemotherapy Trial (MINDACT), investigators are studying genomic profiling compared with clinical assessment to determine the need for chemotherapy in women with node-negative breast cancer (cancer that has not spread to the axillary lymph nodes). The investigators will use both a 70-gene signature test and clinical assessment to determine the women's risk of recurrence. Women eligible to receive chemotherapy who have a high risk of recurrence according to the clinical criteria and a low risk of recurrence according to the 70-gene signature, or have a low risk of recurrence according to the clinical criteria and a high risk of recurrence according to the 70-gene signature, will be randomly assigned to receive treatment based on either the genetic or clinical criteria to determine which better predicts the need for chemotherapy.

Women with breast cancer who are interested in taking part in a clinical trial should talk with their doctor.

Chapter 44

Surgical Treatments for Breast Cancer

Chapter Contents

289

Section 44.1

Overview of Surgeries for Early-Stage Breast Cancer

This section includes text excerpted from "Surgery Choices for Women with Ductal Carcinoma in Situ or Breast Cancer," National Cancer Institute (NCI), November 2012. Reviewed February 2019.

Surgery as an Option for Treatment Women with for Ductal Carcinoma in Situ
Talk with Surgeons

Talk with a breast-cancer surgeon about your choices. Find out what happens during surgery, the types of problems that sometimes occur, and any treatment you might need after surgery. Ask a lot of questions and learn as much as you can. You may also wish to talk with family members, friends, or others who have had breast-cancer surgery. After talking with a surgeon, think about getting a second opinion. A second opinion means getting the advice of another surgeon. This surgeon might tell you about other treatment options. Or, she or he may agree with the advice you got from the first doctor. Some people worry about hurting their surgeon's feelings if they get a second opinion. But it is very common and good surgeons don't mind. Also, some insurance companies require it. It is better to get a second opinion than worry that you made the wrong choice. If you think you might have a mastectomy, this is also a good time to learn about breast reconstruction. Think about meeting with a reconstructive plastic surgeon to learn about this surgery and if it seems like a good option for you.

Learn about Your Surgery Choices

Most women who have ductal carcinoma *in situ* (DCIS) or breast cancer that can be treated with surgery have three surgery choices. They are:

- Breast-sparing surgery, followed by radiation therapy

- Mastectomy

- Mastectomy with breast-reconstruction surgery

290

Think about What Is Important to You

After you have talked with a breast-cancer surgeon and learned the facts, you may also want to talk with your spouse or partner, family, friends, or other women who have had breast-cancer surgery. Then, think about what is important to you. Thinking about these questions and talking them over with others might help.

Surgery Choices

- If I have breast-sparing surgery, am I willing and able to have radiation therapy five days a week for five to eight weeks?
- If I have a mastectomy, do I also want breast reconstruction surgery?
- If I have breast reconstruction surgery, do I want it at the same time as my mastectomy?
- What treatment does my insurance cover? What do I have to pay for?

Life after Surgery

- How important is it to me how my breast looks after cancer surgery?
- How important is it to me how my breast feels after cancer surgery?
- If I have a mastectomy and do not have reconstruction, will my insurance cover prosthesis and special bras?
- Where can I find a breast prosthesis and special bras?

Learning More

- Do I want a second opinion?
- Is there someone else I should talk with about my surgery choices?
- What else do I want to learn or do before I make my choice about breast cancer surgery?

Make Your Choice

You have talked with your surgeon, learned the facts, and thought about what is important to you—it's time to decide which surgery is best for you.

Section 44.2

Mastectomy and Lumpectomy

What Are Mastectomy and Lumpectomy?

Mastectomy is a type of surgery that involves the complete removal of tissue from one breast (called a unilateral mastectomy) or both breasts (bilateral mastectomy). Mastectomy is usually performed as a form of treatment for breast cancer, although it may also be used as a method of preventing breast cancer in people who are at very high risk of developing it due to strong family history or genetic mutations (known as preventative, prophylactic, or risk-reducing mastectomy).

A lumpectomy is a less-invasive form of surgery that involves removing only the cancerous or abnormal tissue from the breast. The surgery is usually followed by radiation therapy to eliminate any cancerous cells that may remain in the breast. Since only a portion of the breast is removed, lumpectomy is also known as breast-conserving surgery or excisional biopsy. Lumpectomy is also sometimes performed to help confirm or rule out a diagnosis of breast cancer.

Both mastectomy and lumpectomy are often presented as treatment options for women with early-stage breast cancer. Studies have shown that the long-term survival rates for mastectomy are the same as for lumpectomy plus radiation therapy. In addition, the risk of cancer spreading beyond the breast to other organs is the same for the two procedures. However, lumpectomy carries a slightly higher risk of recurrence of cancer in the same area.

The main benefit of lumpectomy is the preservation of breast tissue, although newer mastectomy and breast reconstruction techniques can preserve breast skin and provide a more natural appearance following surgery. A potential benefit of mastectomy is that the patient is less likely to require radiation therapy, which involves side effects and can be time-consuming. The characteristics of the tumor, rather than the type of surgery, determine whether a patient requires chemotherapy or other types of drug therapies. Deciding between the two procedures can be difficult for many patients, and it requires careful consideration of the advantages and disadvantages of each.

Advantages and Disadvantages of Mastectomy

One of the main reasons some women opt for mastectomy is that it offers peace of mind. Removing the entire breast eliminates the possibility of recurrence and also reduces the likelihood of radiation therapy. Some patients simply want to get rid of cancer and be done with it. Mastectomy offers advantages over lumpectomy plus radiation in other situations, as well. It is often recommended for patients who:

- Have multiple or widespread malignancies in separate areas of the breast

- Have previously undergone lumpectomy but still, have cancer cells on the margins of the surgical area

- Have previously undergone radiation treatment but experienced a recurrence of breast cancer

- Have a gene mutation that increases the chance of recurrence

- Have a tumor that is large compared to the overall size of the breast, which reduces the likelihood that lumpectomy will produce acceptable cosmetic results

- Cannot tolerate radiation due to pregnancy, connective tissue disease, or other health conditions

- Live too far from a treatment facility to have radiation treatment for five to seven weeks

For many women, the main disadvantage of mastectomy is that it means a complete and permanent loss of the breast. The surgery is more invasive than lumpectomy, so it requires general anesthesia and an overnight hospital stay. It often involves more postsurgery side effects, and the recovery time tends to be longer. In addition, many patients who undergo mastectomy have further reconstructive surgery to restore the appearance of the breast.

Advantages and Disadvantages of Lumpectomy

Given the option, many women opt for lumpectomy because it preserves as much breast tissue as possible. Some patients feel strongly about keeping their breast and maintaining its normal appearance and sensation. Lumpectomy is also a less-invasive surgery than mastectomy, so the recovery time is likely to be shorter. It is often recommended for patients who have precancerous breast abnormalities or malignancies that are small, localized, and at an early stage.

Lumpectomy also has a few potential disadvantages, however, including the following:

- Most patients require five to seven weeks of daily radiation therapy following surgery

- Additional surgeries may be required following the lumpectomy if the pathologist finds cancer cells in the margins around the tumor that were removed

- It involves a slightly higher risk of recurrence than mastectomy

- If there is a recurrence in the same breast, it will usually require a mastectomy because the breast tissue cannot tolerate additional radiation

Deciding between Mastectomy and Lumpectomy

Patients who are offered a choice between mastectomy and lumpectomy plus radiation must weigh the advantages and disadvantages of each procedure. Personal preferences play an important role in the decision. Some factors to consider include the patient's feelings about keeping her breast and ensuring that her breasts match in size and shape. In addition, the patient must decide whether she will worry about the recurrence of breast cancer if she has a lumpectomy.

The decision of whether to have a mastectomy or lumpectomy may also be influenced by where the patient lives. Research has shown that American women are more likely to have mastectomies than women in other countries. Within the United States, mastectomy is most common in the Midwest and South, while lumpectomy is more prevalent on the East Coast and West Coast. The distance a patient must drive to reach a radiation center may also affect her decision.

Finally, the doctor and hospital that provide the treatment may influence the patient's decision whether to have a lumpectomy or mastectomy. University-based hospitals tend to perform more lumpectomies, while community-based hospitals tend to perform more mastectomies. Likewise, older surgeons who were trained prior to 1980, when mastectomy was the standard treatment for all stages of breast cancer, are less likely to recommend lumpectomy. As a result, patients who feel strongly about one procedure or the other may wish to seek a second opinion to more fully understand their options.

References

1. "Deciding between Mastectomy or Lumpectomy," Susan G. Komen Foundation, July 24, 2015.

2. "Mastectomy versus Lumpectomy," BreastCancer.org, 2016.

3. "Tests and Procedures: Lumpectomy," Mayo Clinic, October 23, 2014.

4. "Tests and Procedures: Mastectomy," Mayo Clinic, October 22, 2014.

Section 44.3

Breast Reconstruction Surgery

This section includes text excerpted from "Breast Implant Surgery," U.S. Food and Drug Administration (FDA), August 28, 2018.

Breast-Implant Surgery

Breast-implant surgery can be performed in a hospital, surgery center or doctor's office. Breast-implant surgery patients may have to stay overnight in the hospital (inpatient surgery) or may be able to go home afterward (outpatient surgery). The surgery can be done under local anesthesia, where the patient remains awake and only the breast is numbed to block the pain, or under general anesthesia, where medicine is given to make the patient sleep. Most women receive general anesthesia for this surgery. Breast-implant surgery can last from one to several hours depending on the procedure and personal circumstances.

If the surgery is done in a hospital, the length of the hospital stay will vary based on the type of surgery, the development of any complications after surgery and your general health. The length of the hospital stay may also depend on the type of coverage your insurance provides.

Surgical Consultation

Before surgery, you should have a consultation with your surgeon. Be prepared to ask questions about the surgeon's experience, your surgery, and expected outcomes. The U.S. Food and Drug Administration (FDA) has provided a list of questions that may help guide your discussion. The surgeon should be able to discuss whether you are a good candidate for breast implants, the different type of implants, options for size, shape, surface texture, and placement based on your particular circumstances, as well as the risks and benefits of implant surgery. The surgeon should also be able to provide you with before and after pictures of other patients to help you better understand your expectations and potential outcomes from surgery.

During the consultation, you will need to discuss your medical history, including any medical conditions or drug allergies you may have. You should also discuss any previous surgeries you've had, especially to the breast, and what drugs you are currently taking, including supplements, herbal and over-the-counter (OTC) medications.

It is important to tell the surgeon if you think you may be pregnant.

If you are undergoing breast-implant surgery for reconstruction, you will also need to speak with your surgeon about your personal circumstances, including being treated with chemotherapy and/or radiation therapy, as these can affect your risks of complication and the appearance of the reconstructed breast. The surgeon should also speak to you about the amount of breast tissue that will remain after surgery and future screening for breast implant ruptures and breast cancer.

During the consultation, be sure to ask the surgeon for a copy of the patient labeling for the breast implant she/he plans to use. You have the right to request this information, and your physician is expected to provide it. Be sure to read the patient labeling entirely prior to surgery. It will provide you with information specific to your breast implants, including how to take care of them. Make sure you read and understand the informed consent form before you sign it.

Breast-implant manufacturers are currently conducting clinical studies to evaluate new types of breast implants and to understand the long-term experiences of women who receive breast implants. If you are interested in participating in a clinical study, be sure to ask your surgeon what specific steps you will need to take.

Before Surgery

Your surgeon may ask that you have a mammogram or breast X-rays prior to surgery in order to identify any breast abnormality and so the surgeon has a preoperative image of your breast tissue.

You will usually be asked to not eat or drink anything after midnight the night before surgery and to bring loose clothing, including a loose-fitting bra without underwire, to wear after surgery. If you are going home the same day as the surgery, you will need to plan for someone to drive you home.

Your surgeon should discuss with you the extent of surgery, the estimated time it will take and how they plan to treat for pain and nausea.

During Surgery

Once you have been given anesthesia and it has taken effect, the surgeon will make an incision (cut) in one of the following areas:

- Along the underside of your breast (inframammary)

- Under your arm (transaxillary)

- Around the nipple (periareolar)

- Through the mastectomy scar (for reconstruction)

The FDA-approved labeling warns surgeons NOT to place breast implants through the belly-button (peri-umbilical approach)

The location of the incision can affect how visible the scars are, as well as any complications you may experience after surgery.

Cutting the underside of the breast is the most common location used since it is where the skin naturally folds. Your scarring with this type of incision may be a bit more visible, especially if you are younger, thin and have not yet had children.

Placing the implant through an incision under the arm will likely require your surgeon to use an endoscope, a tool with a camera and other surgical instruments inserted into the incision site to help the surgeon guide the implant into place. While there will likely be no visible scar around your breast, you may have a scar on the underside of your arm.

Cutting around the edge of the nipple (areola) may cause problems with loss or change of sensation in the nipple.

The surgeon will place the implant above (subglandular) or below (submuscular) the chest wall muscles. Be sure to discuss the pros and cons of the implant placement selected for you with your surgeon prior to surgery.

If you are getting silicone-gel filled implants they will already be filled with silicone gel when inserted. If you are getting saline-filled implants and the implant is not prefilled, the surgeon will insert the silicone shell and then fill the implant to the desired level with saline.

The incision is then closed with stitches. Your surgeon may place temporary drains in the incision prior to closing it to prevent fluid or blood accumulation. Catheters to deliver pain medicine at the site of the incision may also be placed prior to closing the incision. The drains or catheters would be removed during a follow-up visit after surgery.

After Surgery

After surgery, you will be taken to a recovery area to be monitored. Your breasts will be wrapped in gauze or a surgical bra.

Your surgeon should describe the usual after surgery (postoperative) recovery process, the possible complications that may occur, and the recovery period. Following the operation, as with any surgery, you can expect some pain, swelling, bruising, and tenderness. These effects may last for a month or longer but should disappear with time. Scarring is a natural result of surgery. Prior to surgery, ask your surgeon to describe the location, size, and appearance of any expected scars. For most women, scars will fade over time into thin lines. The darker your skin, the more prominent the scars are likely to be.

Your surgeon may prescribe medications for pain and/or nausea. If you experience bleeding, fever, warmth, redness of the breast, or other symptoms of infection, you should immediately report these symptoms to your surgeon. Your surgeon should tell you about wound healing and how to care for your wound.

You may need a postoperative bra, compression bandage or jogging bra for extra support as you heal. At your surgeon's recommendation, you will most likely be able to return to work within one to two weeks, but you should avoid any strenuous activities that could raise your pulse and blood pressure for at least two weeks.

Ask your surgeon about a schedule for follow-up visits, limits on your activities, precautions you should take, and when you can return to your normal activities, including exercising. If you received silicone gel-filled breast implants, the FDA recommends that you receive magnetic resonance imaging (MRI) screening for silent rupture three years after receiving your implant and every two years after that.

Continue to get mammograms to screen for breast cancer. Be sure to tell the person giving your mammogram that you have breast implants. Breast implants may make it difficult to see breast tissue on standard mammograms, so they may need to use different techniques.

If you are enrolled in a clinical study, be sure to ask your surgeon for a schedule of follow-up examinations set by the study plan.

Questions to Ask Your Doctor

When choosing a surgeon for a breast-implant procedure, you may want to consider their years of experience, their board certification, their patient follow-up, and your own comfort level with the surgeon. Most breast-implant procedures are performed by board-certified plastic and reconstructive surgeons. The following questions can help guide your discussion with your surgeon regarding breast-implant surgery.

Questions to Ask Your Surgeon

- How many breast implant procedures do you do each year?

- What percentage of your practice is dedicated to breast augmentation? To breast reconstruction?

- What type of implants do you use? Saline or silicone? What is your experience with each?

- What is the most common complication you encounter with breast implant surgery?

- What is your rate of complications in general (capsule contracture, infection, etc.)?

- What is your reoperation rate?

- What is the most common type of reoperation you perform?

Questions to Ask about Breast Implants and Expected Outcomes

- What shape, size, and surface texture are you recommending for my implants?

- Why are you recommending one type of breast implant over another? Why do you recommend this one for me?

- How long will my breast implants last?

299

- What incision site and placement are you recommending for me?

- Do you have before and after photos I can look at for each procedure?

- What results are reasonable for me to expect?

- How will breast implants feel? Will they alter my breast skin or nipple sensation?

- What are the risks and complications associated with having breast implants?

- Can I still get breast implants for augmentation if I have a strong family history of breast cancer?

- How many additional operations on my breast implants can I expect to have over my lifetime?

- How will I be able to tell if my breast implant has ruptured or if there is a problem with my breast implants?

- How will my breasts look if I decide to have the implants removed and not replaced?

- How easy or difficult is it to remove the implants?

- How easy or difficult is it to increase the size of the implants after the breast implants have been placed?

- What can I expect my breasts to look like over time? What do I need to do to maintain them?

- What kind of additional follow-up will I need?

- What are the long-term consequences of breast implants?

- What will my breasts look like after pregnancy? After breastfeeding?

- Will the breast implants affect my ability to breastfeed a baby?

- What are my options if I am dissatisfied with the outcome of my breast implants?

- Can I still get mammograms with breast implants in place?

- Will the mammogram rupture my breast implant?

- What alternate procedures or products are available besides breast implants?

Questions to Ask about the Breast-Implant Operation

- How long will I be in pain after the surgery?

- What is my expected recovery time?

- Will I need help at home for normal activities after the surgery and if so for about how long?

- How long do you expect my operation to take?

- What (if any) secondary procedures associated with my breast augmentation/breast reconstruction will be required?

- How likely is it that I will get an infection after the surgery?

- How much risk is there from the anesthesia?

- What can I do to minimize the risk of short-term and long-term complications?

- Where will my scar be?

Things to Consider before Getting Breast Implants

There are several important things to consider before deciding to undergo breast-implant surgery, including understanding your own expectations and reasons for having the surgery. Below are some things the FDA thinks you should consider before undergoing breast augmentation, reconstruction, or revision surgery.

- Breast implants are not lifetime devices; the longer you have your implants, the more likely it will be for you to have them removed.

- The longer you have breast implants, the more likely you are to experience local complications and adverse outcomes.

- The most common local complications and adverse outcomes are capsular contractures, reoperation and implant removal. Other complications include rupture or deflation, wrinkling, asymmetry, scarring, pain, and infection at the incision site.

- You should assume that you will need to have additional surgeries (reoperations).

- Many of the changes to your breast following implantation may be cosmetically undesirable and irreversible.

- If you have your implants removed but not replaced, you may experience changes to your natural breasts such as dimpling, puckering, wrinkling, breast tissue loss, or other undesirable cosmetic changes.

- If you have breast implants, you will need to monitor your breasts for the rest of your life. If you notice any abnormal changes in your breasts, you will need to see a doctor promptly.

- If you have silicone gel-filled breast implants, you will need to undergo periodic MRI examinations in order to detect ruptures that do not cause symptoms ("silent ruptures"). For early detection of silent rupture, the FDA recommends that women with silicone gel-filled breast implants receive MRI screenings 3 years after they receive a new implant and every two years after that. MRI screening for implant rupture is costly and may not be covered by your insurance.

- If you have breast implants, you have a risk of developing a type of cancer called breast implant-associated anaplastic large cell lymphoma (BIA-ALCL) in the breast tissue surrounding the implant. BIA-ALCL is not breast cancer. Women diagnosed with BIA-ALCL may need to be treated with surgery, chemotherapy and/or radiation therapy.

Section 44.4

Risks of Breast Implants

This section includes text excerpted from "Risks of Breast Implants,"
U.S. Food and Drug Administration (FDA), August 28, 2018.

Some of the complications and adverse outcomes of breast implants include:

- Additional surgeries, with or without removal of the device

- Capsular contracture, scar tissue that forms around the implant and squeezes the implant

- Breast pain

- Changes in nipple and breast sensation

- Rupture with deflation of saline-filled implants

- Rupture with or without symptoms (silent rupture) of silicone gel-filled implants

Implant Complications

The following is a list of local complications and adverse outcomes that occur in at least one percent of breast-implant patients at any time. You may need nonsurgical treatments or additional surgeries to treat any of these, and you should discuss any complication and necessary treatment with your doctor. These complications are listed alphabetically, not in order of how often they occur.

Table 44.1. List of Complications Associated with Breast Implant

Complication	Description
Asymmetry	The breasts are uneven in appearance in terms of size, shape or breast level
Breast Pain	Pain in the nipple or breast area
Breast Tissue Atrophy	Thinning and shrinking of the skin
Calcification/Calcium Deposits	Hard lumps under the skin around the implant. These can be mistaken for cancer during mammography, resulting in additional surgery.
Capsular Contracture	Tightening of the tissue capsule around an implant, resulting in firmness or hardening of the breast and squeezing of the implant if severe
Chest Wall Deformity	Chest wall or underlying rib cage appears deformed
Deflation	Leakage of the saltwater (saline) solution from a saline-filled breast implant, often due to a valve leak or a tear or cut in the implant shell (rupture), with a partial or complete collapse of the implant
Delayed Wound Healing	Incision site fails to heal normally or takes longer to heal
Extrusion	The skin breaks down and the implant appears through the skin
Hematoma	Collection of blood near the surgical site. May cause swelling, bruising and pain. Hematomas usually occur soon after surgery but can occur any time there is an injury to the breast. The body may absorb small hematomas, but large ones may require medical intervention, such as surgical draining.

Table 44.1. Continued

Complication	Description
Iatrogenic Injury/ Damage	Injury or damage to tissue or implant as a result of implant surgery
Infection, including Toxic Shock Syndrome	Occurs when wounds are contaminated with microorganisms, such as bacteria or fungi. Most infections resulting from surgery appear within a few days to a week, but infection is possible any time after surgery. If an infection does not respond to antibiotics, the implant may need to be removed.
Inflammation/ Irritation	Response by the body to an infection or injury. Demonstrated by redness, swelling, warmth, pain and or/ loss of function.
Lymphedema or Lymphadenopathy	Swollen or enlarged lymph nodes
Malposition/ Displacement	The implant is not in the correct position in the breast. This can happen during surgery or afterward if the implant moves or shifts from its original location. Shifting can be caused by factors such as gravity, trauma or capsular contracture.
Necrosis	Dead skin or tissue around the breast. Necrosis can be caused by infection, use of steroids in the surgical breast pocket, smoking, chemotherapy/radiation, and excessive heat or cold therapy.
Nipple/Breast Sensation Changes	An increase or decrease in the feeling in the nipple and/ or breast. Can vary in degree and may be temporary or permanent. May affect sexual response or breastfeeding.
Palpability	The implant can be felt through the skin.
Ptosis	Breast sagging that is usually the result of normal aging, pregnancy or weight loss.
Redness/Bruising	Bleeding at the time of surgery can cause the skin to change color. This is an expected symptom due to surgery and is likely temporary.
Rupture	A tear or hole in the implant's outer shell.
Seroma	Collection of fluid around the implant. May cause swelling, pain, and bruising. The body may absorb small seromas. Large ones will require a surgical drain.
Skin Rash	A rash on or around the breast
Unsatisfactory Style/ Size	Patient or doctor is not satisfied with the overall look based on the style or size of the implant used
Visibility	The implant can be seen through the skin
Wrinkling/Rippling	Wrinkling of the implant that can be felt or seen through the skin

Additional Surgeries

Breast implants are not lifetime devices. The longer you have breast implants, the more likely it is that complications will occur and you will need to have them removed. There is no guarantee that you will have a satisfactory cosmetic outcome from any reoperation.

The type of surgical procedure performed during a reoperation depends on the complication involved. You may need to have one or more reoperations over the course of your life due to one complication or a combination of local complications. More than one procedure may be performed in a single reoperation. Types of surgical procedures that may be performed in a reoperation include:

- Implant removal, with or without replacement

- Capsule removal or surgical release of the scar tissue around the breast implant

- Scar or wound revision, such as surgical removal of excess scar tissue

- Drainage of a hematoma by inserting a needle or tube through the skin to drain the collection of blood

- Repositioning of the implant by surgically opening the incision and moving the implant

- Biopsy/cyst removal by inserting a needle through the skin or cutting through the skin to remove a lump

Removal of Implants

Removal of the implant(s), with or without replacement, is one type of reoperation. As many as 20 percent of women who receive breast implants for augmentation have to have their implants removed within 8 to 10 years. You may need to have your implant removed at some time over the course of your life because of one or more local complications.

After removal, some women do not choose to replace their implants. These women may have cosmetically undesirable dimpling, puckering, or sagging of their natural breasts.

The photograph below shows a 29-year-old woman one year after having her silicone gel-filled breast implants removed, but not replaced. Women with large breast implants, especially those inserted on top of the chest muscles (subglandularly), may have major cosmetic deformity if they choose not to replace them or to undergo additional reconstructive surgery.

Some insurance companies do not cover implant removal or implant replacement, even if the first implant surgery was covered.

Capsular Contracture

Capsular contracture is the hardening of the breast around the implant. It can occur in the tissue surrounding one or both implants. This hardening causes the tissue to tighten, which can be painful.

Capsular contracture may be a more common following infection, hematoma, and seroma. However, the cause of capsular contracture is not known.

There are four grades of capsular contracture, known as "Baker grades."

Baker Grading Scale

- Grade I: Breast is normally soft and looks natural

- Grade II: Breast is a little firm but looks normal

- Grade III: Breast is firm and looks abnormal

- Grade IV: Breast is hard, painful, and looks abnormal

Grades III and IV capsular contracture are considered severe and may require reoperation. The surgical procedure usually involves removal of the implant with or without replacement of the implant. There is a possibility that capsular contracture could occur again after surgery to correct it.

The FDA has not cleared or approved any devices to treat or reduce the incidence of capsular contracture.

The picture below shows a Grade IV capsular contracture in the right breast of a 29-year- old woman 7 years after placement of silicone gel-filled breast implants.

Rupture

Rupture is a tear or hole in the outer shell of the breast implant. When this occurs in a saline breast implant, it deflates, meaning the saltwater (saline) solution leaks from the shell. Silicone gel is thicker than saline, so when a silicone gel-filled implant ruptures, the gel may remain in the shell or in the scar tissue that forms around the implant (intracapsular rupture). The longer you have a breast implant, the greater the chance of implant rupture.

The FDA recommends removing both saline-filled and silicone gel-filled breast implants if they have ruptured. You and your doctor will need to decide whether or not your implant has ruptured and if you should have it replaced or removed without replacement.

Some possible causes of rupture of breast implants include:

- Capsular contracture

- Compression during a mammogram

- Damage by surgical instruments

- Damage during procedures to the breast, such as biopsies and fluid drainage

- Normal aging of the implant

- Overfilling or underfilling of saline-filled breast implants

- Physical stresses such as trauma or intense physical pressure

- Placement through a non-FDA-approved incision site, for example, the belly button

- Too much handling during surgery

Rupture and Deflation in Saline-Filled Breast Implants

The term rupture is used for all types of breast implants, but the term deflation is only used for saline-filled implants. You and/or your doctor will be able to tell if your saline-filled implant ruptures because the saline solution leaks into your body immediately or over several days. You will notice that your implant loses its original size or shape.

The following surgical procedures are not recommended for FDA-approved saline-filled breast implants because they are known to cause rupture and deflation:

- Closed capsulotomy—a technique used to relieve capsular contracture involving manually squeezing the breast to break the hard capsule

- Placement of drugs or other substances inside the implant other than sterile saline

- Any contact of the implant with Betadine, a povidone-iodine topical antiseptic made by Purdue Frederick Company

- Injection through the implant shell

- Alteration of the implant

- Stacking of the implants (more than one implant per breast pocket)

Rupture in Silicone Gel-Filled Implants

If your silicone gel-filled breast implant ruptures, it is not likely that you or your doctor will immediately notice. Silicone gel is thicker than saline, so when a silicone gel-filled implant ruptures, the gel may remain in the shell or in the scar tissue that forms around the implant (intracapsular rupture).

When a silicone gel-filled implant ruptures, a woman may notice a decrease in breast size, change in breast implant shape, hard lumps over the implant or chest area, an uneven appearance of the breasts, pain or tenderness, tingling, swelling, numbness, burning, or changes in sensation. Ruptures that show symptoms usually happen outside of the capsule. However, some ruptures are called "silent ruptures."

A "silent rupture" doesn't change the way an implant looks or feels to a woman because the rupture occurs within the capsule. Silent ruptures are not usually evident by a physical examination by a doctor. Magnetic resonance imaging (MRI) is the most effective method for detecting silent rupture of silicone gel-filled breast implants. The FDA recommends MRI at three years after implantation and every two years after that to screen for rupture.

Silicone gel that leaks outside the capsule surrounding the implant may travel (migrate) away from the breast. The leaked silicone gel may cause lumps to form in the breast or in other tissue, most often the chest wall, armpit or arm. It may be difficult or impossible to remove the silicone gel that has traveled to other parts of the body.

Breastfeeding

Some women who undergo breast augmentation can successfully breastfeed and some cannot. Women who undergo mastectomies and then have breast implant reconstruction surgeries may not be able to breastfeed on the affected side due to loss of breast tissue and the glands that produce milk.

Effects on Children

At this time, it is not known if a small amount of silicone may pass through from the breast implant silicone shell into breast milk during breastfeeding. Although there are currently no established methods for accurately detecting silicone levels in breast milk, a study measuring silicon (one component in silicone) levels did not indicate higher levels in breast milk from women with silicone gel-filled implants when compared to women without implants.

In addition, concerns have been raised regarding potential damaging effects on children born to mothers with implants. Two studies in humans have found no increased risk of birth defects in children born to mothers who have had breast implant surgery. Although low birth weight, was reported in a third study, other factors (for example, lower prepregnancy weight) may explain this finding.

Chapter 45

Chemotherapy for Breast Cancer

Normally, your cells grow and die in a controlled way. Cancer cells keep growing without control. Chemotherapy is drug therapy for cancer. It works by killing the cancer cells, stopping them from spreading, or slowing their growth. However, it can also harm healthy cells, which causes side effects.

How Chemotherapy Is Administered

Your treatment plan will depend on the cancer type, the chemotherapy drugs used, the treatment goal, and how your body responds. Chemotherapy may be given alone or with other treatments. You may get treatment every day, every week, or every month. You may have breaks between treatments so that your body has a chance to build new healthy cells. You might take the drugs by mouth, in a shot, as a cream, or intravenously (IV).

This chapter contains text excerpted from the following sources: Text in this chapter begins with excerpts from "Cancer Chemotherapy," MedlinePlus, National Institutes of Health (NIH), May 1, 2017; Text under the heading "Long-Term Nerve Damage Possible after Chemotherapy for Breast Cancer" is excerpted from "Long-Term Nerve Damage Possible after Chemotherapy for Breast Cancer," National Cancer Institute (NCI), September 19, 2017.

Side Effects of Chemotherapy

You may have a lot of side effects, some, or none at all. It depends on the type and amount of chemotherapy you get and how your body reacts. Some common side effects are fatigue, nausea, vomiting, pain, and hair loss. There are ways to prevent or control some side effects. Talk with your healthcare provider about how to manage them. Healthy cells usually recover after chemotherapy is over, so most side effects gradually go away.

Long-Term Nerve Damage Possible after Chemotherapy for Breast Cancer

Many women who receive taxane-based chemotherapy to treat breast cancer experience long-term peripheral neuropathy, according to follow-up data from a large clinical trial.

Two years after the start of treatment, more than 40 percent of participants in the trial said they still experienced numbness and tingling in their hands or feet, and 10 percent rated their symptoms as severe. Patients with severe neuropathy reported lower quality of life (QOL) than patients without severe symptoms.

"We want to ensure that patients understand both the benefits and harms of treatment, but typically they're only told about the acute side effects," said the study's senior author, Patricia Ganz, M.D., of the Jonsson Comprehensive Cancer Center (JCCC) at the University of California, Los Angeles. "Patients can be really surprised when they're left with lingering neuropathy, or pain, fatigue, cognitive difficulties (potentially) a whole bunch of stuff that no one's really prepared them for."

"It's now expected that with early-stage breast cancer—or even stage II or III—you're going to live a long time," added Ann O'Mara, Ph.D., Head of Palliative Research in National Cancer Institute (NCI), Division of Cancer Prevention (DCP). "So it's now rising to our attention that we need to be more aware of these chronic toxicities," she said.

The study was published in the *Journal of the National Cancer Institute*.

Chapter 46

Hormone Therapy for Breast Cancer

What Are Hormones?

Hormones are substances that function as chemical messengers in the body. They affect the actions of cells and tissues at various locations in the body, often reaching their targets through the bloodstream.

The hormones estrogen (ER) and progesterone (PR) are produced by the ovaries in premenopausal women and by some other tissues, including fat and skin, in both premenopausal and postmenopausal women (PMW) and men. Estrogen promotes the development and maintenance of female sex characteristics and the growth of long bones. Progesterone plays a role in the menstrual cycle and pregnancy.

Estrogen and progesterone also promote the growth of some breast cancers, which are called "hormone-sensitive (or hormone-dependent)" breast cancers. Hormone-sensitive breast cancer cells contain proteins called "hormone receptors" that become activated when hormones bind to them. The activated receptors cause changes in the expression of specific genes, which can stimulate cell growth.

This chapter includes text excerpted from "Hormone Therapy for Breast Cancer," National Cancer Institute (NCI), February 14, 2017.

What Is Hormone Therapy?

Hormone therapy (HT) (also called "hormonal therapy," "hormone treatment," or "endocrine therapy") slows or stops the growth of hormone-sensitive tumors by blocking the body's ability to produce hormones or by interfering with effects of hormones on breast-cancer cells. Tumors that are hormone insensitive do not have hormone receptors and do not respond to hormone therapy.

To determine whether breast-cancer cells contain hormone receptors, doctors test samples of tumor tissue that have been removed by surgery. If the tumor cells contain estrogen receptors, the cancer is called "estrogen receptor-positive (ER-positive)," "estrogen sensitive," or "estrogen responsive." Similarly, if the tumor cells contain progesterone receptors, the cancer is called "progesterone receptor positive (PR or PgR positive)." Approximately 80 percent of breast cancers are ER-positive. Most ER-positive breast cancers are also PR positive. Breast tumors that contain estrogen and/or progesterone receptors are sometimes called "hormone receptor positive (HR-positive)."

Breast cancers that lack estrogen receptors are called "estrogen receptor-negative (ER-negative)." These tumors are estrogen insensitive, meaning that they do not use estrogen to grow. Breast tumors that lack progesterone receptors are called "progesterone receptor negative (PR or PgR negative)." Breast tumors that lack both estrogen and progesterone receptors are sometimes called "hormone receptor negative (HR-negative)."

Hormone therapy for breast cancer should not be confused with menopausal hormone therapy (MHT)—treatment with estrogen alone or in combination with progesterone to help relieve symptoms of menopause. These two types of therapy produce opposite effects: hormone therapy for breast-cancer blocks the growth of HR-positive breast cancer, whereas MHT can stimulate the growth of HR-positive breast cancer. For this reason, when a woman taking MHT is diagnosed with HR-positive breast cancer she is usually asked to stop that therapy.

What Types of Hormone Therapy Are Used for Breast Cancer?

Several strategies are used to treat hormone-sensitive breast cancer:

Blocking Ovarian Function

Because the ovaries are the main source of estrogen in premenopausal women, estrogen levels in these women can be reduced by eliminating or suppressing ovarian function. Blocking ovarian function is called "ovarian ablation (OA)."

Ovarian ablation can be done surgically in an operation to remove the ovaries (called oophorectomy) or by treatment with radiation. This type of ovarian ablation is usually permanent.

Alternatively, the ovarian function can be suppressed temporarily by treatment with drugs called "gonadotropin-releasing hormone (GnRH) agonists," which are also known as "luteinizing hormone-releasing hormone (LH-RH) agonists." These medicines interfere with signals from the pituitary gland that stimulate the ovaries to produce estrogen.

Examples of ovarian suppression drugs that have been approved by the U.S. Food and Drug Administration (FDA) are goserelin (Zoladex®) and leuprolide (Lupron®).

Blocking Estrogen Production

Drugs called "aromatase inhibitors (AIs)" are used to block the activity of an enzyme called "aromatase," which the body uses to make estrogen in the ovaries and in other tissues. Aromatase inhibitors are used primarily in postmenopausal women because the ovaries in premenopausal women produce too much aromatase for the inhibitors to block effectively. However, these drugs can be used in premenopausal women if they are given together with a drug that suppresses ovarian function.

Examples of aromatase inhibitors approved by the FDA are anastrozole (Arimidex®) and letrozole (Femara®), both of which temporarily inactivate aromatase, and exemestane (Aromasin®), which permanently inactivates aromatase.

Blocking Estrogen's Effects

Several types of drugs interfere with estrogen's ability to stimulate the growth of breast-cancer cells:

- **Selective estrogen receptor modulators (SERMs)** bind to estrogen receptors, preventing estrogen from binding. Examples of SERMs approved by the FDA for treatment of breast cancer are tamoxifen (Nolvadex®) and toremifene (Fareston®). Tamoxifen has been used for more than 30 years to treat HR+ hormone receptor-positive breast cancer.

  Because SERMs bind to estrogen receptors, they can potentially not only block estrogen activity (i.e., serve as estrogen antagonists) but also mimic estrogen effects (i.e., serve as estrogen agonists). SERMs can behave as estrogen antagonists in some tissues and as estrogen agonists in other tissues. For example, tamoxifen blocks the effects of estrogen in breast tissue but acts like estrogen in the uterus and bone.

- **Other antiestrogen drugs**, such as fulvestrant (Faslodex®), work in a somewhat different way to block estrogen's effects. Like SERMs, fulvestrant binds to the estrogen receptor and functions as an estrogen antagonist. However, unlike SERMs, fulvestrant has no estrogen agonist effects. It is a pure antiestrogen. In addition, when fulvestrant binds to the estrogen receptor, the receptor is targeted for destruction.

How Is Hormone Therapy Used to Treat Breast Cancer?

There are three main ways that hormone therapy is used to treat hormone-sensitive breast cancer:

Adjuvant Therapy for Early-Stage Breast Cancer

Research has shown that women who receive at least 5 years of adjuvant therapy with tamoxifen after having surgery for early-stage ER-positive breast cancer have reduced risks of breast-cancer recurrence, including new breast cancer in the other breast, and death at 15 years.

Tamoxifen is approved by the FDA for adjuvant hormone treatment of premenopausal and postmenopausal women (and men) with ER-positive early-stage breast cancer, and the aromatase inhibitors anastrozole and letrozole are approved for this use in postmenopausal women.

A third aromatase inhibitor, exemestane, is approved for adjuvant treatment of early-stage breast cancer in postmenopausal women who have received tamoxifen previously.

Until most women who received adjuvant hormone therapy to reduce the chance of a breast-cancer recurrence took tamoxifen every day for five years. However, with the introduction of newer hormone therapies, some of which have been compared with tamoxifen in clinical trials, additional approaches to hormone therapy have become common. For example, some women may take an aromatase inhibitor every day for five years, instead of tamoxifen. Other women may receive additional treatment with an aromatase inhibitor after five years of tamoxifen. Finally, some women may switch to an aromatase inhibitor after one or three years of tamoxifen, for a total of five or more years of hormone therapy. Research has shown that for post-menopausal women who have been treated for early-stage breast cancer, adjuvant therapy with an aromatase inhibitor reduces the risk of recurrence and improves overall survival, compared with adjuvant tamoxifen.

Decisions about the type and duration of adjuvant hormone therapy must be made on an individual basis. This complicated decision-making process is best carried out by talking with an oncologist, a doctor who specializes in cancer treatment.

Treatment of Advanced or Metastatic Breast Cancer

Several types of hormone therapy are approved to treat metastatic or recurrent hormone-sensitive breast cancer. Hormone therapy is also a treatment option for ER-positive breast cancer that has come back in the breast, chest wall, or nearby lymph nodes after treatment (also called a "locoregional recurrence (LRR)").

Two selective estrogen receptor modulators (SERM) are approved to treat metastatic breast cancer, tamoxifen, and toremifene. The anti-estrogen fulvestrant is approved for postmenopausal women with metastatic ER-positive breast cancer that has spread after treatment with other antiestrogens. It may also be used in premenopausal women who have had ovarian ablation.

The aromatase inhibitors anastrozole and letrozole are approved to be given to postmenopausal women as initial therapy for metastatic or locally advanced hormone-sensitive breast cancer. These two drugs, as well as the aromatase inhibitor exemestane, are used to treat post-menopausal women with advanced breast cancer whose disease has worsened after treatment with tamoxifen.

Some women with advanced breast cancer are treated with a combination of hormone therapy and targeted therapy. For example, the targeted therapy drug lapatinib (Tykerb®) is approved to be used in combination with letrozole to treat hormone receptor-positive, (human epidermal growth factor receptor 2(HER2))-positive metastatic breast cancer in postmenopausal women for whom hormone therapy is indicated.

Another targeted therapy, palbociclib (Ibrance®), has been granted accelerated approval for use in combination with letrozole as initial therapy for the treatment of hormone receptor-positive, HER2-negative advanced breast cancer in postmenopausal women. Palbociclib inhibits two cyclin-dependent kinases (CDK4) and cyclin-Dependent Kinase 6 (CDK6) that appear to promote the growth of hormone receptor-positive breast cancer cells.

Palbociclib is also approved to be used in combination with fulvestrant for the treatment of women with hormone receptor-positive, HER2-negative advanced or metastatic breast cancer whose cancer has gotten worse after treatment with another hormone therapy.

Neoadjuvant Treatment of Breast Cancer

The use of hormone therapy to treat breast cancer before surgery (neoadjuvant therapy) has been studied in clinical trials. The goal of neoadjuvant therapy is to reduce the size of a breast tumor to allow breast-conserving surgery (BCS). Data from randomized controlled trials have shown that neoadjuvant hormone therapy (NET)—in particular, with aromatase inhibitors—can be effective in reducing the size of breast tumors in postmenopausal women. The results in premenopausal women are less clear because only a few small trials involving relatively few premenopausal women have been conducted thus far.

No hormone therapy has yet been approved by the FDA for the neoadjuvant treatment of breast cancer.

Can Hormone Therapy Be Used to Prevent Breast Cancer?

Yes. Most breast cancers are ER-positive, and clinical trials have tested whether hormone therapy can be used to prevent breast cancer in women who are at increased risk of developing the disease.

A large National Cancer Institute (NCI)-sponsored randomized clinical trial called the Breast Cancer Prevention Trial (BCPT) found that tamoxifen, taken for 5 years, reduced the risk of developing invasive-breast cancer by about 50 percent in postmenopausal women who were at increased risk. Long-term follow-up of another randomized trial, the International Breast Cancer Intervention Study I (IBIS-I), found that 5 years of tamoxifen treatment reduces the incidence of breast cancer for at least 20 years. A subsequent large randomized trial, the Study of Tamoxifen and Raloxifene (STAR), which was also sponsored by NCI, found that 5 years of raloxifene (a SERM) reduces breast-cancer risk in such women by about 38 percent.

As a result of these trials, both tamoxifen and raloxifene have been approved by the FDA to reduce the risk of developing breast cancer in women at high risk of the disease. Tamoxifen is approved for this use regardless of menopausal status. Raloxifene is approved for use only in postmenopausal women.

Two aromatase inhibitors—exemestane and anastrozole—have also been found to reduce the risk of breast cancer in postmenopausal women at increased risk of the disease. After 3 years of follow up in a randomized trial, women who took exemestane were 65 percent less likely than those who took a placebo to develop breast cancer. After 7 years of follow up in another randomized trial, women who took anastrozole were 50 percent less likely than those who took placebo to develop breast cancer. Both exemestane and anastrozole are approved by the FDA for treatment of women with ER-positive breast cancer. Although both are also used for breast-cancer prevention, neither is approved for that indication specifically.

What Are the Side Effects of Hormone Therapy?

The side effects of hormone therapy depend largely on the specific drug or the type of treatment. The benefits and harms of taking hormone therapy should be carefully weighed for each woman. A common switching strategy used for adjuvant therapy, in which patients take tamoxifen for two or three years, followed by an aromatase inhibitor for two or three years, may yield the best balance of benefits and harms of these two types of hormone therapy.

Hot flashes, night sweats, and vaginal dryness are common side effects of hormone therapy. Hormone therapy also disrupts the menstrual cycle in premenopausal women.

Less common but serious side effects of hormone therapy drugs are listed below.

Tamoxifen

- Risk of blood clots, especially in the lungs and legs

- Stroke

- Cataracts

- Endometrial and uterine cancers

- Bone loss in premenopausal women

- Mood swings, depression, and loss of libido

- In men: headaches, nausea, vomiting, skin rash, impotence, and decreased-sexual interest

Raloxifene

- Risk of blood clots, especially in the lungs and legs

- Stroke in certain subgroups

Ovarian Suppression

- Bone loss

- Mood swings, depression, and loss of libido

Aromatase Inhibitors

- Risk of heart attack, angina, heart failure, and hypercholesterolemia

- Bone loss

- Joint pain

- Mood swings and depression

Fulvestrant

- Gastrointestinal (GI) symptoms

- Loss of strength

- Pain

Can Other Drugs Interfere with Hormone Therapy?

Certain drugs, including several commonly prescribed antidepressants (those in the category called selective serotonin reuptake inhibitors or SSRIs), inhibit an enzyme called "cytochrome P450 2D6 (CYP2D6)." This enzyme plays a critical role in the use of tamoxifen by the body because it metabolizes, or breaks down, tamoxifen into molecules, or metabolites, that are much more active than tamoxifen itself.

The possibility that SSRIs might, by inhibiting CYP2D6, slow the metabolism of tamoxifen and reduce its effectiveness is a concern given that as many as one-fourth of breast-cancer patients experience clinical depression and may be treated with SSRIs. In addition, SSRIs are sometimes used to treat hot flashes caused by hormone therapy.

Many experts suggest that patients who are taking antidepressants along with tamoxifen should discuss treatment options with their doctors. For example, doctors may recommend switching from an SSRI that is a potent inhibitor of CYP2D6, such as paroxetine hydrochloride (Paxil®), to one that is a weaker inhibitor, such as sertraline (Zoloft®), or that has no inhibitory activity, such as venlafaxine (Effexor®) or citalopram (Celexa®). Or they may suggest that their postmenopausal patients take an aromatase inhibitor instead of tamoxifen.

Other medications that inhibit CYP2D6 include the following:

- Quinidine, which is used to treat abnormal heart rhythms

- Diphenhydramine, which is an antihistamine

- Cimetidine, which is used to reduce stomach acid

People who are prescribed tamoxifen should discuss the use of all other medications with their doctors.

Chapter 47

Targeted (Biologic) Therapies for Breast Cancer

What Are Targeted Cancer Therapies?

Targeted cancer therapies are drugs or other substances that block the growth and spread of cancer by interfering with specific molecules ("molecular targets") that are involved in the growth, progression, and spread of cancer. Targeted cancer therapies are sometimes called "molecularly targeted drugs," "molecularly targeted therapies," "precision medicines," or similar names.

Targeted therapies differ from standard chemotherapy in several ways:

- Targeted therapies act on specific molecular targets that are associated with cancer, whereas most standard chemotherapies act on all rapidly dividing normal and cancerous cells.

- Targeted therapies are deliberately chosen or designed to interact with their target, whereas many standard chemotherapies were identified because they kill cells.

- Targeted therapies are often cytostatic (that is, they block tumor cell proliferation), whereas standard chemotherapy agents are cytotoxic (that is, they kill tumor cells).

This chapter includes text excerpted from "Targeted Cancer Therapies," National Cancer Institute (NCI), December 18, 2018.

Targeted therapies are currently the focus of much anticancer drug development. They are a cornerstone of precision medicine, a form of medicine that uses information about a person's genes and proteins to prevent, diagnose, and treat disease.

Many targeted-cancer therapies have been approved by the U.S. Food and Drug Administration (FDA) to treat specific types of cancer. Others are being studied in clinical trials (research studies with people), and many more are in preclinical testing (research studies with animals).

How Are Targets for Targeted-Cancer Therapies Identified?

The development of targeted therapies requires the identification of good targets—that is, targets that play a key role in cancer-cell growth and survival. (It is for this reason that targeted therapies are sometimes referred to as the product of "rational" drug design.)

One approach to identify potential targets is to compare the amounts of individual proteins in cancer cells with those in normal cells. Proteins that are present in cancer cells but not normal cells or that are more abundant in cancer cells would be potential targets, especially if they are known to be involved in cell growth or survival. An example of such a differentially expressed target is the human epidermal growth factor receptor 2 protein (HER-2). HER-2 is expressed at high levels on the surface of some cancer cells. Several targeted therapies are directed against HER-2, including trastuzumab (Herceptin®), which is approved to treat certain breast and stomach cancers that overexpress HER-2.

Another approach to identify potential targets is to determine whether cancer cells produce mutant (altered) proteins that drive cancer progression. For example, the cell growth signaling protein BRAF is present in an altered form (known as BRAF V600E) in many melanomas. Vemurafenib (Zelboraf®) targets this mutant form of the BRAF protein and is approved to treat patients with inoperable or metastatic melanoma that contains this altered BRAF protein.

Researchers also look for abnormalities in chromosomes that are present in cancer cells but not in normal cells. Sometimes these chromosome abnormalities result in the creation of a fusion gene (a gene that incorporates parts of two different genes) whose product, called a "fusion protein," may drive cancer development. Such fusion proteins are potential targets for targeted-cancer therapies. For example, imatinib mesylate (Gleevec®) targets the *BCR-ABL* fusion protein, which is made from pieces of two genes that get joined together in some leukemia cells and promotes the growth of leukemic cells.

How Are Targeted Therapies Developed?

Once a candidate target has been identified, the next step is to develop a therapy that affects the target in a way that interferes with its ability to promote cancer-cell growth or survival. For example, a targeted therapy could reduce the activity of the target or prevent it from binding to a receptor that it normally activates, among other possible mechanisms.

Most targeted therapies are either small molecules or monoclonal antibodies. Small-molecule compounds are typically developed for targets that are located inside the cell because such agents are able to enter cells relatively easily. Monoclonal antibodies are relatively large and generally cannot enter cells, so they are used only for targets that are outside cells or on the cell surface.

Candidate small molecules are usually identified in what is known as "high-throughput screens (HTS)," in which the effects of thousands of test compounds on a specific target protein are examined. Compounds that affect the target (sometimes called "lead compounds") are then chemically modified to produce numerous closely related versions of the lead compound. These related compounds are then tested to determine which are most effective and have the fewest effects on nontarget molecules.

Monoclonal antibodies are developed by injecting animals (usual mice) with purified target proteins, causing the animals to make many different types of antibodies against the target. These antibodies are then tested to find the ones that bind best to the target without binding to nontarget proteins.

Before monoclonal antibodies are used in humans, they are "humanized" by replacing as much of the mouse antibody molecule as possible with corresponding portions of human antibodies. Humanizing is necessary to prevent the human immune system from recognizing the monoclonal antibody as "foreign" and destroying it before it has a chance to bind to its target protein. Humanization is not an issue for small-molecule compounds because they are not typically recognized by the body as foreign.

What Types of Targeted Therapies Are Available?

Many different targeted therapies have been approved for use in cancer treatment. These therapies include hormone therapies, signal transduction inhibitors (STIs), gene expression modulators, apoptosis inducers, angiogenesis inhibitors, immunotherapies, and toxin delivery molecules.

- **Hormone therapies (HTs)** slow or stop the growth of hormone-sensitive tumors, which require certain hormones to grow. HTs act by preventing the body from producing the hormones or by interfering with the action of the hormones. HTs have been approved for both breast cancer and prostate cancer (PC).

- **Signal transduction inhibitors** block the activities of molecules that participate in signal transduction, the process by which a cell responds to signals from its environment. During this process, once a cell has received a specific signal, the signal is relayed within the cell through a series of biochemical reactions that ultimately produce the appropriate response(s). In some cancers, the malignant cells are stimulated to divide continuously without being prompted to do so by external growth factors. Signal transduction inhibitors interfere with this inappropriate signaling.

- **Gene expression modulators** modify the function of proteins that play a role in controlling gene expression.

- **Apoptosis inducers** cause cancer cells to undergo a process of controlled cell death called "apoptosis." Apoptosis is one method the body uses to get rid of unneeded or abnormal cells, but cancer cells have strategies to avoid apoptosis. Apoptosis inducers can get around these strategies to cause the death of cancer cells.

- **Angiogenesis inhibitors** block the growth of new blood vessels to tumors (a process called tumor angiogenesis). A blood supply is necessary for tumors to grow beyond a certain size because blood provides the oxygen and nutrients that tumors need for continued growth. Treatments that interfere with angiogenesis may block tumor growth. Some targeted therapies that inhibit angiogenesis interfere with the action of vascular endothelial growth factor (VEGF), a substance that stimulates new blood vessel formation. Other angiogenesis inhibitors target other molecules that stimulate new blood vessel growth.

- **Immunotherapies** trigger the immune system to destroy cancer cells. Some immunotherapies are monoclonal antibodies that recognize specific molecules on the surface of cancer cells.

Binding of the monoclonal antibody to the target molecule results in the immune destruction of cells that express that target molecule. Other monoclonal antibodies bind to certain immune cells to help these cells better kill cancer cells.

- **Monoclonal antibodies** that deliver toxic molecules can cause the death of cancer cells specifically. Once the antibody has bound to its target cell, the toxic molecule that is linked to the antibody—such as a radioactive substance or a poisonous chemical—is taken up by the cell, ultimately killing that cell. The toxin will not affect cells that lack the target for the antibody—i.e., the vast majority of cells in the body.

Cancer vaccines and **gene therapy** are sometimes considered targeted therapies because they interfere with the growth of specific cancer cells.

How Is It Determined Whether a Patient Is a Candidate for Targeted Therapy?

For some types of cancer, most patients with that cancer will have an appropriate target for a particular targeted therapy and, thus, will be candidates to be treated with that therapy. Chronic myelogenous leukemia (CML) is an example; most patients have the *BCR-ABL* fusion gene. For other cancer types, however, a patient's tumor tissue must be tested to determine whether or not an appropriate target is present. The use of targeted therapy may be restricted to patients whose tumor has a specific gene mutation that codes for the target; patients who do not have the mutation would not be candidates because the therapy would have nothing to target.

Sometimes, a patient is a candidate for a targeted therapy only if she or he meets specific criteria (for example, their cancer did not respond to other therapies, has spread, or is inoperable). These criteria are set by the FDA when it approves a specific targeted therapy.

What Are the Limitations of Targeted-Cancer Therapies?

Targeted therapies do have some limitations. One is that cancer cells can become resistant to them. Resistance can occur in two ways: the target itself changes through mutation so that the targeted therapy no longer interacts well with it, and/or the tumor finds a new pathway to achieve tumor growth that does not depend on the target.

For this reason, targeted therapies may work best in combination. For example, a study found that using two therapies that target different parts of the cell signaling pathway that is altered in melanoma by the BRAF V600E mutation slowed the development of resistance and disease progression to a greater extent than using just one targeted therapy.

Another approach is to use a targeted therapy in combination with one or more traditional chemotherapy drugs. For example, the targeted therapy trastuzumab (Herceptin®) has been used in combination with docetaxel, a traditional chemotherapy drug, to treat women with metastatic breast cancer that overexpresses the protein HER2/neu.

Another limitation of targeted therapy at present is that drugs for some identified targets are difficult to develop because of the target's structure and/or the way its function is regulated in the cell. One example is RAS, a signaling protein that is mutated in as many as one-quarter of all cancers (and in the majority of certain cancer types, such as pancreatic cancer). To date, it has not been possible to develop inhibitors of RAS signaling with existing drug development technologies. However, promising new approaches are offering hope that this limitation can soon be overcome.

What Are the Side Effects of Targeted-Cancer Therapies?

Scientists had expected that targeted-cancer therapies would be less toxic than traditional chemotherapy drugs because cancer cells are more dependent on the targets that are normal cells. However, targeted-cancer therapies can have substantial side effects.

The most common side effects seen with targeted therapies are diarrhea and liver problems, such as hepatitis and elevated liver enzymes. Other side effects seen with targeted therapies include:

- Skin problems (acneiform rash, dry skin, nail changes, hair depigmentation)
- Problems with blood clotting and wound healing
- High blood pressure
- Gastrointestinal (GI) perforation (a rare side effect of some targeted therapies)

Certain side effects of some targeted therapies have been linked to better patient outcomes. For example, patients who develop acneiform rash (skin eruptions that resemble acne) while being treated with the signal transduction inhibitors erlotinib (Tarceva®) or gefitinib (Iressa®), both of which target the epidermal growth factor receptor (EGFR), have tended to respond better to these drugs than patients who do not develop the rash. Similarly, patients who develop high blood pressure (HBP) while being treated with the angiogenesis inhibitor bevacizumab generally have had better outcomes.

The few targeted therapies that are approved for use in children can have different side effects in children than in adults, including immunosuppression and impaired sperm production.

What Targeted Therapies Have Been Approved for Breast Cancer?

The FDA has approved the following targeted therapies for the treatment of breast-cancer patients:

- Everolimus (Afinitor®)

- Tamoxifen (Nolvadex)

- Toremifene (Fareston®)

- Trastuzumab (Herceptin®)

- Fulvestrant (Faslodex®)

- Anastrozole (Arimidex®)

- Exemestane (Aromasin®)

- Lapatinib (Tykerb®)

- Letrozole (Femara®)

- Pertuzumab (Perjeta®)

- Ado-trastuzumab emtansine (Kadcyla®)

- Palbociclib (Ibrance®)

- Ribociclib (Kisqali®)

- Neratinib maleate (Nerlynx™)

- Abemaciclib (Verzenio™)

- Olaparib (Lynparza™)

Chapter 48

CAM Therapies Used in the Treatment of Breast Cancer

Chapter Contents

Section 48.1

CAM and Cancer Treatment

This section includes text excerpted from
"Complementary and Alternative Medicine," National Cancer
Institute (NCI), April 10, 2015. Reviewed February 2019.

Complementary and alternative medicine (CAM) is the term for medical products and practices that are not part of standard medical care.

Standard medical care is a medicine that is practiced by health professionals who hold a medical doctor (M.D.) or doctor of osteopathy (D.O.) degree. It is also practiced by other health professionals, such as physical therapists, physician assistants, psychologists, and registered nurses. Standard medicine may also be called biomedicine or allopathic, Western, mainstream, orthodox, or regular medicine. Some standard medical care practitioners are also practitioners of CAM.

Complementary medicine is treatments that are used along with standard medical treatments but are not considered to be standard treatments. One example is using acupuncture to help lessen some side effects of cancer treatment.

Alternative medicine is treatments that are used instead of standard medical treatments. One example is using a special diet to treat cancer instead of anticancer drugs that are prescribed by an oncologist.

Integrative medicine is a total approach to medical care that combines standard medicine with the CAM practices that have been shown to be safe and effective. They treat the patient's mind, body, and spirit.

Are Complementary and Alternative Medicine Approaches Safe?

Some CAM therapies have undergone careful evaluation and have been found to be safe and effective. However, there are others that have been found to be ineffective or possibly harmful. Less is known about many CAM therapies, and research has been slower for a number of reasons:

- Time and funding issues

- Problems finding institutions and cancer researchers to work with on the studies

- Regulatory issues

CAM therapies need to be evaluated with the same long and careful research process used to evaluate standard treatments. Standard cancer treatments have generally been studied for safety and effectiveness through an intense scientific process that includes clinical trials with large numbers of patients.

Natural Does Not Mean Safe

CAM therapies include a wide variety of botanicals and nutritional products, such as dietary supplements, herbal supplements, and vitamins. Many of these "natural" products are considered to be safe because they are present in, or produced by, nature. However, that is not true in all cases. In addition, some may affect how well other medicines work in your body. For example, the herb St. John's wort, which some people use for depression, may cause certain anticancer drugs not to work as well as they should.

Herbal supplements may be harmful when taken by themselves, with other substances, or in large doses. For example, some studies have shown that kava, an herb that has been used to help with stress and anxiety, may cause liver damage.

Vitamins can also have unwanted effects in your body. For example, some studies show that high doses of vitamins, even vitamin C, may affect how chemotherapy and radiation work. Too much of any vitamin is not safe, even in a healthy person.

Tell your doctor if you're taking any dietary supplements, no matter how safe you think they are. This is very important. Even though there may be ads or claims that something has been used for years, they do not prove that it's safe or effective.

Supplements do not have to be approved by the federal government before being sold to the public. Also, a prescription is not needed to buy them. Therefore, it's up to consumers to decide what is best for them.

National Cancer Institute (NCI) and the National Center for Complementary and Integrative Health (NCCIH) are currently sponsoring or cosponsoring various clinical trials that test CAM treatments and therapies in people. Some study the effects of complementary approaches used in addition to conventional treatments, and some compare alternative therapies with conventional treatments.

What Should Patients Do When Using or Considering Cam Therapies?

Cancer patients who are using or considering using complementary or alternative therapy should talk with their doctor or nurse. Some therapies may interfere with standard treatment or even be harmful. It is also a good idea to learn whether the therapy has been proven to do what it claims to do.

To find a CAM practitioner, ask your doctor or nurse to suggest someone. Or ask if someone at your cancer center, such as a social worker or physical therapist can help you. Choosing a CAM practitioner should be done with as much care as choosing a primary care provider.

Patients, their families, and their healthcare providers can learn about CAM therapies and practitioners from the following government agencies:

- National Center for Complementary and Integrative Health

- NCI Office of Cancer Complementary and Alternative Medicine (OCCAM)

- Office of Dietary Supplements (ODS)

Section 48.2

Soy

This section includes text excerpted from "Soy," National Center for Complementary and Integrative Health (NCCIH), September 2016. Reviewed February 2019.

What Is Known about Soy and Soy Products?

Soy, a plant in the pea family, has been common in Asian diets for thousands of years. Soy is also present in modern Western diets as a food and food ingredient. Soy products are used for menopausal symptoms, bone health, improving memory, high blood pressure (HBP), and high cholesterol levels.

In addition to its food uses, soy is available in dietary supplements, in forms such as tablets, capsules, and powders. Soy supplements may contain soy protein, isoflavones (compounds that have effects in the body similar to those of the female hormone estrogen (ER)), or other soy components.

What Does the Research Say about Soy and Soy Products?

Although there have been many studies on soy products, there are still uncertainties about soy's health effects. Consuming soy protein in place of other proteins may lower levels of low-density lipoprotein (LDL) ("bad") cholesterol to a small extent.

Current evidence indicates that it's safe for women who have had breast cancer or who are at risk for breast cancer to eat soy foods. However, it's uncertain whether soy isoflavone supplements are safe for these women. Soy isoflavone supplements may help to reduce the frequency and severity of menopausal hot flashes, but the effect may be small. It's uncertain whether soy supplements can relieve cognitive problems associated with menopause. Current evidence suggests that soy isoflavone mixtures do not slow bone loss in Western women during or after menopause.

Diets containing soy protein may slightly reduce blood pressure. There's not enough scientific evidence to determine whether soy supplements are effective for any other health uses.

Current National Center for Complementary and Integrative Health (NCCIH)-funded studies on soy and its components are investigating a variety of topics, including stroke outcomes, anti-inflammatory effects, and effects on diabetes.

Except for people with soy allergies, soy is believed to be safe when consumed in normal dietary amounts. However, the safety of long-term use of high doses of soy extracts has not been established.

Side Effects of Soy

The most common side effects of soy are digestive upsets, such as stomach pain and diarrhea.

Long-term use of soy isoflavone supplements might increase the risk of endometrial hyperplasia (EH) (a thickening of the lining of the uterus that may lead to cancer). Soy foods do not appear to increase the risk of endometrial hyperplasia.

Check with Your Healthcare Provider

Tell all your healthcare providers about any complementary or integrative health approaches you use. Give them a full picture of what you do to manage your health. This will help ensure coordinated and safe care.

Section 48.3

Turmeric

This section includes text excerpted from "Turmeric," National Center for Complementary and Integrative Health (NCCIH), September 2016. Reviewed February 2019.

What Is Known about Turmeric?

Turmeric, a plant related to ginger, is grown throughout parts of Asia (especially in India) and Central America. Historically, turmeric has been used in Ayurvedic medicine, primarily in South Asia, for many conditions, including breathing problems, rheumatism, serious pain, and fatigue.

Nowadays, turmeric is used as a dietary supplement for inflammation; arthritis; stomach, skin, liver, and gallbladder problems; cancer; and other conditions. It is a common spice and a major ingredient in curry powder. Its primary active ingredients, curcuminoids, are yellow and used to color foods and cosmetics. Turmeric's underground stems (rhizomes) are dried and made into capsules, tablets, teas, or extracts. Turmeric powder is also made into a paste for skin conditions.

What Are the Health Effects of Turmeric?

A lot of research, including studies, has been done in people on turmeric for a variety of health conditions. Claims that curcuminoids found in turmeric help to reduce inflammation aren't supported by strong studies. Preliminary studies found that curcuminoids may:

- Reduce the number of heart attacks bypass patients had after surgery

- Control knee pain from osteoarthritis, as well as ibuprofen

- Reduce the skin irritation that often occurs after radiation treatments for breast cancer

Other preliminary studies in people have looked at curcumin, a type of curcuminoid, for different cancers, colitis, diabetes, surgical pain, and as an ingredient in mouthwash for reducing plaque.

Is Turmeric Safe?

Turmeric in amounts tested for health purposes is generally considered safe when taken by mouth or applied to the skin. However, high doses or long-term use of turmeric may cause gastrointestinal (GI) problems.

Check with Your Healthcare Provider

Tell all your healthcare providers about any complementary or integrative health approaches you use. Give them a full picture of what you do to manage your health. This will help ensure coordinated and safe care.

Chapter 49

Treating Breast Cancer during Pregnancy

Treatment Option Overview
Factors for Consideration

Treatment options for pregnant women depend on the stage of the disease and the age of the unborn baby. Three types of standard treatment that are used are described below.

Surgery

Most pregnant women with breast cancer have surgery to remove the breast. Some of the lymph nodes under the arm may be removed so they can be checked under a microscope by a pathologist for signs of cancer.

Types of surgery to remove the cancer include:

- **Modified-radical mastectomy (MRM).** Surgery to remove the whole breast that has cancer, many of the lymph nodes under the arm, the lining over the chest muscles, and sometimes, part of the chest wall muscles. This type of surgery is most common in pregnant women.

This chapter includes text excerpted from "Breast Cancer Treatment during Pregnancy (PDQ®)—Patient Version," National Cancer Institute (NCI), December 28, 2018.

- **Breast-conserving surgery (BCS).** Surgery to remove cancer and some normal tissue around it, but not the breast itself. Part of the chest wall lining may also be removed if the cancer is near it. This type of surgery may also be called "lumpectomy," "partial mastectomy," "segmental mastectomy," "quadrantectomy," or "breast-sparing surgery."

After the doctor removes all of the cancer that can be seen at the time of surgery, some patients may be given chemotherapy or radiation therapy after surgery to kill any cancer cells that are left. For pregnant women with early-stage breast cancer, radiation therapy and hormone therapy (HT) are given after the baby is born. Treatment given after surgery, to lower the risk that cancer will come back, is called "adjuvant therapy."

Radiation Therapy

Radiation therapy is a cancer treatment that uses high-energy X-rays or other types of radiation to kill cancer cells or keep them from growing. There are two types of radiation therapy:

- **External radiation therapy** uses a machine outside the body to send radiation toward cancer

- **Internal radiation therapy** uses a radioactive substance sealed in needles, seeds, wires, or catheters that are placed directly into or near cancer

The way the radiation therapy is given depends on the type and stage of the cancer being treated.

External radiation therapy may be given to pregnant women with early stage (stage I or II) breast cancer after the baby is born. Women with late stage (stage III or IV) breast cancer may be given external radiation therapy after the first three months of pregnancy or, if possible, radiation therapy is delayed until after the baby is born.

Chemotherapy

Chemotherapy is a cancer treatment that uses drugs to stop the growth of cancer cells, either by killing the cells or by stopping the cells from dividing. When chemotherapy is taken by mouth or injected into a vein or muscle, the drugs enter the bloodstream and can reach cancer cells throughout the body (systemic chemotherapy). When chemotherapy is placed directly into the cerebrospinal fluid (CBF), an organ or a body cavity such as the abdomen, the drugs mainly affect cancer cells in those areas (regional chemotherapy).

The way the chemotherapy is given depends on the type and stage of the cancer being treated. Systemic chemotherapy is used to treat breast cancer during pregnancy.

Chemotherapy is usually not given during the first-three months of pregnancy. Chemotherapy given after this time does not usually harm the unborn baby but may cause early labor or low birth weight.

Ending the Pregnancy Does Not Seem to Improve the Mother's Chance of Survival

Because ending the pregnancy is not likely to improve the mother's chance of survival, it is not usually a treatment option.

Treatment Options for Breast Cancer during Pregnancy
Early-Stage Breast Cancer

Pregnant women with early-stage breast cancer (stage I and stage II) are usually treated in the same way as patients who are not pregnant, with some changes to protect the unborn baby. Treatment may include the following:

- **MRM**, if the breast cancer was diagnosed early in pregnancy

- **BCS**, if breast cancer is diagnosed later in pregnancy. Radiation therapy may be given after the baby is born.

- **MRM or BCS during pregnancy.** After the first-three months of pregnancy, certain types of chemotherapy may be given before or after surgery.

HT and trastuzumab should not be given during pregnancy.

Late-Stage Breast Cancer

There is no standard treatment for patients with late-stage breast cancer (stage III or stage IV) during pregnancy. Treatment may include the following:

- Radiation therapy
- Chemotherapy

341

Radiation therapy and chemotherapy should not be given during the first-three months of pregnancy.

Special Issues about Breast Cancer during Pregnancy
Lactation (Breast Milk Production) and Breastfeeding Should Be Stopped If Surgery or Chemotherapy Is Planned

If surgery is planned, breastfeeding should be stopped to reduce blood flow in the breasts and make them smaller. Many chemotherapy drugs, especially cyclophosphamide and methotrexate, may occur in high levels in breast milk and may harm the nursing baby. Women receiving chemotherapy should not breastfeed.

Stopping lactation does not improve the mother's prognosis.

Breast Cancer Does Not Appear to Harm the Unborn Baby

Breast cancer cells do not seem to pass from the mother to the unborn baby.

Pregnancy Does Not Seem to Affect the Survival of Women Who Have Had Breast Cancer in the Past

For women who have had breast cancer, pregnancy does not seem to affect their survival. However, some doctors recommend that a woman wait two years after treatment for breast cancer before trying to have a baby, so that any early return of cancer would be detected. This may affect a woman's decision to become pregnant. The unborn baby does not seem to be affected if the mother has had breast cancer.

Chapter 50

Treating Male Breast Cancer

Treatment Option Overview
There Are Different Types of Treatment for Men with Breast Cancer

Different types of treatment are available for men with breast cancer. Some treatments are standard (the currently used treatment), and some are being tested in clinical trials. A treatment clinical trial is a research study meant to help improve current treatments or obtain information on new treatments for patients with cancer. When clinical trials show that a new treatment is better than the standard treatment, the new treatment may become the standard treatment.

For some patients, taking part in a clinical trial may be the best treatment choice. Many of nowadays standard treatments for cancer are based on earlier clinical trials. Patients who take part in a clinical trial may receive the standard treatment or be among the first to receive a new treatment.

Patients who take part in clinical trials also help improve the way cancer will be treated in the future. Even when clinical trials do not lead to effective new treatments, they often answer important questions and help move research forward.

This chapter includes text excerpted from "Male Breast Cancer Treatment (PDQ®)—Patient Version," National Cancer Institute (NCI), December 28, 2018.

Some clinical trials only include patients who have not yet received treatment. Other trials test treatments for patients whose cancer has not gotten better. There are also clinical trials that test new ways to stop cancer from recurring (coming back) or reduce the side effects of cancer treatment.

Clinical trials are taking place in many parts of the country. Information about clinical trials is available from the National Cancer Institute (NCI) www.cancer.gov website. Choosing the most appropriate cancer treatment is a decision that ideally involves the patient, family, and healthcare team.

Standard Treatment for Men with Breast Cancer

Five types of standard treatment are used to treat men with breast cancer which are described below.

Surgery

Surgery for men with breast cancer is usually a modified radical mastectomy (MRM) (removal of the breast, many of the lymph nodes under the arm, the lining over the chest muscles, and sometimes part of the chest wall muscles).

Breast-conserving surgery (BCS), an operation to remove cancer but not the breast itself, is also used for some men with breast cancer. A lumpectomy is done to remove the tumor (lump) and a small amount of normal tissue around it. Radiation therapy is given after surgery to kill any cancer cells that are left.

Chemotherapy

Chemotherapy is a cancer treatment that uses drugs to stop the growth of cancer cells, either by killing the cells or by stopping them from dividing. When chemotherapy is taken by mouth or injected into a vein or muscle, the drugs enter the bloodstream and can reach cancer cells throughout the body (systemic chemotherapy). When chemotherapy is placed directly into the cerebrospinal fluid (CSF), an organ or a body cavity such as the abdomen, the drugs mainly affect cancer cells in those areas (regional chemotherapy).

The way the chemotherapy is given depends on the type and stage of the cancer being treated. Systemic chemotherapy is used to treat breast cancer in men.

Hormone Therapy

Hormone therapy (HT) is a cancer treatment that removes hormones or blocks their action and stops cancer cells from growing. Hormones are substances made by glands in the body and circulated in the bloodstream. Some hormones can cause certain cancers to grow. If tests show that the cancer cells have places where hormones can attach (receptors), drugs, surgery, or radiation therapy is used to reduce the production of hormones or block them from working.

HT with tamoxifen is often given to patients with estrogen-receptor (ER) and progesterone receptor (PR) positive breast cancer and to patients with metastatic breast cancer (MBC) (cancer that has spread to other parts of the body).

HT with an aromatase inhibitor (AI) is given to some men who have MBC. AIs decrease the body's estrogen by blocking an enzyme called "aromatase" from turning androgen into estrogen. Anastrozole, letrozole, and exemestane are types of AIs.

HT with a luteinizing hormone-releasing hormone (LHRH) agonist is given to some men who have MBC. LHRH agonists affect the pituitary gland, which controls how much testosterone is made by the testicles. In men who are taking LHRH agonists, the pituitary gland tells the testicles to make less testosterone. Leuprolide and goserelin are types of LHRH agonists.

Other types of HT include megestrol acetate or antiestrogen therapy, such as fulvestrant.

Radiation Therapy

Radiation therapy is a cancer treatment that uses high-energy X-rays or other types of radiation to kill cancer cells or keep them from growing. There are two types of radiation therapy:

- **External radiation therapy** uses a machine outside the body to send radiation toward cancer

- **Internal radiation therapy** uses a radioactive substance sealed in needles, seeds, wires, or catheters that are placed directly into or near cancer

The way the radiation therapy is given depends on the type and stage of the cancer being treated. external radiation therapy is used to treat Male breast cancer.

Targeted Therapy

Targeted therapy is a type of treatment that uses drugs or other substances to identify and attack specific cancer cells without harming normal cells. Monoclonal antibody therapy, tyrosine kinase inhibitors (TKI), cyclin-dependent kinase inhibitors (CDKI), and mammalian target of rapamycin (mTOR) inhibitors are types of targeted therapies used to treat men with breast cancer.

Monoclonal antibody therapy uses antibodies made in the laboratory from a single type of immune system cell. These antibodies can identify substances on cancer cells or normal substances that may help cancer cells grow. The antibodies attach to the substances and kill the cancer cells, block their growth, or keep them from spreading. Monoclonal antibodies are given by infusion. They may be used alone or to carry drugs, toxins, or radioactive material directly to cancer cells. Monoclonal antibodies are also used with chemotherapy as adjuvant therapy (treatment given after surgery to lower the risk that cancer will come back).

Types of monoclonal antibody therapy include the following:

- **Trastuzumab** is a monoclonal antibody that blocks the effects of the growth factor protein human epidermal growth factor receptor 2 (HER2).

- **Pertuzumab** is a monoclonal antibody that may be combined with trastuzumab and chemotherapy to treat breast cancer.

- **Ado-trastuzumab emtansine** is a monoclonal antibody linked to an anticancer drug. This is called an antibody-drug conjugate (ADC). It may be used to treat men with hormone receptor-positive breast cancer that has spread to other parts of the body.

- **Tyrosine kinase inhibitors** are targeted therapy drugs that block signals needed for tumors to grow. Lapatinib is a tyrosine kinase inhibitor that may be used to treat men with MBC.

- **Cyclin-dependent kinase inhibitors** are targeted therapy drugs that block proteins called cyclin-dependent kinases, which cause the growth of cancer cells. Palbociclib is a cyclin-dependent kinase inhibitor used to treat men with MBC.

- **Mammalian target of rapamycin (mTOR) inhibitors** blocks a protein called mTOR, which may keep cancer cells from growing and prevent the growth of new blood vessels that tumors need to grow.

Chapter 51

Treating Advanced and Recurrent Breast Cancer

Locally Advanced or Inflammatory Breast Cancer

Treatment of locally advanced or inflammatory breast cancer is a combination of therapies that may include the following:

- Surgery (breast-conserving surgery (BCS) or total mastectomy) with lymph node dissection

- Chemotherapy before and/or after surgery

- Radiation therapy after surgery

- Hormone therapy (HT) after surgery for tumors that are estrogen receptor (ER) positive or ER-unknown

- Clinical trials testing new anticancer drugs, new drug combinations, and new ways of giving treatment

This chapter includes text excerpted from "Breast Cancer Treatment (PDQ®)—Patient Version," National Cancer Institute (NCI), December 28, 2018.

Locoregional Recurrent Breast Cancer

Treatment of locoregional recurrent breast cancer (cancer that has come back after treatment in the breast, in the chest wall, or in nearby lymph nodes), may include the following:

- Chemotherapy

- HT for tumors that are hormone receptor positive

- Radiation therapy

- Surgery

- Targeted therapy (trastuzumab)

- A clinical trial of a new treatment

Metastatic Breast Cancer

Treatment options for metastatic breast cancer (cancer that has spread to distant parts of the body) may include the following:

Hormone Therapy

In postmenopausal women who have just been diagnosed with metastatic breast cancer that is hormone receptor positive or if the hormone receptor status is not known, treatment may include:

- Tamoxifen therapy

- Aromatase inhibitor therapy (AI) (anastrozole, letrozole, or exemestane). Sometimes cyclin-dependent kinase (CDK) inhibitor therapy (palbociclib, ribociclib, or abemaciclib) is also given.

In premenopausal women who have just been diagnosed with metastatic breast cancer that is hormone receptor positive, treatment may include tamoxifen, a luteinizing hormone-releasing hormone (LHRH) agonist, or both.

In women whose tumors are hormone receptor positive or hormone receptor unknown, with spread to the bone or soft tissue only, and who have been treated with tamoxifen, treatment may include:

- Aromatase inhibitor therapy

- Other HT such as megestrol acetate (MGA), estrogen or androgen therapy, or antiestrogen therapy such as fulvestrant

Targeted Therapy

In women with metastatic breast cancer that is hormone receptor positive and has not responded to other treatments, options may include targeted therapy such as:

- Trastuzumab, lapatinib, pertuzumab, or mammalian target of rapamycin (mTOR) inhibitors
- Antibody-drug conjugate (ADC) therapy with ado-trastuzumab emtansine
- Cyclin-dependent kinase inhibitor therapy (palbociclib, ribociclib, or abemaciclib) which may be combined with HT

In women with metastatic breast cancer that is HER2/neu positive, treatment may include targeted therapy such as trastuzumab, pertuzumab, ado-trastuzumab emtansine, or lapatinib.

Chemotherapy

In women with metastatic breast cancer that is hormone receptor negative, has not responded to HT, has spread to other organs or has caused symptoms, treatment may include chemotherapy with one or more drugs.

Surgery

- Total mastectomy for women with open or painful breast lesions—radiation therapy may be given after surgery
- Surgery to remove cancer that has spread to the brain or spine—radiation therapy may be given after surgery
- Surgery to remove cancer that has spread to the lung
- Surgery to repair or help support weak or broken bones—radiation therapy may be given after surgery
- Surgery to remove fluid that has collected around the lungs or heart

Radiation Therapy

- Radiation therapy to the bones, brain, spinal cord, breast, or chest wall to relieve symptoms and improve quality of life (QOL)

349

- Strontium-89 (a radionuclide) to relieve pain from cancer that has spread to bones throughout the body

Other Treatment Options

Other treatment options for metastatic breast cancer include:

- Drug therapy with bisphosphonates or denosumab to reduce bone disease and pain when cancer has spread to the bone

- A clinical trial of high-dose chemotherapy with stem cell transplant

- Clinical trials testing new anticancer drugs, new drug combinations, and new ways of giving treatment

Chapter 52

Drugs Approved for Breast Cancer

This chapter lists cancer drugs approved by the U.S. Food and Drug Administration (FDA) for breast cancer. The list includes generic and brand names. This chapter also lists common drug combinations used in breast cancer. The individual drugs in the combinations are FDA-approved. However, the drug combinations themselves usually are not approved, although, they are widely used.

Note: There may be drugs used in breast cancer that are not listed here.

Drugs Approved to Prevent Breast Cancer

Drugs that have been approved for preventing breast cancer are listed below.

Evista (Raloxifene Hydrochloride)

Raloxifene hydrochloride is approved to prevent breast cancer. It is used to decrease the chance of invasive breast cancer in postmenopausal women (PMW) who have a high risk for developing the disease or who have osteoporosis.

This chapter includes text excerpted from "Drugs Approved for Breast Cancer," National Cancer Institute (NCI), June 5, 2018.

Tamoxifen Citrate

Tamoxifen citrate is approved to treat

- Breast cancer in women and men. It is used:

  - In patients whose cancer has metastasized (spread to other parts of the body)

  - In women whose cancer was treated with surgery and radiation therapy

- Ductal carcinoma *in situ* (DCIS). It is used to decrease the chance of invasive breast cancer in patients who have had surgery and radiation therapy for DCIS.

Tamoxifen citrate is also approved to prevent:

- Breast cancer in women who are at high risk for the disease

Drugs Approved to Treat Breast Cancer

Drugs that have been approved for breast-cancer treatment are listed below.

Abemaciclib (Verzenio)

- Abemaciclib is approved to treat breast cancer that is hormone receptor-positive (HR+) and human epidermal growth factor receptor 2 negative (HER2-) and is advanced or has metastasized.

  - It is used with fulvestrant in women whose disease got worse after treatment with hormone therapy (HT).

  - It is used alone in women and men whose disease got worse after treatment with HT and previous chemotherapy given for metastatic disease.

  - It is used with an aromatase inhibitor (AI) given as first-line HT in PMW.

Abemaciclib is also being studied in the treatment of other types of cancer.

Abraxane (Paclitaxel Albumin-Stabilized Nanoparticle Formulation)

Paclitaxel albumin-stabilized nanoparticle formulation is approved to be used alone or with other drugs to treat breast cancer that has recurred (come back) or metastasized.

Paclitaxel albumin-stabilized nanoparticle formulation is a form of paclitaxel contained in nanoparticles (very tiny particles of protein). The drug is also called "nanoparticle paclitaxel" and "protein-bound paclitaxel." This form may work better than other forms of paclitaxel and have fewer side effects.

Ado-Trastuzumab Emtansine

Ado-trastuzumab emtansine is approved to treat breast cancer that is HER2 positive and has metastasized. It is used in patients who have already been treated with trastuzumab and a taxane. It is also used in these patients if cancer recurs after adjuvant therapy.

Afinitor (Everolimus)

Everolimus is approved to treat breast cancer. It is used in combination with exemestane in PMW with advanced HR+ breast cancer that is also HER2– and has not gotten better after treatment with letrozole or anastrozole.

The use of everolimus to treat cancer is approved for the Afinitor and Afinitor Disperz brands. Everolimus is also approved to treat transplant rejection. This use is approved for the Zortress brand.

Anastrozole (Arimidex)

Anastrozole is approved to treat breast cancer in PMW who have any of the following types of breast cancer:

- **Early-stage, HR+ breast cancer.** It is used in women who have already received other treatment.

- **Locally advanced or metastatic breast cancer that is HR+ or HR unknown (it is not known whether it is HR+ or HR–).** It is used as first-line therapy in these patients.

- **Advanced breast cancer** that has gotten worse after treatment with tamoxifen citrate.

Aredia (Pamidronate Disodium)

Pamidronate disodium is approved to be given with chemotherapy to treat bone damage caused by breast cancer that has metastasized to bone.

Aromasin (Exemestane)

Exemestane is approved to treat:

- Advanced breast cancer

- Breast cancer that is early stage and estrogen receptor positive (ER+)

Exemestane is used in PMW who have already been treated with tamoxifen citrate.

Capecitabine (Xeloda)

Capecitabine is approved to be used alone or with other drugs to treat breast cancer that has metastasized in patients whose disease has not gotten better with other chemotherapy.

Cyclophosphamide

Cyclophosphamide is approved to be used alone or with other drugs to treat breast cancer.

Docetaxel (Taxotere)

Docetaxel is approved to be used alone or with other drugs to treat breast cancer that is locally advanced or has metastasized and has not gotten better with other chemotherapy. It is also used to treat breast cancer that is node-positive and can be removed by surgery.

Doxorubicin Hydrochloride

Doxorubicin hydrochloride is approved to be used alone or with other drugs to treat breast cancer. It is also used as adjuvant therapy for breast cancer that has spread to the lymph nodes after surgery.

Doxorubicin hydrochloride is also available in a different form called doxorubicin hydrochloride liposome.

Ellence (Epirubicin Hydrochloride)

Epirubicin hydrochloride is approved to be used with other drugs to treat breast cancer. It is used after surgery in patients whose cancer has spread to the lymph nodes under the arm.

Eribulin Mesylate

Eribulin mesylate is approved to treat breast cancer that has metastasized. It is used in patients who have already been treated with an anthracycline and a taxane.

Everolimus

Everolimus is approved to treat breast cancer. It is used in combination with exemestane in PMW with advanced HR+ breast cancer that is also HER2– and has not gotten better after treatment with letrozole or anastrozole.

The use of everolimus to treat cancer is approved for the Afinitor and Afinitor Disperz brands. Everolimus is also approved to treat transplant rejection. This use is approved for the Zortress brand.

Exemestane

Exemestane is approved to treat

- Advanced breast cancer

- Breast cancer that is early stage and ER+

Exemestane is used in PMW who have already been treated with tamoxifen citrate.

Five-Fu (Fluorouracil Injection)

Fluorouracil injection is approved to treat breast cancer. It is also called "five-FU." It is also available in a topical form.

Fareston (Toremifene)

Toremifene is approved to treat breast cancer that has metastasized. It is used in PMW whose cancer is ER or when it is not known if the cancer is ER+ or ER–.

355

Faslodex (Fulvestrant)

Fulvestrant is approved to treat breast cancer. It is used:

- In PMW with HR+ and HER2− advanced cancer that has not been treated with HT

- In PMW with HR+ advanced cancer that got worse after treatment with HT

- With palbociclib or abemaciclib in women with HR+ and HER2− advanced or metastatic cancer that got worse after treatment with HT

Femara (Letrozole)

Letrozole is approved to be used alone or with other drugs to treat breast cancer in PMW who have any of the following types of breast cancer:

- Early-stage, HR+ breast cancer in women who have already received other treatment

- Early-stage breast cancer that has been treated with tamoxifen citrate for at least five years

- Breast cancer that is locally advanced or has metastasized, is HER2 positive (HER2+) and HR+

- Breast cancer that is locally advanced or has metastasized and it is not known whether the cancer is HR+ or hormone receptor negative (HR−)

- Advanced breast cancer that has gotten worse after antiestrogen therapy

Gemcitabine Hydrochloride

Gemcitabine hydrochloride is approved to be used alone or with other drugs to treat breast cancer that has metastasized and has not gotten better with other chemotherapy. It is used with paclitaxel.

Goserelin Acetate (Zoladex)

Goserelin acetate is approved to treat breast cancer that is advanced. It is used as palliative treatment in premenopausal and perimenopausal women.

Halaven (Eribulin Mesylate)

Eribulin mesylate is approved to treat breast cancer that has metastasized. It is used in patients who have already been treated with an anthracycline and a taxane.

Herceptin (Trastuzumab)

Trastuzumab is approved to be used to treat breast cancer that is HER2+. It is used in patients with:

- Hormone receptor-negative or high-risk cancer. It is given:
  - Alone after combination therapy that included anthracycline chemotherapy.
  - As combination therapy with:
    - Doxorubicin, cyclophosphamide, and either paclitaxel or docetaxel, or
    - Docetaxel and carboplatin
- Metastatic cancer.

It is given:

- With paclitaxel as first-line treatment for metastatic disease, or
- Alone in patients who have received at least one chemotherapy treatment for metastatic disease

This use is approved for the Herceptin, Ogivri, and Herzuma brands of trastuzumab.

Ibrance (Palbociclib)

Palbociclib is approved to be used with other drugs to treat breast cancer that is HR+ and HER2– and is advanced or has metastasized.

- It is used with fulvestrant in women whose disease has gotten worse after treatment with HT.
- It is used with an AI in PMW who have not been treated with HT.

Palbociclib is also being studied in the treatment of other types of cancer.

Ixabepilone (Ixempra)

Ixabepilone is approved to be used alone or with capecitabine to treat breast cancer that is locally advanced or has metastasized. It is used in patients who have not gotten better with other chemotherapy.

Kadcyla (Ado-Trastuzumab Emtansine)

Ado-trastuzumab emtansine is approved to treat breast cancer that is HER2+ and has metastasized. It is used in patients who have already been treated with trastuzumab and a taxane. It is also used in these patients if cancer recurs after adjuvant therapy.

Kisqali (Ribociclib)

Ribociclib is approved to be used with other drugs to treat breast cancer that is HR+ and HER2– and is advanced or has metastasized. It is used:

- With an AI in women who have not been treated with HT

- With fulvestrant in PMW who have not been treated with HT or whose disease get worse during treatment with HT

Ribociclib is also being studied in the treatment of other types of cancer.

Lapatinib Ditosylate (Tykerb)

Lapatinib ditosylate is approved to be used with other drugs to treat breast cancer that is advanced or has metastasized. It is used with:

- Capecitabine in women with HER2+ breast cancer whose disease has not gotten better with other chemotherapy

- Letrozole in PMW with HER2+ and HR+ breast cancer who need HT

Lynparza (Olaparib)

Olaparib is approved to treat breast cancer that is HER2–, has certain germline mutations in the *BRCA1* or *BRCA2* gene, and has metastasized. It is used in patients with cancer that has been treated with chemotherapy given before or after surgery or for metastatic disease.

Megestrol Acetate

Megestrol acetate in tablet form is approved for palliative treatment of advanced disease in breast cancer.

Methotrexate (Trexall)

Methotrexate is approved to be used alone or with other drugs to treat breast cancer.

Neratinib Maleate

Neratinib maleate is approved to treat breast cancer that is early stage and HER2+. It is used as extended adjuvant therapy in patients who have already been treated with trastuzumab after surgery.

Paclitaxel (Taxol)

Paclitaxel is approved to be used alone or with other drugs to treat breast cancer.

Paclitaxel Albumin-Stabilized Nanoparticle Formulation

Paclitaxel albumin-stabilized nanoparticle formulation is approved to be used alone or with other drugs to treat breast cancer that has recurred or metastasized.

Paclitaxel albumin-stabilized nanoparticle formulation is a form of paclitaxel contained in nanoparticles (very tiny particles of protein). The drug is also called "nanoparticle paclitaxel" and "protein-bound paclitaxel." This form may work better than other forms of paclitaxel and have fewer side effects.

Pamidronate Disodium

Pamidronate disodium is approved to be given with chemotherapy to treat bone damage caused by breast cancer that has metastasized to bone.

Perjeta (Pertuzumab)

Pertuzumab is approved to be used with trastuzumab and docetaxel or other drugs to treat breast cancer that is HER2+. It is used:

- In patients with metastatic disease that has not been treated with HT or chemotherapy

- As neoadjuvant therapy (to shrink the tumor before surgery) in patients with locally advanced, inflammatory, or early-stage breast cancer

- As adjuvant therapy in patients with early-stage breast cancer who have a high risk that cancer will recur

Tamoxifen Citrate

Tamoxifen citrate is approved to treat breast cancer in women and men. It is used:

- In patients whose cancer has metastasized

- In women whose cancer was treated with surgery and radiation therapy

Tamoxifen citrate is approved to treat DCIS. It is used to decrease the chance of invasive breast cancer in patients who have had surgery and radiation therapy for DCIS. It is also approved to prevent breast cancer in women who are at high risk for the disease.

Thiotepa

Thiotepa is approved to treat breast cancer.

Toremifene

Toremifene is approved to treat breast cancer that has metastasized. It is used in PMW whose cancer is ER+ or when it is not known if the cancer is ER+ or ER–.

Trastuzumab

Trastuzumab is approved to be used alone or with other drugs to treat:

- Adenocarcinoma of the stomach or gastroesophageal junction. It is used for HER2 positive (HER2+) disease that has metastasized in patients who have not already been treated for metastatic cancer. This use is approved for the Herceptin and Ogivri brands of trastuzumab.

- Breast cancer that is HER2+. It is used in patients with:

- Hormone receptor-negative or high-risk cancer. It is given:
  - Alone after combination therapy that included anthracycline chemotherapy
  - As combination therapy with:
    - Doxorubicin, cyclophosphamide, and either paclitaxel or docetaxel or
    - Docetaxel and carboplatin
- Metastatic cancer.

  It is given:

- With paclitaxel as first-line treatment for metastatic disease, or
- Alone in patients who have received at least one chemotherapy treatment for metastatic disease.

This use is approved for the Herceptin, Ogivri, and Herzuma brands of trastuzumab.

Vinblastine Sulfate

Vinblastine sulfate is approved to treat breast cancer that has not gotten better with other treatment.

Part Six

Managing Side Effects and Complications of Breast-Cancer Treatment

Chapter 53

Anemia

What Is Anemia?

Anemia is a condition that can make you feel very tired, short of breath, and lightheaded. Other signs of anemia may include feeling dizzy or faint, headaches, a fast heartbeat, and/or pale skin.

Cancer treatments, such as chemotherapy and radiation therapy, can cause anemia. When you are anemic, your body does not have enough red blood cells. Red blood cells are the cells that that carry oxygen from the lungs throughout your body to help it work properly. You will have blood tests to check for anemia. Treatment for anemia is also based on your symptoms and on what is causing the anemia.

What Are the Ways to Manage Anemia?

Here are some steps you can take if you have fatigue caused by anemia:

Save your energy and ask for help. Choose the most important things to do each day. When people offer to help, let them do so. They can take you to the doctor, make meals, or do other things you are too tired to do.

This chapter includes text excerpted from "Anemia," National Cancer Institute (NCI), April 29, 2015. Reviewed February 2019.

Balance rest with activity. Take short naps during the day, but keep in mind that too much bed rest can make you feel weak. You may feel better if you take short walks or exercise a little every day.

Eat and drink well. Talk with your doctor, nurse, or a registered dietitian to learn what foods and drinks are best for you. You may need to eat foods that are high in protein or iron.

Talking with Your Healthcare Team

Prepare for your visit by making a list of questions to ask. Consider adding these questions to your list:

- What is causing the anemia?

- What problems should I call you about?

- What steps can I take to feel better?

- Would medicine, iron pills, a blood transfusion, or other treatments help me?

- Would you give me the name of a registered dietitian who could also give me advice?

Chapter 54

Appetite Loss

Cancer treatments may lower your appetite or change the way food tastes or smells. Side effects such as mouth and throat problems, or nausea and vomiting can also make eating difficult. Cancer-related fatigue can also lower your appetite.

Talk with your healthcare team if you are not hungry or if you find it difficult to eat. Don't wait until you feel weak, have lost too much weight, or are dehydrated, to talk with your doctor or nurse. It's important to eat well, especially during treatment for breast cancer.

What Is Appetite Loss?

Appetite loss is when you do not want to eat or do not feel like eating very much. It is a common problem that occurs with cancer and its treatment. You may have appetite loss for just one or two days, or throughout your course of treatment.

Why Appetite Loss Happens

No one knows just what causes appetite loss. Reasons may include:

- Cancer itself

- Fatigue

This chapter contains text excerpted from the following sources: Text in this chapter begins with excerpts from "Appetite Loss and Cancer Treatment," National Cancer Institute (NCI), September 14, 2018; Text beginning with the heading "What Is Appetite Loss?" is excerpted from "Eating Hints: Before, during, and after Cancer Treatment," National Cancer Institute (NCI), January 2018.

- Pain

- Medicines

- Feelings such as stress, fear, depression, and anxiety

- Cancer treatment side effects such as nausea, vomiting, constipation, or changes in how foods taste or smell

Ways to Manage Appetite Loss with Food

Appetite loss can be managed with food by adapting the following ways:

- Drink a liquid or powdered meal replacement, such as "instant breakfast," when it is hard to eat.

- Eat five or six smaller meals each day, instead of three large meals. Many people find that it is easier to eat smaller amounts more often. Doing so can also keep you from feeling too full.

- Keep snacks nearby for when you feel like eating. Take easy-to-carry snacks such as peanut-butter crackers, nuts, granola bars, or dried fruit when you go out.

- Add extra protein and calories to your diet.

- Drink liquids throughout the day—especially when you do not want to eat. If you have trouble remembering to drink, set a timer to remind you to take frequent sips.

- Choose liquids that add calories and other nutrients. Examples include juice, soup, and milk- and soy-based drinks with protein.

- Eat a bedtime snack. Doing so will provide extra calories, but won't affect your appetite for the next meal.

- Change the form of food. For instance, you might make a fruit milkshake instead of eating a piece of fruit.

- Eat soft, cool, or frozen foods. Examples include yogurt, milkshakes, and popsicles.

- Eat larger meals when you feel well and are rested. For many people, a good time to eat is in the morning after a good night's sleep.

- During meals, sip only small amounts of liquids. Many people feel too full if they eat and drink at the same time. If you want more than just small sips, have a larger drink at least 30 minutes before or after meals.

Recipe to Help with Appetite Loss

Table 54.1. Banana Milkshake

Yield: 1 serving	Serving Size: Approximately 2 Cups	
If Made With	Calories per Serving	Protein per Serving
Whole Milk	255	9 grams
2% Milk	226	10 grams
Skim Milk	190	11 grams

Directions. Put all ingredients into a blender. Blend at high speed until smooth.

Ingredients

- One whole ripe banana, sliced
- Vanilla extract (a few drops)
- One cup of milk

Other Ways to Manage

Besides food, there are other ways to manage appetite loss.

- **Talk with a dietitian.** She or he can discuss ways to get enough calories and protein even when you do not feel like eating.

- **Try to have relaxed and pleasant meals.** Examples might include being with people you enjoy and having foods that look good to eat.

- **Exercise.** Being active can help improve your appetite. Studies show that many people with cancer feel better when they get some exercise each day.

- **Talk with your nurse or social worker** if fear, depression, or other feelings affect your appetite or interest in food. He or she can suggest ways to help.

- **Talk to your doctor** if you are having nausea, vomiting, constipation, or changes in how foods taste or smell. Your doctor can help control these problems so that you feel more like eating.

Chapter 55

Bleeding and Bruising

Some cancer treatments, such as chemotherapy and targeted therapy, can increase your risk of bleeding and bruising. These treatments can lower the number of platelets in the blood. Platelets are the cells that help your blood to clot and stop bleeding. When your platelet count is low, you may bruise or bleed a lot or very easily and have tiny purple or red spots on your skin. This condition is called "thrombocytopenia." It is important to tell your doctor or nurse if you notice any of these changes, especially during treatment for breast cancer.

- **Bleeding** that doesn't stop after a few minutes; bleeding from your mouth, nose, or when you vomit; bleeding from your vagina when you are not having your period (menstruation); urine that is red or pink; stools that are black or bloody; or bleeding during your period that is heavier or lasts longer than normal.

- **Head or vision changes** such as bad headaches or changes in how well you see, or if you feel confused or very sleepy.

Ways to Manage Bleeding and Bruising

Steps to take if you are at increased risk of bleeding and bruising:

- **Avoid certain medicines.** Many over-the-counter (OTC) medicines contain aspirin or ibuprofen, which can increase your

This chapter includes text excerpted from "Bleeding and Bruising (Thrombocytopenia) and Cancer Treatment," National Cancer Institute (NCI), September 14, 2018.

risk of bleeding. When in doubt, be sure to check the label. Get a list of medicines and products from your healthcare team that you should avoid taking. You may also be advised to limit or avoid alcohol if your platelet count is low.

- **Take extra care to prevent bleeding.** Brush your teeth gently, with a very soft toothbrush. Wear shoes, even when you are inside. Be extra careful when using sharp objects. Use an electric shaver, not a razor. Use lotion and a lip balm to prevent dry, chapped skin and lips. Tell your doctor or nurse if you are constipated or notice bleeding from your rectum.

- **Care for bleeding or bruising.** If you start to bleed, press down firmly on the area with a clean cloth. Keep pressing until the bleeding stops. If you bruise, put ice on the area.

Talking with Your Healthcare Team about Bleeding and Bruising

Prepare for your visit by making a list of questions to ask. Consider adding these questions to your list:

- What steps can I take to prevent bleeding or bruising?

- How long should I wait for the bleeding to stop before I call you or go to the emergency room?

- Do I need to limit or avoid things that could increase my risk of bleeding, such as alcohol or sexual activity?

- What medicines, vitamins, or herbs should I avoid? Could I get a list from you of medicines to avoid?

Chapter 56

Constipation

What Is Constipation?

Constipation is when you have infrequent bowel movements and stool that may be hard, dry, and difficult to pass. You may also have stomach cramps, bloating, and nausea when you are constipated.

Cancer treatments such as chemotherapy can cause constipation. Certain medicines (such as pain medicines), changes in diet, not drinking enough fluids, and being less active may also cause constipation.

There are steps you can take to prevent constipation. It is easier to prevent constipation than to treat its complications, which may include fecal impaction or bowel obstruction.

What Are the Ways to Prevent or Treat Constipation?

Take these steps to prevent or treat constipation:

- **Eat high-fiber foods.** Adding bran to foods such as cereals or smoothies is an easy way to get more fiber in your diet. Ask your healthcare team how many grams of fiber you should have each day. If you have had an intestinal obstruction or intestinal surgery, you should not eat a high-fiber diet.

- **Drink plenty of liquids.** Most people need to drink at least eight cups of liquid each day. You may need more based on your

---

This chapter includes text excerpted from "Constipation," National Cancer Institute (NCI), April 29, 2015. Reviewed February 2019.

treatment, medications you are taking, or other health factors. Drinking warm or hot liquids may also help.

- **Try to be active every day.** Ask your healthcare team about exercises that you can do. Most people can do light exercise, even in a bed or chair. Other people choose to walk or ride an exercise bike for 15 to 30 minutes each day.

- **Learn about medicine.** Use only medicines and treatments for constipation that are prescribed by your doctor, since some may lead to bleeding, infection, or other harmful side effects in people being treated for cancer. Keep a record of your bowel movements to share with your doctor or nurse.

Talking with Your Healthcare Team

Prepare for your visit by making a list of questions to ask. Consider adding these questions to your list:

- What problems should I call you about?

- What information should I keep track of and share with you? (For example, you may be asked to keep track of your bowel movements, meals that you have, and exercise that you do each day.)

- How much liquid should I drink each day?

- What steps can I take to feel better?

- Would you give me the name of a registered dietitian who can tell me about foods that might help?

- Should I take medicine for constipation? If so, what medicine should I take? What medicine should I avoid?

Chapter 57

Delirium

What Is Delirium?

Delirium is a confused mental state that includes changes in awareness, thinking, judgment, sleeping patterns, as well as behavior. Although delirium can happen at the end of life, many episodes of delirium are caused by medicine or dehydration and are reversible.

The symptoms of delirium usually occur suddenly (within hours or days) over a short period of time and may come and go. Although delirium may be mistaken for depression or dementia, these conditions are different and have different treatments.

What Are the Types of Delirium?

The three main types of delirium include:

1. **Hypoactive delirium:** The patient seems sleepy, tired, or depressed.

2. **Hyperactive delirium:** The patient is restless, anxious, or suddenly agitated and uncooperative.

3. **Mixed delirium:** The patient changes back and forth between hypoactive delirium and hyperactive delirium.

This chapter includes text excerpted from "Delirium," National Cancer Institute (NCI), April 29, 2015. Reviewed February 2019.

What Are the Causes of Delirium?

Your healthcare team will work to find out what is causing delirium so that it can be treated. Causes of delirium may include:

- Advanced cancer
- Older age
- Brain tumors
- Dehydration
- Infection
- Taking certain medicines, such as high doses of opioids
- Withdrawal from or stopping certain medicines
- Early monitoring of someone with these risk factors for delirium may prevent it or allow it to be treated more quickly

Changes caused by delirium can be upsetting for family members and dangerous to the person with cancer, especially if the judgment is affected. People with delirium may be more likely to fall, unable to control their bladder and/or bowels, and more likely to become dehydrated. Their confused state may make it difficult to talk with others about their needs and make decisions about care. Family members may need to be more involved in decision-making.

What Are the Ways to Treat Delirium?

Steps that can be taken to treat symptoms related to delirium include:

Treat the causes of delirium: If medicines are causing delirium, then reducing the dose or stopping them may treat delirium. If conditions such as dehydration, poor nutrition, and infections are causing the delirium, then treating these may help.

Control surroundings: If the symptoms of delirium are mild, it may help to keep the room quiet and well lit, with a clock or calendar and familiar possessions. Having family members around and keeping the same caregivers, as much as possible, may also help.

Consider medicines: Medicines are sometimes given to treat the symptoms of delirium. However, these medicines have serious side effects and patients receiving them require careful observation by a doctor.

Sometimes sedation may help: After discussion with family members, sedation is sometimes used for delirium at the end of life, if it does not get better with other treatments. The doctor will discuss the decisions involved in using sedation to treat delirium with the family.

Talking with Your Healthcare Team

Prepare for the visit by making a list of questions to ask. Consider adding these questions to your list:

- Is my family member at risk for delirium?
- What is causing the delirium?
- What problems should we call you about?
- What treatments are advised for my family member?

Chapter 58

Diarrhea

Diarrhea means having bowel movements that are soft, loose, or watery more often than normal. If diarrhea is severe or lasts a long time, the body does not absorb enough water and nutrients. This can cause you to become dehydrated or malnourished. Cancer treatments, or cancer itself, may cause diarrhea or make it worse. Some medicines, infections, and stress can also cause diarrhea. Tell your healthcare team if you have diarrhea, especially during treatment for breast cancer.

Drink plenty of fluids, to prevent dehydration. It may also help to avoid certain foods, such as dairy products. Diarrhea that leads to dehydration (the loss of too much fluid from the body) and low levels of salt and potassium (important minerals needed by the body) can be life-threatening. Call your healthcare team if you feel dizzy or light-headed, have dark yellow urine or are not urinating, or have a fever of 100.5°F (38°C) or higher.

Ways to Manage Diarrhea

You may be advised to take steps to prevent complications from diarrhea:

- **Drink plenty of fluid each day.** Most people need to drink 8 to 12 cups of fluid each day. Ask your doctor or nurse how much fluid

This chapter includes text excerpted from "Diarrhea and Cancer Treatment," National Cancer Institute (NCI), August 9, 2018.

you should drink each day. For severe diarrhea, only clear liquids or IV (intravenous) fluids may be advised for a short period.

- **Eat small meals that are easy on your stomach.** Eat 6 to 8 small meals throughout the day, instead of 3 large meals. Foods high in potassium and sodium (minerals you lose when you have diarrhea) are good food choices, for most people. Limit or avoid foods and drinks that can make your diarrhea worse.

- **Check before taking medicine.** Check with your doctor or nurse before taking medicine for diarrhea. Your doctor will prescribe the correct medicine for you.

- **Keep your anal area clean and dry.** Try using warm water and wipes to stay clean. It may help to take warm, shallow baths. These are called "sitz baths." A sitz bath typically consists of a plastic tub that you fill with warm water and place under your toilet seat. Sitting in this water for 15 to 20 minutes several times a day offers relief from genital itching, perineum pain or discomfort, and the pain associated with fistulas, hemorrhoids, anal fissures, or an episiotomy. While it is possible to achieve the same result by sitting in a shallow bathtub of warm water, most users prefer the convenience of these inexpensive plastic tubs instead. Drug stores, medical-supply stores, and hospital pharmacies all sell sitz baths, and some provide a salt solution with the tubs. Be sure to confirm with your doctor whether you should use the salt solution. When you're done with your sitz bath, apply gentle pats to your affected area with a clean towel until the area is dry, then wash and dry your sitz bath after each use to avoid bacteria.

Talking with Your Healthcare Team about Diarrhea

Prepare for your visit by making a list of questions to ask. Consider adding these questions to your list:

- What is causing diarrhea?

- What symptoms should I call you about?

- How much liquid should I drink each day?

- Can I speak to a registered dietitian to learn more about foods and drinks that are best for me?

- What medicine or other steps can I take to prevent diarrhea and to decrease rectal pain?

Chapter 59

Fatigue

Fatigue is a common side effect of many cancer treatments, including chemotherapy, immunotherapy, radiation therapy, bone-marrow transplant, and surgery. Conditions such as anemia, as well as pain, medications, and emotions, can also cause or worsen fatigue.

People often describe cancer-related fatigue as feeling extremely tired, weak, heavy, run down, and having no energy. Resting does not always help with cancer-related fatigue. Cancer-related fatigue is one of the most difficult side effects with which many people must cope.

Tell your healthcare team if you feel extremely tired and are not able to do your normal activities or are very tired even after resting or sleeping. There are many causes of fatigue. Keeping track of your levels of energy throughout the day will help your doctor to assess your fatigue. Write down how fatigue affects your daily activities and what makes the fatigue better or worse.

Ways to Manage Fatigue

You may be advised to take these and other steps to feel better:

- **Make a plan that balances rest and activity.** Choose activities that are relaxing for you. Many people choose to listen to music, read, meditate, practice guided imagery or spend time with people they enjoy. Relaxing can help you save your energy

---

This chapter includes text excerpted from "Fatigue and Cancer Treatment," National Cancer Institute (NCI), September 14, 2018.

and lower stress. Light exercise may also be advised by your doctor to give you more energy and help you feel better.

- **Plan time to rest.** If you are tired, take short naps of less than one hour during the day. However, too much sleep during the day can make it difficult to sleep at night. Choose the activities that are most important to you and do them when you have the most energy. Ask for help with important tasks such as making meals or driving.

- **Eat and drink well.** Meet with a registered dietitian to learn about foods and drinks that can increase your level of energy. Foods high in protein and calories will help you keep up your strength. Some people find it easier to eat many small meals throughout the day instead of three big meals. Stay well hydrated. Limit your intake of caffeine and alcohol.

- **Meet with a specialist.** It may help to meet with a counselor, psychologist, or psychiatrist. These experts help people to cope with difficult thoughts and feelings. Lowering stress may give you more energy. Since pain that is not controlled can also be major source of fatigue, it may help to meet with pain or palliative care specialist.

Talking with Your Healthcare Team about Fatigue

Prepare for your visit by making a list of questions to ask. Consider adding these questions to your list:

- What is most likely causing my fatigue?

- What should I keep track of and share so we can develop a plan to help me feel better?

- What types of exercise (and how much) do you recommend for me?

- How much rest should I have during the day? How much sleep should I get at night?

- What food and drinks are best for me?

- Are there treatments or medicines that could help me feel better?

Chapter 60

Hair Loss

Some types of chemotherapy cause the hair on your head and other parts of your body to fall out. Radiation therapy can also cause hair loss on the part of the body that is being treated. Hair loss is called "alopecia." Talk with your healthcare team to learn if the breast cancer treatment you will be receiving causes hair loss. Your doctor or nurse will share strategies that have help others, including those listed below.

Hair Regrowth after Therapy

After chemotherapy. Hair growth typically begins two to three months after treatment has ended. Your hair will be very fine when it starts to grow back. Sometimes your new hair can be curlier or straighter—or even a different color. In time, it may go back to how it was before treatment.

After radiation therapy. Hair often grows back in three to six months after treatment has ended. If you received a very high dose of radiation your hair may grow back thinner or not at all on the part of your body that received radiation.

This chapter includes text excerpted from "Hair Loss (Alopecia) and Cancer Treatment," National Cancer Institute (NCI), December 4, 2017.

Ways to Manage Hair Loss

Talk with your healthcare team about ways to manage before and after hair loss. Some of the ways to manage it is listed below:

- **Treat your hair gently.** You may want to use a hair brush with soft bristles or a wide-tooth comb. Do not use hair dryers, irons, or products such as gels or clips that may hurt your scalp. Wash your hair with a mild shampoo. Wash it less often and be very gentle. Pat it dry with a soft towel.

- **You have choices.** Some people choose to cut their hair short to make it easier to deal with when it starts to fall out. Others choose to shave their heads. If you choose to shave your head, use an electric shaver so you won't cut yourself. If you plan to buy a wig, get one while you still have hair so you can match it to the color of your hair. If you find wigs to be itchy and hot, try wearing a comfortable scarf or turban.

- **Protect and care for your scalp.** Use a sunscreen or wear a hat when you are outside. Choose a comfortable scarf or hat that you enjoy and that keeps your head warm. If your scalp itches or feels tender, using lotions and conditioners can help it feel better.

- **Talk about your feelings.** Many people feel angry, depressed, or embarrassed about hair loss. Sharing these feelings with someone who understands can help. Some people find it helpful to talk with other people who have lost their hair during cancer treatment. Talking openly and honestly with your children and close family members can also help you all. Tell them that you expect to lose your hair during treatment.

Ways to Care for Your Hair When It Grows Back

Be gentle. When your hair starts to grow back, you will want to be gentle with it. Avoid too much brushing, curling, and blow-drying. You may not want to wash your hair as frequently.

Talking with Your Healthcare Team about Hair Loss

Prepare for your visit by making a list of questions to ask. Consider adding these questions to your list:

- Is treatment likely to cause my hair to fall out?

- How should I protect and care for my head? Are there products that you recommend? Ones I should avoid?

- Where can I get a wig or hairpiece?

- What support groups could I meet with that might help?

- When will my hair grow back?

Chapter 61

Hot Flashes and Night Sweats

Hot flashes and night sweats may be side effects of breast cancer or its treatment.

Sweating is the body's way of lowering body temperature by causing heat loss through the skin. In patients with cancer, sweating may be caused by fever, a tumor, or cancer treatment.

Hot flashes can also cause too much sweating. They may occur in natural menopause or in patients who have been treated for breast cancer or prostate cancer.

Hot flashes combined with sweats that happen while sleeping is often called "night sweats" or "hot flushes."

Hot flashes and night sweats affect the quality of life (QOL) in many patients with cancer. A treatment plan to help manage hot flashes and night sweats is based on the patient's condition and goals of care. For some patients, relieving symptoms and improving QOL is the most important goal.

Causes of Hot Flashes and Night Sweats in Breast-Cancer Patients

In patients with cancer, hot flashes and night sweats may be caused by the tumor, its treatment, or other conditions. Sweating happens

This chapter includes text excerpted from "Hot Flashes and Night Sweats (PDQ®)—Patient Version," National Cancer Institute (NCI), March 16, 2018.

with disease conditions such as fever and may occur without disease in warm climates, during exercise, and during hot flashes in menopause. Sweating helps balance body temperature by allowing heat to evaporate through the skin.

Hot flashes and night sweats are common in patients with cancer and in cancer survivors. They are more common in women but can also occur in men. Many patients treated for breast cancer and prostate cancer have hot flashes.

Menopause in women can have natural, surgical, or chemical causes. Chemical menopause in women with cancer is caused by certain types of chemotherapy, radiation, or hormone therapy (HT) with androgen (a male hormone).

"Male menopause" in men with cancer can be caused by orchiectomy (surgery to remove one or both testicles) or HT with gonadotropin-releasing hormone or estrogen. Treatment for breast cancer and prostate cancer can cause menopause or menopause-like effects, including severe hot flashes.

Certain types of drugs can cause night sweats. Drugs that may cause night sweats include the following:

- Tamoxifen
- Aromatase inhibitors (AI)
- Opioids
- Tricyclic antidepressants
- Steroids

Drug Treatment for Hot Flashes and Night Sweats in Breast-Cancer Patients

Sweats are controlled by treating their cause. It is caused by fever are controlled by treating the cause of the fever. Sweats caused by a tumor are usually controlled by treatment of the tumor.

Hot flashes may be controlled with estrogen-replacement therapy. Hot flashes during natural or treatment-related menopause can be controlled with estrogen-replacement therapy. However, many women are not able to take estrogen replacement (for example, women who have or had breast cancer). Hormone-replacement therapy (HRT) that combines estrogen with progestin may increase the risk of breast cancer or breast-cancer recurrence.

Other drugs may be useful in some patients. Studies of nonestrogen drugs to treat hot flashes in women with a history of breast cancer have reported that many of them do not work as well as estrogen replacement or have side effects. Megestrol (a drug like progesterone), certain antidepressants, anticonvulsants, and clonidine (a drug used to treat high blood pressure) are nonestrogen drugs used to control hot flashes. Some antidepressants may change how other drugs, such as tamoxifen, work in the body. Side effects of drug therapy may include the following:

- **Antidepressants** used to treat hot flashes over a short period of time may cause nausea, drowsiness, dry mouth, and changes in appetite.

- **Anticonvulsants** used to treat hot flashes may cause drowsiness, dizziness, and trouble concentrating.

- **Clonidine** may cause dry mouth, drowsiness, constipation, and insomnia.

Patients may respond in different ways to drug therapy. It is important that the patient's healthcare providers know about all medicines, dietary supplements, and herbs the patient is taking.

Drugs that may relieve nighttime hot flashes or night sweats and improve sleep at the same time are being studied in clinical trials.

If one medicine does not improve symptoms, switching to another medicine may help.

Nondrug Treatment for Hot Flashes and Night Sweats in Breast-Cancer Patients

Treatments that change how patients deal with stress, anxiety, and negative emotions may help manage hot flashes. These are called "psychological interventions." Psychological interventions help patients gain a sense of control and develop coping skills to manage symptoms. Staying calm and managing stress may lower levels of a hormone called serotonin that can trigger hot flashes.

Psychological interventions may help hot flashes and related problems when used together with drug treatment.

Hypnosis may help relieve hot flashes. It is a trance-like state that allows a person to be more aware, focused, and open to suggestion. Under hypnosis, the person can concentrate more clearly on a specific thought, feeling, or sensation without becoming distracted.

Hypnosis is a newer treatment for hot flashes that has been shown to be helpful. In hypnosis, a therapist helps the patient to deeply relax and focus on calming thoughts. This may lower stress levels, balance body temperature, and calm the heart rate and breathing rate.

Comfort measures may help relieve night sweats related to cancer. It may be used to treat night sweats related to cancer. Since body temperature goes up before a hot flash, doing the following may control body temperature and help control symptoms:

- Wear loose-fitting clothes made of cotton

- Use fans and open windows to keep air moving

- Practice relaxation training and slow, deep breathing

Herbs and dietary supplements should be used with caution. Studies of vitamin E for the relief of hot flashes show that it is only slightly better than a placebo (pill that has no effect). Most studies of soy and black cohosh show they are no better than a placebo in reducing hot flashes. Soy contains estrogen-like substances; the effect of soy on the risk of breast-cancer growth or recurrence is not clear. Studies of ground flaxseed to treat hot flashes have shown mixed results.

Claims are made about several other plant-based and natural products as remedies for hot flashes. These include dong quai, milk thistle, red clover, licorice root extract, and chaste tree berry. Since little is known about how these products work or whether they affect the risk of breast cancer, women should be cautious about using them.

Acupuncture has been studied in the treatment of hot flashes. Pilot studies of acupuncture and randomized clinical trials that compare true acupuncture and sham (inactive) treatment have been done in patients with hot flashes and results are mixed. A review of many studies combined showed that acupuncture had slight or no effects in breast-cancer patients with hot flashes.

Chapter 62

Infection and Neutropenia

An infection is the invasion and growth of germs in the body, such as bacteria, viruses, yeast, or other fungi. An infection can begin anywhere in the body, may spread throughout the body, and can cause one or more of these signs:

- Fever of 100.5°F (38°C) or higher or chills

- A cough or a sore throat

- Diarrhea

- Ear pain, headache or sinus pain, or a stiff or sore neck

- Skin rash

- Sores or white coating in your mouth or on your tongue

- Swelling or redness, especially where a catheter enters your body

- Urine that is bloody or cloudy, or pain when you urinate

Call your healthcare team if you have signs of an infection. Infections during cancer treatment can be life-threatening and require urgent medical attention. Be sure to talk with your doctor or nurse before taking medicine—even aspirin, acetaminophen (such as Tylenol®),

---

This chapter includes text excerpted from "Infection and Neutropenia during Cancer Treatment," National Cancer Institute (NCI), September 14, 2018.

or ibuprofen (such as Advil®) for a fever. These medicines can lower a fever but may also mask or hide signs of a more serious problem.

Some types of cancer and treatments such as chemotherapy may increase your risk of infection. This is because they lower the number of white blood cells (WBCs), the cells that help your body to fight infection. During chemotherapy, there will be times in your treatment cycle when the number of WBCs (called "neutrophils") is particularly low and you are at increased risk of infection. Stress, poor nutrition, and not enough sleep can also weaken the immune system, making infection more likely.

You will have blood tests to check for neutropenia (a condition in which there is a low number of neutrophils). Medicine may sometimes be given to help prevent infection or to increase the number of WBCs.

Ways to Prevent Infection

Your healthcare team will talk with you about these and other ways to prevent infection:

- **Wash your hands often and well.** Use soap and warm water to wash your hands well, especially before eating. Have people around you wash their hands well too.

- **Stay extra clean.** If you have a catheter, keep the area around it clean and dry. Clean your teeth well and check your mouth for sores or other signs of infection each day. If you get a scrape or cut, clean it well. Let your doctor or nurse know if your bottom is sore or bleeds, as this could increase your risk of infection.

- **Avoid germs.** Stay away from people who are sick or have a cold. Avoid crowds and people who have just had a live vaccine, such as one for chicken pox, polio, or measles. Follow food-safety guidelines; make sure the meat, fish, and eggs you eat are well cooked. Keep hot foods hot and cold foods cold. You may be advised to eat only fruits and vegetables that can be peeled or to wash all raw fruits and vegetables very well.

Talking with Your Healthcare Team about Infection

Prepare for your visit by making a list of questions to ask regarding infection. Consider adding these questions to your list:

- Am I at increased risk of infection during treatment? When am I at increased risk?

- What steps should I take to prevent infection?

- What signs of infection should I look for?

- Which signs signal that I need urgent medical care at the emergency room? Which should I call you about?

Chapter 63

Lymphedema

Lymphedema is a condition in which the lymph fluid does not drain properly. It may build up in the tissues and causes swelling. This can happen when part of the lymph system is damaged or blocked, such as during surgery to remove lymph nodes or radiation therapy. Cancers that block lymph vessels can also cause lymphedema.

Lymphedema usually affects an arm or leg, but it can also affect other parts of the body, such as the head and neck. You may notice symptoms of lymphedema at the part of your body where you had surgery or received radiation therapy. Swelling usually develops slowly, over time. It may develop during treatment or it may start years after treatment.

At first, lymphedema in an arm or leg may cause symptoms such as:

- Swelling and a heavy or achy feeling in your arms or legs that may spread to your fingers and toes

- A dent when you press on the swollen area

- Swelling that is soft to the touch and is usually not painful at first

Lymphedema that is not controlled may cause:

- More swelling, weakness, and difficulty moving your arm or leg

- Itchy, red, warm skin, and sometimes a rash

This chapter includes text excerpted from "Lymphedema and Cancer Treatment," National Cancer Institute (NCI), April 29, 2015. Reviewed February 2019.

- Wounds that don't heal, and an increased risk of skin infections that may cause pain, redness, and swelling

- Thickening or hardening of the skin

- Tight feeling in the skin; pressing on the swollen area does not leave a dent

- Hair loss

Lymphedema in the head or neck may cause:

- Swelling and a tight uncomfortable feeling on your face, neck, or under your chin

- Difficulty moving your head or neck

Tell your healthcare team as soon as you notice symptoms. Early treatment may prevent or reduce the severity of problems caused by lymphedema.

Ways to Manage Lymphedema

Steps you may be advised to take to prevent lymphedema or to keep it from getting worse:

- **Protect your skin.** Use lotion to avoid dry skin. Use sunscreen. Wear plastic gloves with cotton lining when working in order to prevent scratches, cuts, or burns. Keep your feet clean and dry. Keep your nails clean and short to prevent ingrown nails and infection. Avoid tight shoes and tight jewelry.

- **Exercise.** Work to keep body fluids moving, especially in places where lymphedema has developed. Start with gentle exercises that help you to move and contract your muscles. Ask your doctor or nurse what exercises are best for you.

- **Manual lymph drainage.** See a trained specialist (a certified lymphedema therapist) to receive a type of therapeutic massage called "manual lymph drainage" (MLD). Therapeutic massage works best to lower lymphedema when given early, before symptoms progress.

Ways to Treat Lymphedema

Your doctor or nurse may advise you to take these and other steps to treat lymphedema:

- **Wear compression garments or bandages.** Wear special garments, such as sleeves, stockings, bras, compression shorts, gloves, bandages, and face or neck compression wear. Some garments are meant to be worn during the day, while others are to be worn at night.

- **Other practices.** Your healthcare team may advise you to use compression devices (special pumps that apply pressure periodically) or have laser therapy or other treatments.

Talking with Your Healthcare Team about Lymphedema

Prepare for your visit by making a list of questions to ask. Consider adding these questions to your list:

- What can I do to prevent these problems?

- What symptoms should I call you about?

- What steps can I take to feel better?

- Would you recommend that I see a certified lymphedema therapist?

- If lymphedema advances, what special garments should I wear during the day and during the night?

Chapter 64

Mouth and Throat Problems

Cancer treatments may cause dental, mouth, and throat problems. Radiation therapy to the head and neck may harm the salivary glands and tissues in your mouth and/or make it hard to chew and swallow safely. Some types of chemotherapy and immunotherapy can also harm cells in your mouth, throat, and lips. Drugs used to treat breast cancer and certain bone problems may also cause oral complications.

Mouth and throat problems may include:

- Changes in taste (dysgeusia) or smell

- Dry mouth (xerostomia)

- Infections and mouth sores

- Pain or swelling in your mouth (oral mucositis)

- Sensitivity to hot or cold foods

- Swallowing problems (dysphagia)

- Tooth decay (cavities)

Mouth problems are more serious if they interfere with eating and drinking because they can lead to dehydration and/or malnutrition. It's important to call your doctor or nurse if you have pain in your mouth, lips, or throat that makes it difficult to eat, drink, or sleep or if you have a fever of 100.5°F (38°C) or higher.

This chapter includes text excerpted from "Mouth and Throat Problems during Cancer Treatment," National Cancer Institute (NCI), August 9, 2018.

Ways to Prevent Mouth and Dental Problems

Your doctor or nurse may advise you to take these and other steps:

- **Get a dental check-up before starting treatment.** Before you start treatment, visit your dentist for a cleaning and check-up. Tell the dentist about your cancer treatment and try to get any dental work completed before starting treatment.

- **Check and clean your mouth daily.** Check your mouth every day for sores or white spots. Tell your doctor or nurse as soon as you notice any changes, such as pain or sensitivity. Rinse your mouth throughout the day with a solution of warm water, baking soda, and salt. Ask your nurse to write down the mouth rinse recipe that is recommended for you. Gently brush your teeth, gums, and tongue after each meal and before going to bed at night. Use a very soft toothbrush or cotton swabs. If you are at risk of bleeding, ask if you should floss.

Ways to Manage Mouth Problems and Changes in Taste

Your healthcare team may suggest that you take these and other steps to manage these problems:

- **Sore mouth or throat.** Choose foods that are soft, wet, and easy to swallow. Soften dry foods with gravy, sauce, or other liquids. Use a blender to make milkshakes or blend your food to make it easier to swallow. Ask about pain medicine, such as lozenges or sprays that numb your mouth and make eating less painful. Avoid foods and drinks that can irritate your mouth; foods that are crunchy, salty, spicy, or sugary; and alcoholic drinks. Don't smoke or use tobacco products.

- **Dry mouth.** Drink plenty of liquids because a dry mouth can increase the risk of tooth decay and mouth infections. Keep water handy and sip it often to keep your mouth wet. Suck on ice chips or sugar-free hard candy, have frozen desserts, or chew sugar-free gum. Use a lip balm. Ask about medicines such as saliva substitutes that can coat, protect, and moisten your mouth and throat. Acupuncture may also help with dry mouth.

- **Changes to your sense of taste.** Foods may seem to have no taste or may not taste the way they used to or food may not have much taste at all. Radiation therapy may cause a change in sweet, sour, bitter, and salty tastes. Chemotherapy drugs may cause an unpleasant chemical or metallic taste in your mouth. If you have taste changes it may help to try different foods to find ones that taste best to you. Trying cold foods may also help. Here are some more tips to consider:

- If food tastes bland, marinate foods to improve their flavor or add spices to foods.

- If red meat tastes strange, switch to other high-protein foods such as chicken, eggs, fish, peanut butter, turkey, beans, or dairy products.

- If foods taste salty, bitter, or acidic, try sweetening them.

- If foods taste metallic, switch to plastic utensils and nonmetal cooking dishes.

- If you have a bad taste in your mouth, try sugar-free lemon drops, gum, or mints.

Talking with Your Healthcare Team about Mouth and Throat Problems

Prepare for your visit by making a list of questions to ask. Consider adding these questions to your list:

- When might these problems start to occur? How long might they last?

- What steps can I take to feel better?

- What medicines can help?

- What symptoms or problems should I call the doctor about?

- What pain medicine and/or mouthwashes could help me?

- Would you recommend a registered dietitian who I could see to learn about good food choices?

Chapter 65

Nausea and Vomiting

Nausea is when you feel sick to your stomach as if you are going to throw up. Vomiting is when you throw up. There are different types of nausea and vomiting caused by cancer treatment, including anticipatory, acute, and delayed nausea and vomiting. Controlling nausea and vomiting will help you to feel better and prevent more serious problems such as malnutrition and dehydration.

Your doctor or nurse will determine what is causing your symptoms and advise you on ways to prevent them. Medicines called "antinausea drugs" or "antiemetics" are effective in preventing or reducing many types of nausea and vomiting. The medicine is taken at specific times to prevent and/or control symptoms of nausea and vomiting. There are also practical steps you may be advised to take to feel better, including those listed below.

Ways to Manage Nausea and Vomiting

You may be advised to take these steps to feel better:

- **Take an antinausea medicine.** Talk with your doctor or nurse to learn when to take your medicine. Most people need to take an antinausea medicine even on days when they feel well. Tell your doctor or nurse if the medicine doesn't help. There are different kinds of medicine and one may work better than another for you.

This chapter includes text excerpted from "Nausea and Vomiting in People with Cancer," National Cancer Institute (NCI), August 9, 2018.

- **Drink plenty of water and fluids.** Drinking will help to prevent dehydration, a serious problem that happens when your body loses too much fluid and you are not drinking enough. Try to sip on water, fruit juices, ginger ale, tea, and/or sports drinks throughout the day.

- **Avoid certain foods.** Don't eat greasy, fried, sweet, or spicy foods if you feel sick after eating them. If the smell of food bothers you, ask others to make your food. Try cold foods that do not have strong smells, or let food cool down before you eat it.

- **Try these tips on treatment days.** Some people find that it helps to eat a small snack before treatment. Others avoid eating or drinking right before or after treatment because it makes them feel sick. After treatment, wait at least one hour before you eat or drink.

- **Learn about complementary medicine practices that may help.** Acupuncture relieves nausea and/or vomiting caused by chemotherapy in some people. Deep breathing, guided imagery, hypnosis, and other relaxation techniques (such as listening to music, reading a book, or meditating) also help some people.

Talking with Your Healthcare Team about Nausea and Vomiting

Prepare for your visit by making a list of questions to ask. Consider adding these questions to your list:

- What symptoms or problems should I call you about?

- What medicine could help me? When should I take this medicine?

- How much liquid should I drink each day? What should I do if I throw up?

- What foods would be easy on my stomach? What foods should I avoid?

- Could I meet with a registered dietitian to learn more?

- What specialists could I see to learn about acupuncture and other practices that could help to lower my symptoms?

Chapter 66

Nerve Problems and Cancer Treatment

People with nerve problems caused by cancer treatment need to take care to prevent falls. Sometimes integrative medicine practices, advised by your doctor, can also help you to feel better.

Some breast cancer treatments cause peripheral neuropathy, a result of damage to the peripheral nerves. These nerves carry information from the brain to other parts of the body. Side effects depend on which peripheral nerves (sensory, motor, or autonomic) are affected.

Damage to sensory nerves (nerves that help you feel pain, heat, cold, and pressure) can cause:

- Tingling, numbness, or a pins-and-needles feeling in your feet and hands that may spread to your legs and arms

- Inability to feel a hot or cold sensation, such as a hot stove

- Inability to feel pain, such as from a cut or sore on your foot

Damage to motor nerves (nerves that help your muscles to move) can cause:

- Weak or achy muscles. You may lose your balance or trip easily. It may also be difficult to button shirts or open jars.

This chapter includes text excerpted from "Nerve Problems (Peripheral Neuropathy) and Cancer Treatment," National Cancer Institute (NCI), August 9, 2018.

- Muscles that twitch and cramp or muscle wasting (if you don't use your muscles regularly).

- Swallowing or breathing difficulties (if your chest or throat muscles are affected)

Damage to autonomic nerves (nerves that control functions such as blood pressure, digestion, heart rate, temperature, and urination) can cause:

- Digestive changes such as constipation or diarrhea

- Dizzy or faint feeling, due to low blood pressure

- Sexual problems; men may be unable to get an erection and women may not reach orgasm

- Sweating problems (either too much or too little sweating)

- Urination problems, such as leaking urine or difficulty emptying your bladder

If you start to notice any of the problems listed above, talk with your doctor or nurse. Getting these problems diagnosed and treated early is the best way to control them, prevent further damage, and to reduce pain and other complications.

Ways to Prevent or Manage Problems Related to Nerve Changes

You may be advised to take these steps:

- **Prevent falls.** Have someone help you prevent falls around the house. Move rugs out of your path so you will not trip on them. Put rails on the walls and in the bathroom, so you can hold on to them and balance yourself. Put bathmats in the shower or tub. Wear sturdy shoes with soft soles. Get up slowly after sitting or lying down, especially if you feel dizzy.

- **Take extra care in the kitchen and shower.** Use potholders in the kitchen to protect your hands from burns. Be careful when handling knives or sharp objects. Ask someone to check the water temperature, to make sure it's not too hot.

- **Protect your hands and feet.** Wear shoes, both inside and outside. Check your arms, legs, and feet for cuts or scratches every day. When it's cold, wear warm clothes to protect your hands and feet.

- **Ask for help and slow down**. Let people help you with difficult tasks. Slow down and give yourself more time to do things.

- **Ask about pain medicine and integrative medicine practices.** You may be prescribed pain medicine. Sometimes practices such as acupuncture, massage, physical therapy, yoga, and others may also be advised to lower pain. Talk with your healthcare team to learn what is advised for you.

Talking with Your Healthcare Team

Prepare for your visit by making a list of questions to ask. Consider adding these questions to your list:

- What symptoms or problems might I have? Which ones should I call you about?

- When will these problems start? How long might they last?

- What medicine, treatments, and integrative medicine practices could help me to feel better?

- What steps can I take to feel better? What precautions should I take to stay safe?

- Could you refer me to a specialist who could give me additional advice?

Chapter 67

Osteoporosis

The Impact of Breast Cancer

Other than skin cancer, breast cancer is the most common cancer in women. It can occur in both men and women, but it is very rare in men. Although the exact cause is not known, the risk of developing breast cancer increases with age. The risk is particularly high in women age 60 and older. Because of their age, these women are already at increased risk for osteoporosis. Given the rising incidence of breast cancer and the improvement of long-term survival rates, bone health and fracture prevention have become important health issues among breast cancer survivors.

Facts about Osteoporosis

Osteoporosis is a condition in which the bones become less dense and more likely to fracture. Fractures from osteoporosis can result in significant pain and disability. In the United States, more than 53 million people either already have osteoporosis or are at high risk due to low bone mass.

Risk factors for developing osteoporosis include:

- Thinness or small frame

- Family history of the disease

This chapter includes text excerpted from "What Breast Cancer Survivors Need to Know about Osteoporosis," NIH Osteoporosis and Related Bone Diseases— National Resource Center (NIH ORBD—NRC), April 2016.

- Being postmenopausal and particularly having had early menopause

- Abnormal absence of menstrual periods (amenorrhea)

- Prolonged use of certain medications, such as those used to treat lupus, asthma, thyroid deficiencies, and seizures

- Low calcium intake

- Lack of physical activity

- Smoking

- Excessive alcohol intake

Osteoporosis often can be prevented. It is known as a silent disease because, if undetected, bone loss can progress for many years without symptoms until a fracture occurs. Osteoporosis has been called a "childhood disease with old age consequences" because building healthy bones in youth helps prevent osteoporosis and fractures later in life. However, it is never too late to adopt new habits for healthy bones.

The Link between Breast Cancer and Osteoporosis

Women who have had breast-cancer treatment may be at increased risk for osteoporosis and fracture. Estrogen has a protective effect on bone, and reduced levels of the hormone trigger bone loss. Because of treatment medications or surgery, many breast-cancer survivors experience a loss of ovarian function and, consequently, a drop in estrogen levels. Women who were premenopausal before their cancer treatment may go through menopause earlier than those who have not had breast cancer. Results from the National Institutes of Health (NIH)-supported Women's Health Initiative Observational Study (WHI-OS) found an increase in fracture risk among breast-cancer survivors.

Ways to Manage Osteoporosis

Several strategies can reduce one's risk for osteoporosis or lessen the effects of the disease in women who have already been diagnosed.

Nutrition. Some studies have found a link between diet and breast cancer. However, it is not yet clear which foods or supplements may play a role in reducing breast cancer risk. As far as bone health is concerned, a well-balanced diet rich in calcium and vitamin D is important. Good sources of calcium include low-fat dairy products; dark green, leafy vegetables; and calcium-fortified foods and beverages. Supplements can help ensure that the calcium requirement is met each day, especially in people with a proven milk allergy. The Institute of Medicine (IOM) recommends a daily calcium intake of 1,000 mg (milligrams) for men and women up to age 50. Women over age 50 and men over age 70 should increase their intake to 1,200 mg daily.

Vitamin D plays an important role in calcium absorption and bone health. Food sources of vitamin D include egg yolks, saltwater fish, and liver. Many people, especially those who are older or housebound, may need vitamin D supplements to achieve the recommended intake of 600 to 800 IU (International Units) each day.

Exercise. Like muscle, bone is living tissue that responds to exercise by becoming stronger. The best activity for your bones is weight-bearing exercise that forces you to work against gravity. Some examples include walking, climbing stairs, weight training, and dancing. Regular exercise, such as walking, may help prevent bone loss and will provide many other health benefits. Research suggests that exercise also may reduce breast-cancer risk in younger women.

Healthy lifestyle. Smoking is bad for bones as well as the heart and lungs. Women who smoke tend to go through menopause earlier, resulting in earlier reduction in levels of the bone-preserving hormone estrogen and triggering earlier bone loss. In addition, smokers may absorb less calcium from their diets. Some studies have found a slightly higher risk of breast cancer in women who drink alcohol, and evidence suggests that alcohol can have a negative effect on bone health. Those who drink heavily are more prone to bone loss and fracture, because of both poor nutrition and an increased risk of falling.

Bone density test. A bone mineral density (BMD) test measures bone density in various parts of the body. This safe and painless test can detect osteoporosis before a fracture occurs and can predict one's chances of fracturing in the future. The BMD test can help determine whether medication should be considered. A woman recovering from breast cancer should ask her doctor whether she might be a candidate for a bone density test.

Medication. There is no cure for osteoporosis. However, several medications are available to prevent and treat this disease. Bisphosphonates, a class of osteoporosis treatment medications, have demonstrated some success in their ability to treat breast cancers that have spread to bone.

Another osteoporosis treatment medication, raloxifene, is a selective estrogen receptor modulator (SERM) that has been shown to reduce the risk of breast cancer in women with osteoporosis. The NIH's Study of Tamoxifen and Raloxifene (STAR) found that raloxifene was as effective as tamoxifen in reducing the risk of postmenopausal breast cancer in high-risk women.

Chapter 68

Pain

Cancer itself and the side effects of cancer treatment can sometimes cause pain. Pain is not something that you have to "put up with." Controlling pain is an important part of your cancer treatment plan. Pain can suppress the immune system, increase the time it takes your body to heal, interfere with sleep, and affect your mood.

Talk with your healthcare team about pain, especially if:

- The pain isn't getting better or going away with pain medicine
- The pain comes on quickly
- The pain makes it hard to eat, sleep, or perform your normal activities
- You feel new pain
- You have side effects from the pain medicine such as sleepiness, nausea, or constipation

Your doctor will work with you to develop a pain control plan that is based on your description of the pain. Taking pain medicine is an important part of the plan. Your doctor will talk with you about using drugs to control pain and prescribe medicine (including opioids and nonopioid medicines) to treat the pain.

This chapter includes text excerpted from "Pain in People with Cancer," National Cancer Institute (NCI), August 9, 2018.

Ways to Treat or Lessen Pain

Here are some steps you can take, as you work with your healthcare team to prevent, treat, or lessen pain:

- **Keep track of your pain levels.** Each day, write about any pain you feel. Writing down answers to the questions below will help you describe the pain to your doctor or nurse.

  - What part of your body feels painful?

  - What does the pain feel like (is it sharp, burning, shooting, or throbbing) and where do you feel the pain?

  - When does the pain start? How long does the pain last?

  - What activities (such as eating, sleeping, or other activities) does pain interfere with?

  - What makes the pain feel better or worse? For example, do ice packs, heating pads, or exercises help? Does pain medicine help? How much do you take? How often do you take it?

  - How bad is the pain, on a scale of 1 to 10, where "10" is the most pain and "1" is the least pain?

- **Take the prescribed pain medicine.** Take the right amount of medicine at the right time. Do not wait until your pain gets too bad before taking pain medicine. Waiting to take your medicine could make it take longer for the pain to go away or increase the amount of medicine needed to lower pain. Do not stop taking the pain medicine unless your doctor advises you to. Tell your doctor or nurse if the medicine no longer lowers the pain, or if you are in pain, but it's not yet time to take the pain medicine.

- **Meet with a pain specialist.** Specialists who treat pain often work together as part of pain or palliative care team. These specialists may include a neurologist, surgeon, physiatrist, psychiatrist, psychologist, or pharmacist. Talk with your healthcare team to find a pain specialist.

- **Ask about integrative medicine.** Treatments such as acupuncture, biofeedback, hypnosis, massage therapy, and physical therapy may also be used to treat pain.

Talking with Your Healthcare Team about Pain

Prepare for your visit by making a list of questions to ask. Consider adding these questions to your list:

- What problems or levels of pain should I call you about?

- What is most likely causing the pain?

- What can I do to lessen the pain?

- What medicine should I take? If the pain doesn't go away, how much more medicine can I take, and when can I take it?

- What are the side effects of this pain medicine? How long will they last?

- Is there a pain specialist I could meet with to get more support to lower my pain?

Chapter 69

Complementary and Alternative Medicine Therapies Used for the Side Effects of Breast Cancer and Its Treatment

Chapter Contents

Section 69.1

Acupuncture May Reduce Treatment-Related Joint Pain for Breast-Cancer Patients

This section includes text excerpted from "Acupuncture
May Reduce Treatment-Related Joint Pain for Breast Cancer
Patients," National Cancer Institute (NCI), January 8, 2018.

Acupuncture can reduce joint pain caused by drugs called "aromatase inhibitors" (AI), according to results from a large, rigorous study of this approach in postmenopausal women (PMW) with early-stage breast cancer.

Many women with hormone receptor (HR)-positive early breast cancers, which rely on estrogen (ER) to fuel tumor growth, take AIs after surgery to reduce their risk of cancer recurring. These drugs, which block estrogen (ER) production, are also used to prevent breast cancer in PMW at high risk for the disease and to treat HR-positive metastatic breast cancer.

"About 50 percent of patients on these medications complain of some joint pain or stiffness, and about half of those patients describe the pain as severe," causing some women to stop taking the drugs, said the trial's lead investigator, Dawn Hershman, M.D., of Columbia University Medical Center (CUMC).

Several small studies have suggested that acupuncture may alleviate aromatase inhibitor-related joint pain and stiffness, although others have shown no benefit, said Dr. Hershman, who presented the findings of the new study at the San Antonio Breast Cancer Symposium (SABCS). She and her colleagues designed their large study to get a clearer answer to the question of whether acupuncture can relieve AI-related pain.

"Identifying interventions to address AI-induced joint pain is essential but has been lacking to date. This trial demonstrated that, compared with a placebo, acupuncture may provide a durable, non-pharmacologic option for improving the musculoskeletal symptoms (MSD) experienced by these patients," said Raquel Reinbolt, M.D., a medical oncologist specializing in breast cancer with The Ohio State University Comprehensive Cancer Center (OSUCCC), who was not involved with the study.

"Reducing the drug toxicity experience may then translate into improved adherence (to therapy), and ultimately, improved breast cancer outcomes," Dr. Reinbolt said.

And, having acupuncture, along with engaging with the acupuncturist, as an alternative or in addition to taking prescription pain medications may help patients feel empowered to manage joint pain that can occur as a side effect of their cancer treatment, said Ann O'Mara, Ph.D., R.N., head of palliative care research in National Cancer Institute's (NCI), Division of Cancer Prevention (DCP).

"A major strength of the study is that it was a multisite trial and included many patients from general oncology practices, not just from university medical centers," Dr. O'Mara noted. This means the results are likely to be broadly generalizable to women in the community.

Pain Relief Continued after Treatments Ended

The clinical trial was led by the NCI-funded Southwest Oncology Group (SWOG) and carried out at 11 sites that participate in the NCI's Community Oncology Research Program (NCORP). The 226 women in the trial were all taking a third-generation aromatase inhibitor—anastrozole (Arimidex®), letrozole (Femara®), or exemestane (Aromasin®)—after surgery for early-stage HR-positive breast cancer and were randomly assigned to receive true acupuncture, sham acupuncture (placebo), or no treatment. Sham acupuncture involves shallow insertion of short, thin needles at nonacupuncture points.

All acupuncturists involved in the study were licensed and were rigorously trained on site by an acupuncturist on the study team. They were monitored for quality of care throughout the study.

To be enrolled in the study, women could not have taken opioid or corticosteroid drugs or received any alternative or physical therapy for AI-related joint pain in the past four weeks. Notably, Dr. Hershman said, 80 percent of the patients in the study were taking over-the-counter (OTC) acetaminophen or ibuprofen for joint pain without experiencing relief.

Roughly half of the study participants (110) received true acupuncture twice a week for six weeks, followed by once-a-week maintenance sessions for 6 more weeks. The other half were in one of two control groups: 59 received sham acupuncture on the same schedule as the true acupuncture group, and the remaining 57 received no treatment.

The no-treatment group was included to control for any possible benefits or possible negative effects of the sham acupuncture, Dr. Hershman explained.

Study investigators followed the women for another 12 weeks after treatments ended. Patients reported on their pain before, during, and after treatment using various methods, including a questionnaire on

419

which women could indicate a rating of "worst pain" on a scale of 0 to 10.

After 6 weeks, "we saw a mean two-point reduction of worst pain (in the true-acupuncture group compared with worst pain before treatment), which is a major reduction," and these effects were maintained after 12 weeks, Dr. Hershman said.

Moreover, "even at 24 weeks, women in the true-acupuncture group had less pain overall than women in either (control) group," Dr. Hershman added.

The main side effect of true and sham acupuncture was mild bruising, which was more common in the true-acupuncture group than in the sham-acupuncture group.

Patients in both the sham-acupuncture and no-treatment groups reported a roughly one-point mean reduction in worst pain at six weeks. Although it's not clear why the control groups also saw an improvement, Dr. Hershman said that, in symptom-management studies where patients are monitored and assessed over time, researchers often see an improvement of symptoms in the control group.

More Investigations Planned

The new findings should make healthcare providers more likely to suggest acupuncture to their patients, Dr. Hershman said.

"Acupuncture is a safe and effective alternative approach for managing aromatase inhibitor-induced joint pain. The primary limitations of this treatment at the current time are cost and availability. Hopefully, this (new) data will generate additional discussion regarding reimbursement (by medical insurance) and access to treatment," Dr. Reinbolt said.

One possible limitation of the study, Dr. O'Mara said, is that most participants (88%) were white, despite the inclusion of patients from across the United States. Only 5 percent and 7 percent of participants, respectively, were black or Asian.

As usual, some questions remain. "If you start having aches and pains, should you go back (for more acupuncture sessions)? Should you continue with, say, once-a-week treatments until you finish taking aromatase inhibitors?" Dr. O'Mara asked.

The team is not planning to pursue those questions. But, Dr. Hershman said, "We offered everybody 10 acupuncture sessions at the end of 24 weeks, regardless of which group they were in, and we'll be doing a separate analysis to see how many patients in each group accepted the offer."

The team also plans to use tissue samples that they collected from patients throughout the trial to gain a better understanding of what causes aromatase inhibitor-related joint symptoms, "and what the mechanism of acupuncture may be in terms of providing pain relief," Dr. Hershman said.

Section 69.2

Hypnosis May Reduce Hot Flashes in Breast-Cancer Survivors

This section includes text excerpted from "Hypnosis May Reduce Hot Flashes in Breast Cancer Survivors," National Cancer Institute (NCI), February 2, 2015. Reviewed February 2019.

Hot flashes are a problem for many menopausal women and a common side effect of breast cancer treatment. For many breast cancer survivors, vasomotor symptoms result in discomfort, disrupted sleep, anxiety, and decreased the quality of life (QOL). Hormonal (estrogen (ER)) drugs have been used to treat hot flashes, but because estrogens are associated with an increased risk of breast cancer, they usually are avoided by breast cancer survivors. Since nonhormonal treatments do not work for some women and may have adverse effects, new interventions for hot flashes are needed. Previous research has indicated that hypnosis may be a promising alternative.

In a study, researchers funded by the National Cancer Institute (NCI) and National Center for Complementary and Alternative Medicine (NCCAM) investigated the effects of hypnosis on hot flashes among women with a history of primary breast cancer, no current evidence of detectable disease, and at least 14 hot flashes per week over a 1-month period. Sixty women were assigned to receive either hypnosis (weekly 50-minute sessions, plus instructions for at-home self-hypnosis) or no treatment; 51 women completed the 5-week study.

The women who received hypnosis had a 68-percent reduction in self-reported hot flash frequency/severity and experienced an average of 4.39 fewer hot flashes per day. Compared with controls, they also had significant improvements in self-reported anxiety, depression, interference with daily activities, and sleep.

The researchers concluded that hypnosis appears to reduce perceived hot flashes in breast cancer survivors and may have additional benefits such as improved mood and sleep. They recommend long-term, randomized, placebo-controlled studies to further explore the benefits of hypnosis for breast cancer survivors. The researchers are currently conducting a randomized clinical trial (RCT) with 200 participants.

Section 69.3

Yoga for Relief from Fatigue

This section includes text excerpted from "Iyengar Yoga May Improve Fatigue in Breast Cancer Survivors," National Cancer Institute (NCI), September 24, 2017.

Yoga may help improve fatigue and vigor in breast cancer survivors, according to a National Center for Complementary and Integrative Health (NCCIH)-funded study published in the journal Cancer. Data from the National Cancer Institute (NCI) suggest that fatigue may be a significant issue long into cancer survivorship.

Researchers from the University of California at Los Angeles (LA) randomly assigned 31 breast-cancer survivors (all postmenopausal women (PMW)) with persistent, cancer-related fatigue to participate for 12 weeks in either Iyengar yoga classes targeted at improving fatigue or health education classes. Iyengar yoga is a type of hatha yoga involving body postures and breath control; the yoga classes were conducted for 90 minutes twice a week. The health education classes consisted of lectures on topics such as cancer-related fatigue and psychosocial issues in cancer survivorship and were conducted for 120 minutes once a week. Neither group was instructed to do home practice or reading.

At 12 weeks, and 3 months after the treatment was completed, participants in the yoga group reported significant improvements in the severity of fatigue, compared with those in the health education group. Similar benefits were observed for participants' vigor; the yoga group had a significant increase in vigor compared with the health education group during this time period. Both groups also had comparable declines in depressive symptoms and perceived stress by the 3-month follow-up; however, no significant changes in sleep or physical performance were observed.

The researchers noted several limitations of the study, including the small number of participants and the restriction of participants to women with a diagnosis of early-stage disease and who had completed cancer treatment. Therefore, the beneficial effects from this study may not necessarily apply to breast cancer survivors with more advanced disease or who are currently undergoing treatment. Further, the researchers suggested that because the total number of class hours for yoga (36 hours) was greater than that for health education (24 hours), it is possible that the benefits observed in the yoga group may be attributable in part to the higher number of participation hours. The researchers concluded that future studies are needed and noted that yoga's effects on the immune and neuroendocrine systems are currently being investigated among the participants in this study.

Section 69.4

Spirituality in Cancer Care

This section includes text excerpted from "Spirituality in Cancer Care (PDQ®)—Patient Version," National Cancer Institute (NCI), May 18, 2015. Reviewed February 2019.

Coping with Cancer and the Role of Spirituality

Studies have shown that religious and spiritual values are important to Americans. Most American adults say that they believe in a higher power and that their religious beliefs affect how they live their lives. However, people have different ideas about life after death, belief in miracles, and other religious beliefs. Such beliefs may be based on gender, education, and ethnic background.

Many patients with cancer rely on spiritual or religious beliefs and practices to help them cope with their disease. This is called "spiritual coping." Many caregivers also rely on spiritual coping. Each person may have different spiritual needs, depending on cultural and religious traditions. For some seriously ill patients, spiritual well-being may affect how much anxiety they feel about death. For others, it may affect what they decide about end-of-life treatments. Some patients and their family caregivers may want doctors to talk about spiritual concerns but may feel unsure about how to bring up the subject.

Some studies show that doctors' support of spiritual well-being in very ill patients helps improve their quality of life (QOL). Healthcare providers who treat patients coping with cancer are looking at new ways to help them with religious and spiritual concerns. Doctors may ask patients which spiritual issues are important to them during treatment as well as near the end-of-life. When patients with advanced cancer receive spiritual support from the medical team, they may be more likely to choose hospice care and less aggressive treatment at the end-of-life.

Spirituality and Religion May Have Different Meanings

The terms "spirituality" and "religion" are often used in place of each other, but for many people, they have different meanings. Religion may be defined as a specific set of beliefs and practices, usually within an organized group. Spirituality may be defined as an individual's sense of peace, purpose, and connection to others, and beliefs about the meaning of life. Spirituality may be found and expressed through an organized religion or in other ways. Patients may think of themselves as spiritual or religious or both.

Serious Illness, Such as Cancer, May Cause Spiritual Distress

Serious illnesses such as cancer may cause patients or family caregivers to have doubts about their beliefs or religious values and cause much spiritual distress. Some studies show that patients with cancer may feel that they are being punished by God or may have a loss of faith after being diagnosed. Other patients may have mild feelings of spiritual distress when coping with cancer.

Spirituality and Quality of Life

It is not known for sure how spirituality and religion are related to health. Some studies show that spiritual or religious beliefs and practices create a positive mental attitude that may help a patient feel better and improve the well-being of family caregivers. Spiritual and religious well-being may help improve health and quality of life (QOL) in the following ways:

- Decrease anxiety, depression, anger, and discomfort
- Decrease the sense of isolation (feeling alone) and the risk of suicide
- Decrease alcohol and drug abuse
- Lower blood pressure and the risk of heart disease
- Help the patient adjust to the effects of cancer and its treatment
- Increase the ability to enjoy life during cancer treatment
- Give a feeling of personal growth as a result of living with cancer
- Increase positive feelings, including:
  - Hope and optimism
  - Freedom from regret
  - Satisfaction with life
  - A sense of inner peace

Spiritual and religious well-being may also help a patient live longer.

Spiritual distress may also affect health. Spiritual distress may make it harder for patients to cope with cancer and cancer treatment. Healthcare providers may encourage patients to meet with experienced spiritual or religious leaders to help deal with their spiritual issues. This may improve their health, QOL, and ability to cope.

Chapter 70

Sexual Health Issues in Women

Women being treated for breast cancer may experience changes that affect their sexual life during, and sometimes after, treatment. While you may not have the energy or interest in sexual activity that you did before treatment, feeling close to and being intimate with your spouse or partner is probably still important.

Your doctor or nurse may talk with you about how cancer treatment might affect your sexual life, or you may need to be proactive and ask questions such as: What sexual changes or problems are common among women receiving this type of treatment? What methods of birth control or protection are recommended during treatment?

Whether or not your sexual health will be affected by treatment depends on factors such as:

- The type of cancer
- The type of treatment(s)
- The amount (dose) of treatment
- The length (duration) of treatment
- Your age at the time of treatment

This chapter includes text excerpted from "Sexual Health Issues in Women with Cancer," National Cancer Institute (NCI), August 9, 2018.

- The amount of time that has passed since treatment

- Other personal health factors

Cancer Treatments May Cause Sexual Problems in Women

Some problems that affect a woman's sexual health during treatment are temporary and improve once treatment has ended. Other side effects may be long-term or may start after treatment. Your doctor will talk with you about side effects you may have based on your treatment(s):

- **Chemotherapy** can lower estrogen levels and cause primary ovarian insufficiency. This means the ovaries aren't producing hormones and releasing eggs. Symptoms may include hot flashes, irregular or no periods, and vaginal dryness, which can make sexual intercourse difficult or painful. Chemotherapy can also affect vaginal tissue, which may cause sores.

- **Hormone therapy** (also called endocrine therapy) may cause low estrogen levels, which can lead to symptoms such as hot flashes, irregular or no periods, and vaginal dryness.

- **Radiation therapy** to the pelvis (such as to the bladder, cervix, colon, ovaries, rectum, uterus, or vagina) can cause low estrogen levels and, therefore, vaginal dryness. Vaginal stenosis (less elastic, narrow, and shorter vagina), vaginal atrophy (weak vaginal muscles and thin vaginal wall), and vaginal itching, burning, and inflammation can also cause pain and discomfort during sex.

- **Surgery for gynecologic cancers** may affect your sexual life. Treatment for other cancers can also bring about physical changes that may affect the way you view your body. Your healthcare team will talk with you about what to expect and teach you how to adjust after surgery, such as after a mastectomy or an ostomy, for example.

- **Medicines** such as opioids and some drugs used to treat depression may lower your interest in sex.

Ways to Manage Sexual-Health Issues

People on your healthcare team have helped others to cope during this difficult time and can offer valuable suggestions. You may also want to talk with a sexual-health expert to get answers to any questions or concerns.

Most women can be sexually active during treatment, but you'll want to confirm this with your doctor. For example, there may be times during treatment when you are at increased risk of infection or bleeding and may be advised to abstain from sexual intercourse.

Your healthcare team can help you:

- **Learn about medicine and exercises to make sex more comfortable, including:**

  - Vaginal gels or creams to stop a dry, itchy, or burning feeling

  - Vaginal lubricants or moisturizers

  - Vaginal estrogen cream that may be appropriate for some types of cancer

  - A dilator to help prevent or reverse scarring, if radiation therapy or graft-versus-host disease has affected your vagina

  - Exercises for pelvic muscles to lower pain, improve bladder retention, improve bowel function, and increase the flow of blood to the area, which can improve your sexual health

- **Manage related side effects:** Talk with your doctor or nurse about problems such as pain, fatigue, hair loss, loss of interest in activities, sadness, or trouble sleeping, that may affect your sex life. Speaking up about side effects can help you get the treatment and support you need to feel better.

- **Learn about condoms and/or contraceptives:** Condoms may be advised to prevent your partner's exposure to some types of chemotherapy that may remain in vaginal secretions. If you are of childbearing age, contraceptives may be advised to prevent pregnancy while you are receiving treatment and for a period of time following treatment.

- **Get support and counseling:** During this time, you can gain strength and support by sharing your concerns with people you are close to. You may also benefit from participating in a professionally moderated or led support group. Your nurse or social worker can recommend support groups and counselors in your area.

Talking with Your Healthcare Team about Sexual-Health Issues

As you think about the changes that treatment has brought into your life, make a list of questions to discuss with your doctor, nurse, or social worker. Consider adding these to your list:

- What sexual problems are common among women receiving this treatment?

- What sexual problems might I have during treatment?

- When might these changes occur?

- How long might these problems last? Will any of these problems be permanent?

- How can these problems be prevented, treated, or managed?

- What specialist(s) would you suggest that I talk with to learn more?

- Is there a support group that you recommend?

- What method(s) of birth control are advised?

- What precautions do I need to take during treatment? For example, should my partner use a condom? Are there times when I should avoid sexual activity?

- Manage related side effects: Talk with your doctor or nurse about problems such as pain, fatigue, hair loss, loss of interest in activities, sadness, or trouble sleeping, that may affect your sex life. Speaking up about side effects can help you get the treatment and support you need to feel better.

Chapter 71

Sleep Problems

Sleeping well is important for your physical and mental health. A good night's sleep not only helps you to think clearly, it also lowers your blood pressure, helps your appetite, and strengthens your immune system.

Sleep problems such as being unable to fall asleep and/or stay asleep, also called "insomnia," are common among people being treated for cancer. Studies show that as many as half of all patients have sleep-related problems. These problems may be caused by the side effects of treatment, medicine, long hospital stays, or stress.

Talk with your healthcare team if you have difficulty sleeping, so you can get the help you need. Sleep problems that go on for a long time may increase the risk of anxiety or depression. Your doctor will do an assessment, which may include a polysomnogram (recordings taken during sleep that show brain waves, breathing rate, and others activities such as heart rate) to correctly diagnose and treat sleep problems. Assessments may be repeated from time to time, since sleeping problems may change over time.

Ways to Manage Sleep Problems

There are steps that you and your healthcare team can take to help you sleep well again.

This chapter includes text excerpted from "Sleep Problems (Insomnia) and Cancer Treatment," National Cancer Institute (NCI), August 9, 2018.

- **Tell your doctor about problems that interfere with sleep.**
  Getting treatment to lower side effects such as pain or bladder
  or gastrointestinal problems may help you sleep better.

- **Cognitive behavioral therapy (CBT) and relaxation
  therapy may help.** Practicing these therapies can help you
  to relax. For example, a CBT therapist can help you learn to
  change negative thoughts and beliefs about sleep into positive
  ones. Strategies such as muscle relaxation, guided imagery, and
  self-hypnosis may also help you.

- **Set good bedtime habits.** Go to bed only when sleepy, in a
  quiet and dark room, and in a comfortable bed. If you do not fall
  asleep, get out of bed and return to bed when you are sleepy.
  Stop watching television or using electronic devices a couple
  of hours before going to bed. Don't drink or eat a lot before
  bedtime. While it's important to keep active during the day with
  regular exercise, exercising a few hours before bedtime may
  make sleep more difficult.

- **Sleep medicine may be prescribed.** Your doctor may
  prescribe sleep medicine for a short period if other strategies
  don't work. The sleep medicine prescribed will depend on your
  specific problem (such as trouble falling asleep or trouble staying
  asleep) as well as other medicines you are taking.

Talking with Your Healthcare Team about Sleep Problems

Prepare for your visit by making a list of questions to ask. Consider
adding these questions to your list:

- Why am I having trouble sleeping?

- What problems should I call you about?

- What steps can I take to sleep better?

- Would you recommend a sleep therapist who could help with the
  problems I am having?

- Would sleep medicine be advised for me?

Chapter 72

Urinary and Bladder Problems

For urinary and bladder problems caused by cancer treatments, drink plenty of water. Ask your doctor what symptoms to call about—such as fever or pain, for example.

Symptoms of a Urinary Problem

Talk with your doctor or nurse to learn what symptoms you may experience and ask which ones to call about. Some urinary or bladder changes may be normal, such as changes to the color or smell of your urine caused by some types of chemotherapy. Your healthcare team will determine what is causing your symptoms and will advise on steps to take to feel better.

Irritation of the bladder lining (radiation cystitis):

- Pain or a burning feeling when you urinate
- Blood in your urine
- Trouble starting to urinate
- Trouble emptying your bladder completely
- Feeling that you need to urinate urgently or frequently

This chapter includes text excerpted from "Urinary and Bladder Problems," National Cancer Institute (NCI), August 9, 2018.

- Leaking a little urine when you sneeze or cough

- Bladder spasms, cramps, or discomfort in the pelvic area

Urinary tract infection (UTI):

- Pain or a burning feeling when you urinate

- Urine that is cloudy or red

- A fever of 100.5 °F (38 °C) or higher, chills, and fatigue

- Pain in your back or abdomen

- Difficulty urinating or not being able to urinate

In people being treated for cancer, a UTI can turn into a serious condition that needs immediate medical care. Antibiotics will be prescribed if you have a bacterial infection.

Symptoms that may occur after surgery:

- Leaking urine (incontinence)

- Trouble emptying your bladder completely

Ways to Prevent or Manage Urinary and Bladder Problems

Here are some steps you may be advised to take to feel better and to prevent problems:

- **Drink plenty of liquids.** Most people need to drink at least 8 cups of fluid each day, so that urine is light yellow or clear. You'll want to stay away from things that can make bladder problems worse. These include caffeine, drinks with alcohol, spicy foods, and tobacco products.

- **Prevent urinary tract infections.** Your doctor or nurse will talk with you about ways to lower your chances of getting a urinary tract infection. These may include going to the bathroom often, wearing cotton underwear and loose-fitting pants, learning about safe and sanitary practices for catheterization, taking showers instead of baths, and checking with your nurse before using products such as creams or lotions near your genital area.

Talking with Your Healthcare Team

Prepare for your visit by making a list of questions to ask. Consider adding these questions to your list:

- What symptoms or problems should I call you about?
- What steps can I take to feel better?
- How much should I drink each day? What liquids are best for me?
- Are there certain drinks or foods that I should avoid?

Part Seven

Living with Breast Cancer

Chapter 73

Life after Cancer Treatment

The end of cancer treatment is often a time to rejoice. Most likely you're relieved to be finished with the demands of treatment. You may be ready to put the experience behind you and have life return to the way it used to be. Or you may be ready to have a fresh start at something new.

Yet at the same time, you may feel sad and worried. It can take time to recover. Many are uncertain about how to move forward, feeling anxious about the future. It's very common to be thinking about whether cancer will come back and what happens now. Often this time is called adjusting to a "new normal." You will have many different feelings during this time.

One of the hardest things after treatment is not knowing what happens next. Those who have gone through cancer treatment describe the first few months as a time of change. It's not so much "getting back to normal" as it is finding out what's normal for you now. People often say that life has new meaning or that they look at things differently.

Your new normal may include:

- Making changes in the way you eat and what you do

- New or different sources of support

- Permanent scars on your body

- Not being able to do some things you used to do more easily

---

This chapter includes text excerpted from "A New Normal," National Cancer Institute (NCI), September 12, 2018.

- New routines than you had before

- Emotional scars from going through so much

You may see yourself in a different way, or find that others think of you differently now. Whatever your new normal may be, give yourself time to adapt to the changes. Take it one day at a time.

Coping with Fear of Cancer Recurrence

When cancer treatment is over, patients are often faced with mixed emotions. While happiness and relief accompany the end of treatment, survivors may also feel fear and anxiety. Probably the most common fear is that cancer will come back (a cancer recurrence).

Fear of recurrence is normal and often lessens over time. However, even years after treatment, some events may cause you to become worried. Follow-up visits, certain symptoms, the illness of a loved one, or the anniversary date of the date you were diagnosed can all trigger concern.

One step you can take is to be informed. Understand what you can do for your health now, and find out about the services available to you. Doing so can give you a greater sense of control.

Even though you can't control whether or not your cancer recurs, there are steps you can take to help cope with your fears.

Talk to Your Healthcare Team

- **Let your healthcare team know your concerns.** Be honest about the fears of your cancer coming back so they can address your worries. The risk of recurrence differs in each patient. Your healthcare team can give you the facts about your type of cancer and the chances of recurrence. They can assure you that they're looking out for you.

- **Know that it's common for cancer survivors to have fears about every ache and pain.** Talk to your healthcare team if you're having a symptom that worries you. You can get advice about whether or not to schedule an appointment. Just having a conversation with them about your symptoms may help calm your fears. And, over time, you may start to recognize certain feelings in your body as normal.

- **Keep notes about any symptoms you have.** Also, take notes about any anxiety you feel. Write down questions for your

440

healthcare team before follow-up visits so you can be prepared to tell them what you've been going through since your last check-up or conversation.

- **Talk to a counselor.** If you find that your fears are more than you can handle, ask for a referral for someone to talk to. If thoughts about cancer recurrence interfere with your daily life, you might feel better seeing a counselor or therapist. A professional may help you put your concerns in perspective.

- **Make sure you have a follow-up care plan.** Having a plan may give you a sense of control and a way to feel proactive with your health after treatment.

Take Care of Your Mind and Body

Even though you can't control whether or not your cancer recurs, you can use your energy to focus on wellness and manage stress. Here are some things you can do to take care of your mind and body:

- **Find ways to help yourself relax**. Relaxation exercises have been proven to help people with stress and may help you relax when you feel worried. Meditation and yoga also help reduce stress.

- **Talk to others**. Sharing your feelings with friends and family may help you feel better and realize that you're not alone. You can also join a support group to talk to others who are having the same fears.

- **Exercise**. Moderate exercise (examples: walking, biking, and swimming) can help reduce anxiety and depression. It also may improve your mood and boost your self-esteem.

- **Eat a healthy diet**. Talk to a dietician or nutritionist about the foods you should eat to stay healthy and maintain your strength.

- **Write your feelings down**. It may help you to express your feelings by writing in a journal or a notebook. Many people find that getting their thoughts on paper helps them to let go of worries and fears.

- **Seek comfort from spirituality**. Many survivors have found their faith, religion, or sense of spirituality to be a source of strength.

- **Give back.** Some people like to channel their energy by volunteering and helping others. Being productive in this way gives them a sense of meaning and lets them turn their attention on others.

- **Take part in clubs, classes, or social gatherings**. Getting out of the house may help you focus on other things besides cancer and the worries it brings.

Chapter 74

Nutrition and Cancer

Overview of Nutrition in Cancer Care
Good Nutrition Is Important for Cancer Patients

Nutrition is a process in which food is taken in and used by the body for growth, to keep the body healthy, and to replace tissue. Good nutrition is important for good health. Eating the right kinds of foods before, during, and after cancer treatment can help the patient feel better and stay stronger. A healthy diet includes eating and drinking enough of the foods and liquids that have important nutrients (vitamins, minerals, protein, carbohydrates, fat, and water) the body needs.

Healthy Eating Habits Are Important during and after Cancer Treatment

Nutrition therapy is used to help cancer patients keep a healthy body weight, maintain strength, keep body tissue healthy, and decrease side effects both during and after treatment.

A Registered Dietitian Is an Important Part of the Healthcare Team

A registered dietitian (or nutritionist) is a part of the team of health professionals that help with cancer treatment and recovery. A dietitian

This chapter includes text excerpted from "Nutrition in Cancer Care (PDQ®)—Patient Version," National Cancer Institute (NCI), March 16, 2018.

will work with patients, their families, and the rest of the medical team to manage the patient's diet during and after cancer treatment.

Cancer and Cancer Treatments May Cause Side Effects That Affect Nutrition

For many patients, the effects of cancer and cancer treatments make it hard to eat well. Cancer treatments that affect nutrition include:

- Chemotherapy

- Hormone therapy (HT)

- Radiation therapy

- Surgery

- Immunotherapy

- Stem-cell transplant

When the head, neck, esophagus, stomach, intestines, pancreas, or liver are affected by the cancer treatment, it is hard to take in enough nutrients to stay healthy.

Cancer and Cancer Treatments May Cause Malnutrition

Cancer and cancer treatments may affect taste, smell, appetite, and the ability to eat enough food or absorb the nutrients from food. This can cause malnutrition, which is a condition caused by a lack of key nutrients. Alcohol abuse and obesity may increase the risk of malnutrition.

Malnutrition can cause the patient to be weak, tired, and unable to fight infection or finish cancer treatment. Malnutrition may be made worse if cancer grows or spreads.

Eating the right amount of protein and calories is important for healing, fighting infection, and having enough energy.

Anorexia and Cachexia Are Common Causes of Malnutrition in Cancer Patients

Anorexia is the loss of appetite or desire to eat. It is a common symptom in patients with cancer. Anorexia may occur early in the disease or later if cancer grows or spreads. Some patients already have anorexia when they are diagnosed with cancer. Most patients who have advanced cancer will have anorexia. Anorexia is the most common cause of malnutrition in cancer patients.

Cachexia is a condition marked by weakness, weight loss, and fat and muscle loss. It is common in patients with tumors that affect eating and digestion. It can occur in cancer patients who are eating well but are not storing fat and muscle because of tumor growth.

Some tumors change the way the body uses certain nutrients. The body's use of protein, carbohydrates, and fat may be affected, especially by tumors of the stomach, intestines, or head and neck. A patient may seem to be eating enough, but the body may not be able to absorb all the nutrients from the food.

Cancer patients may have anorexia and cachexia at the same time.

Side Effects of Cancer Treatment

Cancer treatments and cancer can cause side effects. Side effects are problems that occur when treatment affects healthy tissues or organs. Speak up about any side effects you have, or changes you notice, so your healthcare team can treat or help you to reduce these side effects.

Learn about steps you can take to prevent or manage the side effects listed below:

- Anemia

- Appetite loss

- Bleeding and bruising (Thrombocytopenia)

- Constipation

- Delirium

- Diarrhea

- Edema (Swelling)

- Fatigue

- Fertility issues in boys and men

- Fertility issues in girls and women

- Hair loss (Alopecia)

- Infection and neutropenia

- Lymphedema

- Memory or concentration problems

- Mouth and throat problems
- Nausea and vomiting
- Nerve problems (Peripheral neuropathy)
- Pain
- Sexual-health issues in men
- Sexual-health issues in women
- Skin and nail changes
- Sleep problems
- Urinary and bladder problems

Keep in mind that side effects vary from person to person, even among those receiving the same treatment.

Nutrition Assessment in Cancer Care
The Healthcare Team May Ask Questions about Diet and Weight History

Screening is used to look for health problems that affect the risk of poor nutrition. This can help find out if the patient is likely to become malnourished, and if nutrition therapy is needed.

The healthcare team may ask questions about the following:

- Weight changes over the past year
- Changes in the amount and type of food eaten
- Problems that have affected eating, such as loss of appetite, nausea, vomiting, diarrhea, constipation, mouth sores, dry mouth, changes in taste and smell, or pain
- Ability to walk and do other activities of daily living (dressing, getting into or out of a bed or chair, taking a bath or shower, and using the toilet)

A physical exam is done to check the body for general health and signs of disease. The patient is checked for signs of loss of weight, fat, and muscle, and for fluid buildup in the body.

Counseling and Diet Changes Are Made to Improve the Patient's Nutrition

A registered dietitian can work with patients and their families to counsel them about ways to improve the patient's nutrition. The registered dietitian provides care based on the patient's nutrition and diet needs. Changes to the diet are made to help decrease symptoms from cancer or cancer treatment. These changes may be in the types and amount of food, how often a patient eats, and how food is eaten (for example, at a certain temperature or taken with a straw).

A registered dietitian works with other members of the healthcare team to check the patient's nutritional health during cancer treatment and recovery. In addition to the dietitian, the healthcare team may include the following:

- Physician
- Nurse
- Social worker
- Psychologist

The Goal of Nutrition Therapy for Patients Who Have Advanced Cancer Depends on the Overall Plan of Care

The goal of nutrition therapy in patients with advanced cancer is to give patients the best possible quality of life (QOL) and control the symptoms that cause distress.

Patients with advanced cancer may be treated with anticancer therapy and palliative care, palliative care alone, or may be in hospice care. Nutrition goals will be different for each patient. Some types of treatment may be stopped if they are not helping the patient.

As the focus of care goes from cancer treatment to hospice or end-of-life care, nutrition goals may become less aggressive, and shift to ensuring that the patient is as comfortable as possible.

Treatment of Symptoms Related to Nutrition Intake

When the side effects of cancer or cancer treatment affect normal eating, changes can be made to help the patient get the nutrients they need. Eating foods that are high in calories, protein, vitamins, and minerals is important. Meals should be planned to meet the patient's nutrition needs and tastes in food.

The following are some of the more common symptoms caused by cancer and cancer treatment and ways to treat or control them.

Anorexia

The following may help cancer patients who have anorexia (loss of appetite or desire to eat):

- Eat foods that are high in protein and calories. The following are high-protein food choices:
  - Beans
  - Chicken
  - Fish
  - Meat
  - Yogurt
  - Eggs
- Add extra protein and calories to food, by using such things as protein-fortified milk
- Eat high-protein foods first in your meal when your appetite is strongest
- Sip only small amounts of liquids during meals
- Drink milkshakes, smoothies, juices, or soups if you do not feel like eating solid foods
- Eat foods that smell good
- Try new foods and new recipes
- Try blenderized drinks that are high in nutrients (check with your doctor or registered dietitian first)
- Eat small meals and healthy snacks often throughout the day
- Eat larger meals when you feel well and are rested
- Eat your largest meal when you feel hungriest, whether at breakfast, lunch, or dinner
- Make and store small amounts of favorite foods so they are ready to eat when you are hungry
- Be as active as possible so that you will have a good appetite
- Brush your teeth and rinse your mouth to relieve symptoms and aftertastes
- Talk to your doctor or registered dietitian if you are having eating problems such as nausea, vomiting, or changes in how foods taste and smell

If these diet changes do not help with the anorexia, tube feedings may be needed so that you will get enough nutrients each day. Medicines may be given to increase appetite.

Nausea

The following may help cancer patients control nausea:

- Choose foods that appeal to you. Do not force yourself to eat food that makes you feel sick. Do not eat your favorite foods (to avoid linking them to being sick).
- Eat foods that are bland, soft, and easy-to-digest, rather than heavy meals.
- Eat dry foods such as crackers, bread sticks, or toast throughout the day.
- Eat foods that are easy on your stomach, such as white toast, plain yogurt, and clear broth.
- Eat dry toast or crackers before getting out of bed if you have nausea in the morning.
- Eat foods and drink liquids at room temperature (not too hot or too cold).
- Slowly sip liquids throughout the day.
- Suck on hard candies such as peppermints or lemon drops if your mouth has a bad taste.
- Stay away from food and drink with strong smells.
- Eat five or six small meals every day instead of three large meals.
- Sip on only small amounts of liquid during meals to avoid feeling full or bloated.
- Do not skip meals and snacks. An empty stomach may make your nausea worse.
- Rinse your mouth before and after eating.
- Don't eat in a room that has cooking odors or that is very warm. Keep the living space at a comfortable temperature and well-ventilated.
- Sit up or lie with your head raised for one hour after eating.

- Plan the best times for you to eat and drink.
- Relax before each cancer treatment.
- Wear clothes that are loose and comfortable.
- Keep a record of when you feel nausea and why.
- Talk with your doctor about using antinausea medicine.

Vomiting

The following may help cancer patients control vomiting:

- Do not eat or drink anything until the vomiting stops
- Drink small amounts of clear liquids after vomiting stops
- After you are able to drink clear liquids without vomiting, drink liquids such as strained soups, or milkshakes, that are easy on your stomach
- Eat five or six small meals every day instead of three large meals
- Sit upright and bend forward after vomiting
- Ask your doctor to order medicine to prevent or control vomiting

Dry Mouth

The following may help cancer patients with a dry mouth:

- Eat foods that are easy to swallow.
- Moisten food with sauce, gravy, or salad dressing.
- Eat foods and drinks that are very sweet or tart, such as lemonade, to help make more saliva.
- Chew gum or suck on hard candy, ice pops, or ice chips.
- Sip water throughout the day.
- Do not drink any type of alcohol, beer, or wine.
- Do not eat foods that can hurt your mouth (such as spicy, sour, salty, hard, or crunchy foods).
- Keep your lips moist with lip balm.
- Rinse your mouth every one to two hours. Do not use a mouthwash that contains alcohol.

- Do not use tobacco products and avoid secondhand smoke.
- Ask your doctor or dentist about using artificial saliva or similar products to coat, protect, and moisten your mouth and throat.

Mouth Sores

The following can help patients who have mouth sores:

- Eat soft foods that are easy to chew, such as milkshakes, scrambled eggs, and custards.
- Cook foods until soft and tender.
- Cut food into small pieces. Use a blender or food processor to make food smooth.
- Suck on ice chips to numb and soothe your mouth.
- Eat foods cold or at room temperature. Hot foods can hurt your mouth.
- Drink with a straw to move liquid past the painful parts of your mouth.
- Use a small spoon to help you take smaller bites, which are easier to chew.
- Stay away from the following:
  - Citrus foods, such as oranges, lemons, and limes
  - Spicy foods
  - Tomatoes and ketchup
  - Salty foods
  - Raw vegetables
  - Sharp and crunchy foods
  - Drinks with alcohol
- Do not use tobacco products.
- Check your mouth each day for sores, white patches, or puffy and red areas.
- Rinse your mouth 3 to 4 times a day. Mix ¼ teaspoon baking soda, teaspoon salt, and 1 cup warm water for a mouth rinse. Do not use mouthwash that contains alcohol.
- Do not use toothpicks or other sharp objects.

Taste Changes

The following may help cancer patients who have taste changes:

- Eat poultry, fish, eggs, and cheese instead of red meat.

- Add spices and sauces to foods (marinate foods).

- Eat meat with something sweet, such as cranberry sauce, jelly, or applesauce.

- Try tart foods and drinks.

- Use sugar-free lemon drops, gum, or mints if there is a metallic or bitter taste in your mouth.

- Use plastic utensils and do not drink directly from metal containers if foods have a metal taste.

- Try to eat your favorite foods, if you are not nauseated. Try new foods when feeling your best.

- Find nonmeat, high-protein recipes in a vegetarian or Chinese cookbook.

- Chew food longer to allow more contact with taste buds, if the food tastes dull but not unpleasant.

- Keep foods and drinks covered, drink through a straw, turn a kitchen fan on when cooking, or cook outdoors if smells bother you.

- Brush your teeth and take care of your mouth. Visit your dentist for checkups.

Sore Throat and Trouble Swallowing

The following may help cancer patients who have a sore throat or trouble swallowing:

- Eat soft foods that are easy to chew and swallow, such as milkshakes, scrambled eggs, oatmeal, or other cooked cereals.

- Eat foods and drinks that are high in protein and calories.

- Moisten food with gravy, sauces, broth, or yogurt.

- Stay away from the following foods and drinks that can burn or scratch your throat:

  - Hot foods and drinks

- Spicy foods
- Foods and juices that are high in acid
- Sharp or crunchy foods
- Drinks with alcohol
- Cook foods until soft and tender.
- Cut food into small pieces. Use a blender or food processor to make food smooth.
- Drink with a straw.
- Eat five or six small meals every day instead of three large meals.
- Sit upright and bend your head slightly forward when eating or drinking, and stay upright for at least 30 minutes after eating.
- Do not use tobacco.
- Talk to your doctor about tube feedings if you cannot eat enough to stay strong.

Lactose Intolerance

The following may help patients who have symptoms of lactose intolerance:

- Use lactose- free or low-lactose milk products. Most grocery stores carry food (such as milk and ice cream) labeled "lactose-free" or "low lactose."
- Choose milk products that are low in lactose, such as hard cheeses (such as cheddar) and yogurt.
- Try products made with soy or rice (such as soy and rice milk and frozen desserts). These products do not contain lactose.
- Avoid only the dairy products that give you problems. Eat small portions of dairy products, such as milk, yogurt, or cheese, if you can.
- Try nondairy drinks and foods with calcium added.
- Eat calcium-rich vegetables, such as broccoli and greens.
- Take lactase tablets when eating or drinking dairy products. Lactase breaks down lactose so it is easier to digest.
- Prepare your own low-lactose or lactose-free foods.

Weight Gain

The following may help cancer patients prevent weight gain:

- Eat a lot of fruits and vegetables.

- Eat foods that are high in fiber, such as whole-grain bread, cereals, and pasta.

- Choose lean meats, such as lean beef, pork trimmed of fat, and poultry (such as chicken or turkey) without skin.

- Choose low-fat milk products.

- Eat less fat (eat only small amounts of butter, mayonnaise, desserts, and fried foods).

- Cook with low-fat methods, such as broiling, steaming, grilling, or roasting.

- Eat less salt.

- Eat foods that you enjoy so you feel satisfied.

- Eat only when hungry. Consider counseling or medicine if you eat because of stress, fear, or depression. If you eat because you are bored, find activities you enjoy.

- Eat smaller amounts of food at meals.

- Exercise daily.

- Talk with your doctor before going on a diet to lose weight.

Types of Nutrition Support
Nutrition Support Helps Patients Who Cannot Eat or Digest Food Normally

It is best to take in food by mouth whenever possible. Some patients may not be able to take in enough food by mouth because of problems from cancer or cancer treatment.

Nutrition Support Can Be Given in Different Ways

In addition to counseling by a dietitian, and changes to the diet, nutrition therapy includes nutritional supplement drinks and enteral and parenteral nutrition support. Nutritional supplement drinks help cancer patients get the nutrients they need. They provide energy, protein, fat, carbohydrates, fiber, vitamins, and minerals. They are not meant to be the patient's only source of nutrition.

A patient who is not able to take in the right amount of calories and nutrients by mouth may be fed using the following:

- **Enteral nutrition.** Nutrients are given through a tube inserted into the stomach or intestines.

- **Parenteral nutrition.** Nutrients are infused into the bloodstream.

The nutrients are given in liquid formulas that have water, protein, fats, carbohydrates, vitamins, and/or minerals.

Nutrition support can improve a patient's QOL during cancer treatment, but may cause problems that should be considered before making the decision to use it. The patient and healthcare team should discuss the harms and benefits of each type of nutrition support.

Enteral Nutrition

Enteral nutrition is also called "tube feeding."

Enteral nutrition is giving the patient nutrients in liquid form (formula) through a tube that is placed into the stomach or small intestine. The following types of feeding tubes may be used:

- A **nasogastric tube** is inserted through the nose and down the throat into the stomach or small intestine. This is used when enteral nutrition is only needed for a few weeks.

- A **gastrostomy tube** is inserted into the stomach or a jejunostomy tube is inserted into the small intestine through an opening made on the outside of the abdomen. This is usually used for long-term enteral feeding or for patients who cannot use a tube in the nose and throat.

The type of formula used is based on the specific needs of the patient. There are formulas for patients who have special health conditions, such as diabetes, or other needs, such as religious or cultural diets.

Parenteral Nutrition

Parenteral nutrition carries nutrients directly into the bloodstream. It is used when the patient cannot take food by mouth or by enteral feeding. Parenteral feeding does not use the stomach or intestines to digest food. Nutrients are given to the patient directly into the blood, through a catheter inserted into a vein. These nutrients include proteins, fats, vitamins, and minerals.

The catheter may be placed into a vein in the chest or in the arm. A central venous access catheter is placed beneath the skin and into a large vein in the upper chest. The catheter is put in place by a surgeon. This type of catheter is used for long-term parenteral feeding.

A peripheral venous catheter is placed into a vein in the arm. A peripheral venous catheter is put in place by trained medical staff. This type of catheter is usually used for short-term parenteral feeding for patients who do not have a central venous access catheter.

The patient is checked often for infection or bleeding at the place where the catheter enters the body.

Medicines to Treat Loss of Appetite and Weight Loss

Medicine may be given with nutrition therapy to treat loss of appetite and weight loss. It is important that cancer symptoms and side effects that affect eating and cause weight loss are treated early. Both nutrition therapy and medicine can help lessen the effects that cancer and its treatment have on weight loss.

Different types of medicine may be used to treat loss of appetite and weight loss. Medicines that improve appetite and cause weight-gain, such as prednisone and megestrol, may be used to treat loss of appetite and weight loss. Studies have shown that the effect of these medicines may not last long or there may be no effect. Treatment with a combination of medicines may work better than treatment with one medicine. Patients who are treated with a combination of medicines may have more side effects.

Nutrition Trends in Cancer
Some Cancer Patients Try Special Diets to Improve Their Prognosis

Cancer patients may try special diets to make their treatment work better, prevent side effects from treatment, or to treat cancer itself. However, for most of these special diets, there is no evidence that shows they work.

Vegetarian or vegan diet. It is not known if following a vegetarian or vegan diet can help side effects from cancer treatment or the patient's prognosis. If the patient already follows a vegetarian or vegan diet, there is no evidence that shows they should switch to a different diet.

Macrobiotic diet. A macrobiotic diet is a high-carbohydrate, low-fat, plant-based diet. No studies have shown that this diet will help cancer patients.

Ketogenic diet. A ketogenic diet limits carbohydrates and increases fat intake. The purpose of the diet is to decrease the amount of glucose (sugar) the tumor cells can use to grow and reproduce. It is a hard diet to follow because exact amounts of fats, carbohydrates, and proteins are needed. However, the diet is safe.

Some Cancer Patients May Take Dietary Supplements

A dietary supplement is a product that is added to the diet. It is usually taken by mouth and usually has one or more dietary ingredients. Cancer patients may take dietary supplements to improve their symptoms or treat their cancer.

Vitamin C. Vitamin C is a nutrient that the body needs in small amounts to function and stay healthy. It helps fight infection, heal wounds, and keep tissues healthy. Vitamin C is found in fruits and vegetables. It can also be taken as a dietary supplement.

Probiotics. Probiotics are live microorganisms used as dietary supplements to help with digestion and normal bowel function. They may also help keep the gastrointestinal tract healthy.

Studies have shown that taking probiotics during radiation therapy and chemotherapy can help prevent diarrhea caused by those treatments. This is especially true for patients receiving radiation therapy to the abdomen. Cancer patients who are receiving radiation therapy to the abdomen or chemotherapy that is known to cause diarrhea may be helped by probiotics.

Melatonin. Melatonin is a hormone made by the pineal gland (tiny organ near the center of the brain). Melatonin helps control the body's sleep cycle. It can also be made in a laboratory and taken as a dietary supplement.

Several small studies have shown that taking a melatonin supplement with chemotherapy and/or radiation therapy for treatment of solid tumors may be helpful. It may help reduce side effects of treatment. Melatonin does not appear to have side effects.

Oral glutamine. Oral glutamine is an amino acid that is being studied for the treatment of diarrhea and mucositis (inflammation of the lining of the digestive system, often seen as mouth sores) caused by chemotherapy or radiation therapy. Oral glutamine may help prevent mucositis or make it less severe.

Cancer patients who are receiving radiation therapy to the abdomen may benefit from oral glutamine. Oral glutamine may reduce the severity of diarrhea. This can help the patients continue with their treatment plan.

Chapter 75

Exercise after Cancer

What Is Physical Activity?

Physical activity is defined as any movement that uses skeletal muscles and requires more energy than does resting. Physical activity can include working, exercising, performing household chores, and leisure-time activities such as walking, tennis, hiking, bicycling, and swimming.

Physical activity is essential for people to maintain a balance between the number of calories consumed and the number of calories used. Consistently expanding fewer calories than are consumed leads to obesity, which scientists have convincingly linked to increased risks of 13 different cancers. Additionally, evidence indicates that physical activity may reduce the risks of several cancers through other mechanisms, independent of its effect on obesity.

Is Physical Activity Beneficial for Cancer Survivors?

Research indicates that physical activity may have beneficial effects for several aspects of cancer survivorship—specifically, weight gain, quality of life (QOL), cancer recurrence or progression, and prognosis (likelihood of survival). Most of the evidence for the potential benefits

This chapter includes text excerpted from "Physical Activity and Cancer," National Cancer Institute (NCI), January 27, 2017.

of physical activity in cancer survivors come from people diagnosed with breast, prostate, or colorectal cancer (CRC).

- **Weight gain.** Both reduced physical activity and the side effects of cancer treatment can contribute to weight gain after a cancer diagnosis. In a cohort study (a type of epidemiologic study), weight gain after breast-cancer diagnosis was linked to worse survival. In a 2012 meta-analysis of randomized controlled clinical trials examining physical activity in cancer survivors, physical activity was found to reduce both body mass index (BMI) and body weight.

- **Quality of life.** A 2012 Cochrane Collaboration systematic review of controlled clinical trials of exercise interventions in cancer survivors indicated that physical activity may have beneficial effects on overall health-related QOL and on specific QOL issues, including body image/self-esteem, emotional well-being, sexuality, sleep disturbance, social functioning, anxiety, fatigue, and pain. In a 2012 meta-analysis of randomized controlled trials (RCT) examining physical activity in cancer survivors, physical activity was found to reduce fatigue and depression and to improve physical functioning, social functioning, and mental health.

- **Recurrence, progression, and survival.** Being physically active after a cancer diagnosis is linked to better cancer-specific outcomes. Consistent evidence from epidemiologic studies links physical activity after diagnosis with better breast-cancer outcomes. For example, a large cohort study found that women who exercised moderately (the equivalent of walking 3 to 5 hours per week at an average pace) after a breast-cancer diagnosis had approximately 40 to 50 percent lower risks of breast-cancer recurrence, death from breast cancer, and death from any cause compared with more sedentary women. The potential physical activity benefit with regard to death from breast cancer was most apparent in women with hormone receptor-positive tumors.

Another prospective cohort study found that women who had breast cancer and who engaged in recreational physical activity roughly equivalent to walking at an average pace of 2 to 2.9 mph for 1 hour per week had a 35 to 49 percent lower risk of death from breast cancer compared with women who engaged in less physical activity.

Findings from epidemiologic studies cannot completely exclude reverse causation as a possible explanation of the link between physical activity and better cancer outcomes. That is, people who feel good are more likely to exercise and be physically active than people who do not feel good.

Chapter 76

Breast Cancer and Your Emotions: Tips for Coping

Just as cancer treatment affects your physical health, it can affect the way you feel, think, and do the things you like to do. It's normal to have many different feelings after treatment ends. Just as you need to take care of your body after treatment, you need to take care of your emotions.

Each person's experience with cancer is different, and the feelings, emotions, and fears that you have are unique. The values you grew up with may affect how you think about and deal with cancer. Some people may feel they have to be strong and protect their friends and families. Others seek support from loved ones or other cancer survivors or turn to their faith to help them cope. Some seek help from counselors and others outside the family, while others don't feel comfortable with this approach.

Whatever you decide, it's important to do what's right for you and try not to compare yourself with others.

Worrying about Your Health

Worrying about cancer coming back is normal, especially during the first year after treatment. This is one of the most common fears

This chapter includes text excerpted from "Facing Forward—Life after Cancer Treatment," National Cancer Institute (NCI), March 2018.

people have after cancer treatment. For some, the fear is so strong that they no longer enjoy life, sleep well, eat well, or even go to follow-up visits. "If I get it again, what am I going to do?" one woman said. "I never thought I'd make it through the first time." Others may react in a more positive way. As one survivor put it, "Cancer is just part of life, and we always have hope."

As time goes by, many survivors report that they think about their cancer less often. However, even years after treatment, some events may cause you to become worried. Follow-up visits, symptoms similar to the ones you had before, the illness of a family member, or the anniversary of the date you were diagnosed can trigger concern.

Coping with Fear of Cancer Returning

Be informed. Learning about your cancer, understanding what you can do for your health now, and finding out about the services available to you can give you a greater sense of control. Some studies even suggest that people who are well-informed about their illness and treatment are more likely to follow their treatment plans and recover from cancer more quickly than those who are not.

Express your feelings of fear, anger, or sadness. People have found that when they express strong feelings like anger or sadness, they're more able to let go of them. Some sort out their feelings by talking to friends or family, other cancer survivors, or a counselor. But even if you prefer not to discuss your cancer with others, you can still sort out your feelings by thinking about them or writing them down.

Look for the positive. Sometimes this means looking for the good even in a bad time or trying to be hopeful instead of thinking the worst. Try to use your energy to focus on wellness and what you can do now to stay as healthy as possible.

Don't blame yourself for your cancer. Some people believe that they got cancer because of something they did or did not do. Remember, cancer can happen to anyone.

You don't have to be upbeat all the time. Many people say they want to have the freedom to give in to their feelings sometimes. As one woman said, "When it gets really bad, I just tell my family I'm having a bad cancer day and go upstairs and crawl into bed."

Find ways to help yourself relax. The exercises have been proven to help others and may help you relax when you feel worried.

Be as active as you can. Getting out of the house and doing something can help you focus on other things besides cancer and the worries it brings.

Look at what you can control. Some people say that putting their lives in order helps. Being involved in your healthcare, keeping your appointments, and making changes in your lifestyle are among the things you can control. Even setting a daily schedule can give you a sense of control. And while no one can control every thought, some say that they try not to dwell on the fearful ones.

Feeling Stress

When you were diagnosed, you may have put concerns such as family, work, or finances aside. Now that treatment is over, these issues may begin to resurface.

Many cancer survivors also worry that stress may have played a role in their illness. It's important to remember that the exact cause of many cancers is still unknown. No research shows that stress causes cancer, but we do know that stress can cause other health problems. Finding ways to reduce or control the stress in your life may help you feel better. Devoting time to any activities that make you feel calm or relaxed may help.

Reducing Stress

Many survivors have found activities such as the ones below useful in dealing with their worries after treatment ends. Ask your doctor, nurse, social worker, or local cancer organization about taking part in activities like these.

Exercise. Exercise is a known way to reduce stress and feel less tense—whether you've had cancer or not. As one man put it, "I can feel down a little bit, and it is a fine line with depression, but when I walk 30 or 45 minutes in the fresh air, I feel like I can take on the world sometimes." See your doctor before making an exercise plan, and be careful not to overdo it. If you can't walk, ask about other types of movement that may be helpful, such as chair exercises or stretching.

Mind–body methods. Activities such as meditation or relaxation may help you lower stress by quieting your mind. Try focusing on your breathing or repeating words or phrases to yourself. Other methods include hypnosis, yoga, or imagery.

Creative outlets. Art, music, or dance gives people the chance to express themselves in different ways. Even people who have never danced, painted, or drawn before have found these activities helpful and fun.

Sharing personal stories. Telling and hearing stories about living with cancer can help people air their concerns, solve problems, and find meaning in what they've been through.

Finding Humor and Laughing

Laughter can help you relax. When you laugh, your brain releases chemicals that produce pleasure and relax your muscles. Even a smile can fight off stressful thoughts. Of course, you may not always feel like laughing, but other people have found that these ideas can help:

- Ask people to send you funny cards.

- Enjoy the funny things children and pets do.

- Watch funny movies or TV shows.

- Listen to comedy recordings.

- Buy a funny desk calendar.

- Read joke books or check out jokes on the Internet. If you don't own a computer, use one at your local library.

You may even find that you can laugh at yourself. "I went by to help a friend this summer, and it was really hot, so I took my wig off," one woman said. "I got ready to go and I couldn't find it. After searching high and low, I found it hanging from her dog's mouth. But I just stuck it on my head and went home. My husband said, 'What happened?' Needless to say, that wig has never been the same."

Coping with Depression and Anxiety

After treatment, you may still feel angry, tense, or sad. For most people, these feelings go away or lessen over time. For some people though, these emotions can become more severe. The painful feelings do not get any better, and they get in the way of daily life. These people may have a medical condition called depression. For some, cancer treatment may have added to this problem by changing the way the brain works.

Getting Help

Talk with your doctor. If your doctor thinks that you suffer from depression, She or he may treat it or refer you to other experts. Many survivors get help from therapists who are experts in both depression and helping people recovering from cancer. Your doctor may also give you medicine to help you feel less tense.

If you find it hard to talk about your feelings, you may want to show your doctor this booklet. It can help you explain what you're going through. Don't feel that you should have to control these feelings on your own. Getting the help you need is important for your life and your health.

Do You Need Help?

If you have any of the following signs for more than two weeks, talk to your doctor about treatment. Some symptoms could be due to physical problems, so it's important to be willing to talk about them with your doctor.

Emotional signs:

- Feelings of worry, anxiety, or sadness that don't go away

- Feeling emotionally numb

- Feeling overwhelmed, out of control, or shaky

- Having a sense of guilt or feeling unworthy

- Feeling helpless or hopeless

- Feeling short-tempered or moody

- Having a hard time concentrating, or feeling scatterbrained

- Crying for long periods of time or many times each day

- Focusing on worries or problems

- Having a hard time getting certain thoughts out of your mind

- Finding it hard to enjoy everyday things, such as food or being with friends

- Finding yourself avoiding situations or things that you know are really harmless

- Thinking about hurting or killing yourself

Body changes:

- Unintended weight gain or loss not due to illness or treatment

- Sleep problems, such as not being able to sleep, having nightmares, or sleeping too much

- Racing heart, dry mouth, increased perspiration, upset stomach, diarrhea

- Physically slowing down

- Fatigue that doesn't go away, headaches, or other aches and pains

Feeling Angry

Many people find themselves feeling angry about having cancer or about things that happened to them during their diagnosis or treatment. They may have had a bad experience with a healthcare provider or with an unsupportive friend or relative.

Feeling angry is normal. And sometimes it can motivate you to take action. But hanging on to it can get in the way of taking care of yourself or moving on. If you can, look at what's causing your anger and what you can do to lessen it.

Feeling Alone

After treatment, you may miss the support you got from your healthcare team. You may feel as if your safety net has been pulled away and that you get less attention and support from healthcare providers now that treatment is over. Feelings like these are normal anytime your regular contact with people who mean a lot to you comes to an end.

It's also normal to feel somewhat cut off from other people—even family and friends—after cancer treatment. Often, friends and family want to help, but they don't know how. Others may be scared of the disease. You may also feel that only others who have had cancer can understand your feelings.

Getting Help

What can you do to make yourself feel better? Try to think about how you could replace the emotional support you used to receive from your healthcare team, such as:

- Asking one of your nurses or doctors if you could call sometimes. This could help you stay connected and help you feel less alone. Even just knowing you can call them may help.

- Finding support services offered over the phone or Internet.

- Finding new sources of support for your recovery. Friends, family, other cancer survivors, and clergy members are a few ideas.

- Joining a cancer support group. People who have had cancer meet in groups to talk about their feelings and concerns. Besides sharing their own stories, they hear what others have gone through and how other people have dealt with the same problems they are facing. A support group may also help members of your family cope with their concerns.

Joining a Support Group

Support groups can have many benefits. Even though a lot of people receive support from friends and family, the number one reason they join a support group is to be with others who have had similar cancer experiences. Some research shows that joining a support group improves quality of life (QOL) and enhances survival.

Support groups can:

- Give you a chance to talk about your feelings and work through them

- Help you deal with practical problems, such as problems at work or school

- Help you cope with side effects of treatment

Types of Support Groups and Where to Find Them

There are many different types of support groups. Some may be for one type of cancer only, while others may be open to those with any cancer. Some may be for women or for men only. Support groups may be led by health professionals or fellow cancer survivors. Support groups aren't just for people who have had cancer.

Support groups can be helpful for children or family members of survivors. These groups focus on family concerns such as role changes, relationship changes, financial worries, and how to support the person who had cancer. Some groups include both cancer survivors and family members.

Not only do support groups meet in person, they also meet online. Internet support groups can be a big help to people with computers who live in rural areas or who have trouble getting to meetings. Some Internet groups are sponsored by cancer organizations, while others are not monitored. With informal chat groups, you can seek support at any time of the day or night. While these online groups can provide valuable emotional support, they may not always offer correct medical information. Be careful about any cancer information you get from the Internet, and check with your doctor before making any changes that are based on what you read.

Is a Support Group Right for Me?

A support group may not be right for everyone. For some people, hearing about others' problems can make them feel worse. Or you may find that your need for a support group changes over time.

If you are thinking about joining a support group, here are some questions you may want to ask the group's contact person:

- How large is the group?
- Who attends (survivors, family members, types of cancer, age range)?
- How long are the meetings?
- How often does the group meet?
- How long has the group been together?
- Who leads the meetings—a professional or a survivor?
- What is the format of the meetings?
- Is the main purpose to share feelings, or do people also offer tips to solve common problems?
- If I go, can I just sit and listen?

Before joining a group, here are questions you may want to ask yourself:

- Am I comfortable talking about personal issues?
- Do I have something to offer to the group?
- What do I hope to gain by joining a group?

Support groups vary greatly, and if you have one bad experience, it doesn't mean support groups are not a good option for you. You may also want to find another cancer survivor with whom you can discuss your cancer experience. Many organizations can pair you with someone who had your type of cancer and is close to your age and background.

Finding Meaning after Cancer Treatment

Survivors often express the need to understand what having had cancer means to their lives now. In fact, many find that cancer causes them to look at life in new ways. They may reflect on spirituality, the purpose of life, and what they value most.

These changes can be very positive. Many reports feeling lucky or blessed to have survived treatment and take new joy in each day. For some, the meaning of their illness becomes clear only after they have been living with cancer for a long time; for others, the meaning changes over time. It's also common to view the cancer experience both negatively and positively at the same time.

Often, people make changes in their lives to reflect what matters most to them now. You might spend more time with your loved ones, place less focus on your job, or enjoy the pleasures of nature. You might also find that going through a crisis like cancer gives you renewed strength.

"I feel good that I've found ways to cope," one colon cancer survivor said. "I also feel better able to handle any future problems that might come up. I have the strength that I didn't know I had."

Faith, Religion, or Spirituality

Having a serious illness can affect your spiritual outlook, regardless of whether you feel connected to traditional religious beliefs. After treatment, you and your loved ones may struggle to understand why cancer has entered your lives. You may wonder why you had to endure such a trial in your life.

Cancer survivors often report that they look at their faith or spirituality in a new way. For some, their faith may get stronger or seem more vital. Others may question their faith and wonder about the meaning of life or their purpose in it. Many say they have a new focus on the present and try to live each day to the fullest.

Many survivors have found that their faith, religion, or sense of spirituality is a source of strength. They say that through their faith, they have been able to find meaning in their lives and make sense of their cancer experience. Faith or religion can also be a way for survivors to connect with others in their community who may share similar experiences or outlooks or who can provide support. Studies have also shown that for some, religion can be an important part of both coping with and recovering from cancer.

The way cancer affects faith or spirituality is different for everyone. It's common to question your beliefs after cancer. These questions can be difficult, but for some, seeking answers and searching for personal meaning in spirituality helps them cope.

Finding Comfort and Meaning

- Read uplifting stories about the human spirit.

- Pray or meditate to help you gain perspective.

- Take part in community or social gatherings for your own support and to support others.

- Talk with others who have had similar experiences.

- Find resources at a place of worship for people dealing with chronic illnesses like cancer.

- Grieve for your losses. Recognize that you have been through a lot, and it's normal to be sad over the way life was before cancer.

How Can You Find New Meaning in Your Life after Cancer?

Assess your life. Some survivors say their cancer gave them a wakeup call and a second chance to make life what they want it to be. Ask yourself: do your roles in your family fulfill you, or are you doing what people expect of you? What are things you've always wanted to try? Are you happy in your job, or are you just used to it?

Seek spiritual support. A trusted clergy member or professional counselor may be able to help you with life questions.

Keep a journal. Write down your thoughts about what gives meaning to your life now.

Think about helping others who have had cancer. For some, reaching out and helping others helps them find meaning. Others want to get cancer out of their minds and prefer to focus their energy in other ways. If you want to help, many local and national cancer groups need volunteers. Or you may prefer to reach out to people you know and spread the word through family and friends.

Think about taking part in a research study. Research studies are trying to identify the effects of cancer and its treatment on survivors. Joining a research study is always voluntary, and it could benefit both you and others. If you want to learn more about studies that involve cancer survivors, talk with your doctor.

Chapter 77

Talking to Family and Loved Ones about Your Cancer

Family Matters

Families are not all alike. Your family may include a spouse (husband or wife), children, and parents. Or maybe you think of your partner or close friends as your family.

Cancer affects the whole family, not just the person with the disease. How are the people in your family dealing with your cancer? Maybe they are afraid or angry, just like you.

When you first find out you have cancer and are going through treatments, day-to-day routines may change for everyone. For example, someone in your family may need to take time off work to drive you to treatments. You may need help with chores and errands.

How your family reacts to your cancer may depend a lot on how you've faced hard times in the past.

Some families find it easy to talk about cancer. They may easily share their feelings about the changes that cancer brings to their lives. Other families find it harder to talk about cancer. The people in these families may be used to solving problems alone and not want to talk about their feelings.

This chapter includes text excerpted from "Taking Time: Support for People with Cancer," National Cancer Institute (NCI), January 19, 2011. Reviewed February 2019.

Families that have gone through a divorce or had other losses may have even more trouble talking about cancer.

If your family is having trouble talking about feelings, think about getting some help. Your doctor or nurse can refer you to a counselor who can help people in your family talk about what cancer means to them. Many families find that, even though it can be hard to do, they feel close to each other when they deal with cancer together.

Changes to Your Roles in the Family

When someone in a family has cancer, everyone takes on new roles and responsibilities. For example, a child may be asked to do more chores or a spouse or partner may need to help pay bills, shop, or do yard work. Family members sometimes have trouble adjusting to these new roles.

Adjusting to Your New Situation

Many families have trouble getting used to the role changes that may be required when a loved one has cancer.

Money: Cancer can reduce the amount of money your family has to spend or save. If you're not able to work, someone else in your family may feel that he or she needs to get a job. You and your family may need to learn more about health insurance and find out what will be covered and what you need to pay for. Most people find it stressful to keep up with money matters.

Living arrangements: People with cancer sometimes need to change where they live or whom they live with. Now that you have cancer, you may need to move in with someone else to get the care you need. This can be hard because you may feel that you are losing your independence, at least for a little while. Or, you may need to travel far from home for treatment. If you have to be away from home for treatments take a few little things from home with you. This way, there will be something familiar even in a strange place.

Daily activities: You may need help with duties such as paying bills, cooking meals, or coaching your children's teams. Asking others to do these things for you can be hard.

Developing a Plan

Even when others offer to help, it's important to let people know that you can still do some things for yourself. As much as you're able, keep up with your normal routine by making a decision, doing household chores, and working on hobbies that you enjoy.

Asking for help is not a sign of weakness. Think about hiring someone or asking for a volunteer. You might be able to find a volunteer through groups in your community.

Paid help or volunteers may be able to help with the following:

- Physical care, such as bathing or dressing

- Household chores, such as cleaning or food shopping

- Skilled care, such as giving you special feedings or medications

Just as you need time for yourself, your family members also need time to rest, have fun, and take care of their other duties. Respite care is a way people can get the time they need. In respite care, someone comes to your home and takes care of you while your family member goes out for a while. Let your doctor or social worker know if you want to learn more about respite care.

Spouses and Partners

Your husband, wife, or partner may feel just as scared by cancer as you do. You both may feel anxious, helpless, or afraid. You may find it hard to be taken care of by someone you love.

People react to cancer in different ways. Some cannot accept that cancer is a serious illness. Others try too hard to be "perfect" caregivers. And some people refuse to talk about cancer. For most people, thinking about the future is scary.

It helps if you and the people close to you can talk about your fears and concerns. You may want to meet with a counselor who can help both of you talk about these feelings.

Sharing Information

Including your spouse or partner in treatment decisions is important. You can meet with your doctor together and learn about your type of cancer. You might want to find out about common symptoms, treatment choices, and their side effects. This information will help both of you plan for the future.

Your spouse or partner will also need to know how to help take care of your body and your feelings. And, even though it's not easy, both of you should think about the future and make plans in case you don't survive your cancer. You may find it helpful to meet with a financial planner or a lawyer.

Staying Close

Everyone needs to feel needed and loved. You may have always been the "strong one" in your family, but now is the time to let your spouse or partner help you. This can be as simple as letting the other person fluff your pillow, bring you a cool drink, or read to you.

Feeling sexually close to your partner is also important. You may not be interested in sex when you're in treatment because you feel tired, sick to your stomach, or in pain. But when your treatment is over, you may feel like having sex again. Until then, you and your spouse or partner may need to find new ways to show that you care about each other. This can include touching, holding, hugging, and cuddling.

Time Away

Your spouse or partner needs to keep a sense of balance in his or her life. He or she needs time to take care of personal chores and errands. Your partner will also need time to sort through his or her own feelings about cancer. And most importantly, everyone needs time to rest. If you don't want to be alone when your loved one is away, think about getting respite care or asking a friend to stay with you.

Children

Even though your children will be sad and upset when they learn about your cancer, do not pretend that everything is OK. Even very young children can sense when something is wrong. They will see that you don't feel well or aren't spending as much time with them as you used to. They may notice that you have a lot of visitors and phone calls or that you need to be away from home for treatment and doctor's visits.

Children as young as 18 months old begin to think about and understand what is going on around them. It is important, to be honest, and tell your children that you are sick and the doctors are working to make you better. Telling them the truth is better than letting them imagine the worst. Give your children time to ask questions and express their feelings. And if they ask questions that you can't answer, let them know that you will find out the answers for them.

When you talk with your children, use words and terms they can understand. For example, say "doctor" instead of "oncologist" or "medicine" instead of "chemotherapy." Tell your children how much you

478

love them and suggest ways they can help with your care. Share books about cancer that are written for children. Your doctor, nurse, or social worker can suggest good ones for your child.

Let other adults in your children's lives know about your cancer. This includes teachers, neighbors, coaches, or other relatives who can spend extra time with them. These other adults may be able to take your children to their activities, as well as listen to their feelings and concerns. Your doctor or nurse can also help by talking with your children and answering their questions. Or you can ask them if there's a child life specialist on staff. This is a person who can help children understand medical issues and also offer psychological and emotional support.

Children can react to cancer in many different ways. For example, they may experience the following:

- Be confused, scared, or lonely

- Feel guilty and think that something they did or said caused your cancer

- Feel angry when they are asked to be quiet or do more chores around the house

- Miss the amount of attention they are used to getting

- Regress and behave as they did when they were much younger

- Get into trouble at school or at home

- Be clingy and afraid to leave the house

Teenagers and a Parent's Cancer

Teens are at a time in their lives when they are trying to break away and be independent from their parents. When a parent has cancer, breaking away can be hard for them to do. They may become angry, act out, or get into trouble.

Try to get your teens to talk about their feelings. Tell them as much as they want to know about your cancer. Ask them for their opinions and, if possible, let them help you make decisions.

Teens may want to talk with other people in their lives. Friends can be a great source of support, especially those who also have a serious illness in their family. Other family members, teachers, coaches, and spiritual leaders can also help. Encourage your teenage children to talk about their fears and feelings with people they trust and feel close to.

479

Some towns even have support groups for teens whose parents have cancer. Also, ask your social worker about Internet resources for this group. Many have online chats and forums for support.

Adult Children

Your relationship with your adult children may change now that you have cancer. You may do the following:

- Ask them to take on new duties, such as making healthcare decisions, paying bills, or taking care of the house.

- Ask them to explain some of the information you've received from your doctor or to go with you to doctor's visits so they can also hear what the doctors are telling you.

- Rely on them for emotional support. For instance, you may ask them to act as "go-betweens" with friends or other family members.

- Want them to spend a lot of time with you. This can be hard, especially if they have jobs or young families of their own.

- Find it hard to receive—rather than give—comfort and support from them.

- Feel awkward when they help with your physical care, such as feeding or bathing.

It is important to talk about cancer with your adult children, even if they get upset or worry about you. Include them when talking about your treatment. Let them know your thoughts and wishes. They should be prepared in case you don't recover from your cancer.

Even adult children worry that their parents will die. When they learn that you have cancer, adult children may realize how important you are to them. They may feel guilty if they haven't been close with you. They may feel bad if they cannot spend a lot of time with you because they live far away or have other duties. Some of these feelings may make it harder to talk to your adult children. If you have trouble talking with your adult children, ask your doctor or nurse to suggest a counselor you can all talk with.

Make the most of the time you have with your adult children. Talk about how much you mean to each other. Express all your feelings—not just love but also anxiety, sadness, and anger. Don't worry about saying the wrong thing. It's better to share your feelings rather than hide them.

Cancer Risk for the Children of People Who Have Cancer

Now that you have cancer, your children may wonder about their chance of getting it as well. A higher risk for some types of cancer is passed from parent to child. However, this is not the case for every type. And everyone's body is different. If concerned, however, children should talk with a doctor about their risk of getting cancer.

Testing for certain genes can be a way to find out if a person is at higher risk of getting cancer. Although some genetic tests can be helpful, they don't always give people the kinds of answers they are seeking. Talk to your doctor if you or someone in your family wants to learn more about genetic changes that increase cancer risk. He or she can refer you to a person who is specially trained in this area.

These experts can help you think through your choices and answer your questions.

Parents

Since people are living much longer these days, many people with cancer may also be caring for their aging parents. For example, you may help your parents with their shopping or take them to a doctor. Your aging parents may even live with you.

You have to decide how much to tell your parents about your cancer. Your decision may depend on how well your parents can understand and cope with the news. If your parents are in good health, think about talking with them about your disease.

Now that you have cancer, you may need extra help caring for your parents. You may need help only while you are in treatment. Or you may need to make long-term changes in your parents' care. Talk with your family members, friends, health professionals, and community agencies to see how they can help.

Close Friends

Once friends learn of your cancer, they may begin to worry. Some will ask you to tell them ways to help. Others will wonder how they can help but may not know how to ask. You can help your friends cope with the news by letting them help you in some way. Think about the things your friends do well and don't mind doing. Make a list of things you think you might need. This way, when they ask you how they can be of help, you'll be able to share your list of needs and allow them to pick something they're willing to do.

Your sample list of needs might include the following:

- Babysit on days that I go to treatment.

- Prepare frozen meals for my "down days."

- Put my name on the prayer list at my place of worship.

- Bring me a few books from the library when you go.

- Visit for tea or coffee when you can.

- Let others know that it is alright to call or visit me (or let others know that I'm not ready for visitors just yet).

Sharing Your Feelings about Cancer

Just as you have strong feelings about cancer, your family or friends will react to it as well. For instance, your friends or family may do the following:

- Hide or deny their sad feelings

- Find someone to blame for your cancer

- Change the subject when someone talks about cancer

- Act mad for no real reason

- Make jokes about cancer

- Pretend to be cheerful all the time

- Avoid talking about your cancer

- Stay away from you, or keep their visits short

Finding a Good Listener

It can be hard to talk about how it feels to have cancer. But talking can help, even though it's hard to do. Many people find that they feel better when they share their thoughts and feelings with their close family and friends.

Friends and family members may not always know what to say to you. Sometimes they can help by just being good listeners. They don't always need to give you advice or tell you what they think. They simply need to show that they care and are concerned about you.

You might find it helpful to talk about your feelings with people who aren't family or friends. Instead, you might want to meet in a support group with others who have cancer or talk with a counselor.

Choosing a Good Time to Talk

Some people need time before they can talk about their feelings. If you aren't ready, you might say, "I don't feel like talking about my cancer right now. Maybe I will later." And sometimes when you want to talk, your family and friends may not be ready to listen.

It's often hard for other people to know when to talk about cancer. Sometimes people send a signal when they want to talk. They might do the following:

- Bring up the subject of cancer
- Talk about things that have to do with cancer, such as a newspaper story about a new cancer treatment that they just read
- Spend more time with you
- Act nervous or make jokes that aren't very funny

You can help people feel more comfortable by asking them what they think or how they feel. Sometimes people can't put their feelings into words. Sometimes, they just want to hug each other or cry together.

Expressing Anger

Many people feel angry or frustrated when they deal with cancer. You might find that you get mad or upset with the people you depend on. You may get upset with small things that never bothered you before.

People can't always express their feelings. Anger sometimes shows up as actions instead of words. You may find that you yell a lot at the kids or the dog. You might slam doors.

Try to figure out why you are angry. Maybe you're afraid of cancer or are worried about money. You might even be angry about your treatment.

Be True to Your Feelings

Some people pretend to be cheerful, even when they're not. They think that they won't feel sad or angry if they act cheerful. Or they want to seem as if they're able to handle cancer themselves. Also, your family and friends may not want to upset you and will act as if nothing is bothering them. You may even think that being cheerful may help your cancer go away.

483

When you have cancer, you have many reasons to be upset. "Down days" are to be expected. You don't have to pretend to be cheerful when you're not. This can keep you from getting the help you need. Be honest and talk about all your feelings, not just the positive ones.

Sharing without Talking

For many, it's hard to talk about being sick. Others feel that cancer is a personal or private matter and find it hard to talk openly about it. If talking is hard for you, think about other ways to share your feelings. For instance, you may find it helpful to write about your feelings. This might be a good time to start a journal or diary if you don't already have one. Writing about your feelings is a good way to sort through them and a good way to begin to deal with them. All you need to get started is something to write with and something to write on.

Journals can be personal or shared. People can use a journal as a way of 'talking' to each other. If you find it hard to talk to someone near to you about your cancer try starting a shared journal. Leave a booklet or pad in a private place that both of you select. When you need to share, write in it and return it to the private place. Your loved one will do the same. Both of you will be able to know how the other is feeling without having to speak aloud.

If you have e-mail, this can also be a good way to share without talking.

People Helping People

No one needs to face cancer alone. When people with cancer seek and receive help from others, they often find it easier to cope.

You may find it hard to ask for or accept help. After all, you are used to taking care of yourself. Maybe you think that asking for help is a sign of weakness. Or perhaps you do not want to let others know that some things are hard for you to do. All these feelings are normal.

People feel good when they help others. However, your friends may not know what to say or how to act when they're with you. Some people may even avoid you. But they may feel more at ease when you ask them something specific like to cook a meal or pick up your children after school. There are many ways that family, friends, other people who have cancer, spiritual or religious leaders, and healthcare providers can help. In turn, there are also ways you can help and support your caregivers.

Family and Friends

Family and friends can support you in many ways. But, they may wait for you to give them hints or ideas about what to do. Someone who is not sure if you want company may call "just to see how things are going." When someone says, "Let me know if there is anything I can do," be honest. For example, tell this person if you need help with an errand or a ride to the doctor's office.

Family members and friends can also do the following:

- Keep you company, give you a hug, or hold your hand
- Listen as you talk about your hopes and fears
- Help with rides, meals, errands, or household chores
- Go with you to doctor's visits or treatment sessions
- Tell other friends and family members ways they can help

Other People Who Have Cancer

Even though your family and friends help, you may also want to meet people who have cancer now or have had it in the past. Often, you can talk with them about things you can't discuss with others. People with cancer understand how you feel and can do the following:

- Talk with you about what to expect
- Tell you how they cope with cancer and live a normal life
- Help you learn ways to enjoy each day
- Give you hope for the future

Let your doctor or nurse know that you want to meet other people with cancer. You can also meet other people with cancer in the hospital, at your doctor's office, or through a cancer support group.

Support Groups

Cancer support groups are meetings for people with cancer and those touched by cancer. They can be in person, by phone, or on the Internet. These groups allow you and your loved ones to talk with others facing the same problems. Some support groups have a lecture as well as time to talk. Almost all groups have a leader who runs the meeting. The leader can be someone with cancer or a counselor or social worker.

You may think that a support group is not right for you. Maybe you think that a group won't help or that you don't want to talk with others about your feelings. Or perhaps you're afraid that the meetings will make you sad or depressed.

Support groups may not be for everyone. Some people choose to find support in other ways. But many people find them very helpful. People in the groups often do the following:

- Talk about what it's like to have cancer

- Help each other feel better, more hopeful, and not so alone

- Learn about what's new in cancer treatment

- Share tips about ways to cope with cancer

Types of Support Groups

Some groups focus on all kinds of cancer. Others talk about just one kind, such as a group for women with breast cancer or a group for men with prostate cancer.

Groups can be open to everyone or just for people of a certain age, sex, culture, or religion. For instance, some groups are just for teens or young children.

Some groups talk about all aspects of cancer. Others focus on only one or two topics such as treatment choices or self-esteem.

Therapy groups focus on feelings such as sadness and grief. Mental health professionals often lead these types of groups.

In some groups, people with cancer meet in one support group and their loved ones meet in another. This way, people can say what they really think and feel and not worry about hurting someone's feelings.

In other groups, patients and families meet together. People often find that meeting in these groups is a good way for each to learn what the other is going through.

Telephone support groups are where everyone dials into a phone line and are linked together to talk. They can share and talk to others with similar experiences from all over the country. There is usually little or no charge.

Online support groups are "meetings" that take place by computer. People meet through chat rooms, listservs, or moderated discussion groups and talk with each other over e-mail. People often like online support groups because they can take part in them any time of the day or night. They're also good for people who can't travel to meetings.

The biggest problem with online groups is that you can't be sure if what you learn is correct. Always talk with your doctor about cancer information you learn from the Internet.

If you have a choice of support groups, visit a few and see what they are like. See which ones make sense for you. Although many groups are free, some charge a small fee. Find out if your health insurance pays for support groups.

Where to Find a Support Group

Many hospitals, cancer centers, community groups, and schools offer cancer support groups. Here are some ways to find groups near you:

- Call your local hospital and ask about its cancer support programs.

- Ask your social worker to suggest groups.

- Do an online search for groups.

- Look in the health section of your local newspaper for a listing of cancer support groups.

Chapter 78

Breast Cancer, Work, and Your Rights

Chapter Contents

Section 78.1

Getting Back to Work after Cancer Treatment

This section includes text excerpted from "Facing Forward—Life after Cancer Treatment," National Cancer Institute (NCI), March 2018.

Your Workplace

Research shows that cancer survivors who continue to work are as productive on the job as other workers. Most cancer survivors who are physically able to work to go back to their jobs. Returning to work can help them feel they are getting back to the life they had before being diagnosed with cancer.

Some cancer survivors change jobs after cancer treatment. If you decide to look for a new job after cancer treatment, remember that you do not need to try to do more—or settle for less—than you are able to handle. If you have a résumé, list your jobs by the skills you have or what you've done, rather than by jobs and dates worked. This way, you don't highlight the time you didn't work due to your cancer treatment.

Whether returning to their old jobs or beginning new ones, some survivors are treated unfairly when they return to the workplace. Employers and employees may have doubts about cancer survivors' ability to work.

Handling Problems at Work

You might face certain problems at your workplace. In such cases:

- Decide how to handle the problem.
  - What are your rights as an employee?
  - Are you willing to take action to correct a problem?
  - Do you still want to work there? Or would you rather look for a new job?
- If necessary, ask your employer to adjust to your needs.
  - Start by talking informally to your supervisor, personnel office, employee assistance counselor (EAP), shop steward, or union representative.

- Ask for a change that would make it easier for you to keep your job (for example, flextime, working at home, special equipment at work).

- Document each request and its outcome for your records.

- Get help working with your employer if you need it.

  - Ask your doctor or nurse to find times for follow-up visits that don't conflict with your other responsibilities.

  - Get your doctor to write a letter to your employer or personnel officer explaining how, if at all, your cancer may affect your work or your schedule.

Friends and Coworkers

The response of friends, coworkers, or people at school after your cancer treatment may differ. Some may be a huge source of support, while others may be a source of anger or frustration. Some people mean well, but they do not know the right things to say. Maybe they just don't know how to offer support. Others don't want to deal with your cancer at all.

If friends and coworkers seem unsupportive, it could be because they are anxious for you or for themselves. Your cancer experience may threaten them because it reminds them that cancer can happen to anyone. Try to understand their fears and be patient as you try to regain a good relationship.

Many survivors say that acting cheerful around others for their comfort is a strain. "I don't want to smile anymore," one melanoma survivor said. "I don't have the energy to be upbeat all the time." A prostate cancer (PC) survivor noted, "You know if you complain sometimes, for some people, it turns them off. So I try not to do that."

As survivors sort out what matters most, they may even decide to let some casual friendships go, to give more time to the meaningful ones. One brain-cancer survivor found that after cancer, "You really know how many true friends you've got. And they don't stop calling just because they hear you're in remission. They really love you and think something of you." A kidney-cancer survivor found that "letting weak friendships go was hard, but I also got the support I didn't expect from people at work and in church."

On the job or where you volunteer, some people may not under-stand about cancer and your ability to perform while recovering from treatment. They may think you aren't able to work as hard as before or that your having had cancer means you are going to die soon. Sometimes, fear and lack of knowledge result in unfair treatment.

Getting Help

If you find that a friend or coworker's feelings about cancer are hurting you, try to resolve the problem with that person face-to-face. If it is still affecting your work after that, your manager, shop steward, company medical department, employee-assistance counselor, or personnel office may be able to help.

When hurtful remarks or actions get you down, talking with a friend, family member, or counselor may help you come up with ideas for handling it. But if coworker attitudes get in the way of doing your job, it is a problem that management should address.

Section 78.2

Women's Health and Cancer Rights Act

This section includes text excerpted from "The Center for Consumer Information and Insurance Oversight," Centers for Medicare & Medicaid Services (CMS), February 2, 2012. Reviewed February 2019.

The Women's Health and Cancer Rights Act of 1998 (WHCRA) is a federal law that provides protections to patients who choose to have breast reconstruction in connection with a mastectomy.

If WHCRA applies to you and you are receiving benefits in connection with a mastectomy and you elect breast reconstruction, coverage must be provided for:

- All stages of reconstruction of the breast on which the mastectomy has been performed

- Surgery and reconstruction of the other breast to produce a symmetrical appearance, and

- Prostheses and treatment of physical complications of all stages of the mastectomy, including lymphedema

This law applies to two different types of coverage:

1. Group health plans (provided by an employer or union)

2. Individual health insurance policies (not based on employment)

Group health plans can either be "insured" plans that purchase health insurance from a health-insurance issuer, or "self-funded" plans that pay for coverage directly. How they are regulated depends on whether they are sponsored by private employers, or state or local ("non-federal") governmental employers. Private group health plans are regulated by the Department of Labor. State and local governmental plans, for purposes of WHCRA, are regulated by the Centers for Medicare & Medicaid Services (CMS). If any group health plan buys insurance, the insurance itself is regulated by the state's insurance department.

Contact your employer's plan administrator to find out if your group coverage is insured or self-funded, to determine what entity or entities regulate your benefits.

Health insurance sold to individuals (not through employment) is primarily regulated by state insurance departments.

WHCRA requires group health plans and health-insurance companies (including Health Maintenance Organizations (HMOs)), to notify individuals regarding the coverage required under the law. Notice about the availability of these mastectomy-related benefits must be given:

1. To participants and beneficiaries of a group health plan at the time of enrollment, and to policyholders at the time an individual health insurance policy is issued, and

2. Annually to group health plan participants and beneficiaries, and to policyholders of individual policies

Contact your state's insurance department to find out whether additional state law protections apply to your coverage if you are in an insured group health plan or have individual (nonemployment based) health-insurance coverage. WHCRA does not apply to

493

high-risk pools since the pool is a means by which individuals obtain health coverage other than through health insurance policies or group health plans.

WHCRA does NOT require group health plans or health-insurance issuers to cover mastectomies in general. If a group health plan or health-insurance issuer chooses to cover mastectomies, then the plan or issuer is generally subject to WHCRA requirements.

Section 78.3

Your Rights after a Mastectomy

This section includes text excerpted from "Your Rights after a Mastectomy," U.S. Department of Labor (DOL), September 2018.

Frequently Asked Questions on Women's Health and Cancer Rights Act of 1998

I've been diagnosed with breast cancer and plan to have a mastectomy, which my plan covers. Will my health plan cover reconstructive surgery too?

If your group health plan or health-insurance company covers mastectomies, it must provide certain reconstructive surgery and other benefits related to the mastectomy, including:

- All stages of reconstruction of the breast on which the mastectomy was performed

- Surgery and reconstruction of the other breast to produce a symmetrical appearance

- Prostheses, and

- Treatment of physical complications of the mastectomy, including lymphedema. The plan must consult with you and your attending physician when determining how this coverage will be provided.

494

I Must Have a Mastectomy for Medical Reasons, Although I Have Not Been Diagnosed with Cancer. Does Women's Health and Cancer Rights Act Apply to Me?

Yes, the law applies if your group health plan or health-insurance company covers mastectomies and you are receiving benefits in connection with a mastectomy—whether or not you have cancer. Despite its name, nothing in the law limits Women's Health and Cancer Rights Act (WHCRA) rights to cancer patients.

Do All Group Health Plans and Health-Insurance Companies Have to Provide Reconstructive Surgery Benefits?

Generally, WHCRA applies to all group health plans that provide coverage for medical and surgical benefits with respect to a mastectomy, as well as their insurance companies. However, there are exceptions for some "church plans" and "government plans." If your coverage is provided by a "church plan" or "governmental plan," check with your plan administrator.

Will I Have to Pay a Deductible or Coinsurance?

Possibly. Group health plans or health-insurance companies may impose deductibles or coinsurance requirements on mastectomies and postmastectomy treatment, but no more than those established for other benefits. In other words, the deductible for postmastectomy reconstructive surgery should be similar to the deductible for any similar procedure covered by the plan.

Before I Changed Jobs, I Had a Mastectomy and Chemotherapy Which Were Covered under My Previous Employer's Plan. Now I Am Enrolled under My New Employer's Plan and Want Reconstructive Surgery. Is My New Employer's Plan Required to Cover It?

If you request reconstructive surgery, your new employer's plan generally must cover it if:

- The plan provides coverage for mastectomies, and

- You are receiving benefits under the plan that are related to your mastectomy

In addition, your new employer's plan generally must cover the other benefits specified in WHCRA, even if you were not enrolled in your new employer's plan when you had the mastectomy. The Patient Protection and Affordable Care Act (PPACA) includes additional protections. A group health plan generally cannot limit or deny benefits relating to a health condition that existed before you enrolled in your new employer's plan.

My Employer's Group Health Plan Provides Coverage through an Insurance Company. after My Mastectomy, My Employer Changed Insurance Companies. The New Insurance Company Refuses to Cover My Reconstructive Surgery. Is That Legal?

Note if:

- The new insurance company provides coverage for mastectomies

- You are receiving benefits under the plan related to your mastectomy, and

- You elect to have reconstructive surgery

If these conditions apply, then the new insurance company must provide coverage for breast reconstruction as well as the other benefits required under WHCRA. It does not matter that you were not covered by the new company when you had the mastectomy.

I Understand That My Group Health Plan Must Provide Me with a Notice of My WHCRA When I Enroll in the Plan. What Information Does This Notice Include?

Plans must provide a notice to all employees when they enroll in the health plan that:

- Describes the benefits that WHCRA requires the plan and its insurance companies to cover, which include:

  - Coverage of all stages of reconstruction of the breast on which the mastectomy was performed

  - Surgery and reconstruction of the other breast to produce a symmetrical appearance

  - Prostheses, and

- Treatment of physical complications of the mastectomy, including lymphedema

- States that mastectomy-related benefits coverage will be provided in a manner determined in consultation with the attending physician and the patient

- Describes any applicable deductibles and coinsurance limitations that apply to the coverage specified under WHCRA. Deductibles and coinsurance limitations may be imposed only if they are consistent with those established for other benefits under the plan or coverage

What Information Does the Annual WHCRA Notice from My Health Plan Include?

Your annual notice should describe the four categories of coverage required under WHCRA and how to obtain a detailed description of the mastectomy-related benefits available under your plan. For example, an annual notice might look like this: "Do you know that your plan, as required by the WHCRA of 1998, provides benefits for mastectomy-related services including all stages of reconstruction and surgery to achieve symmetry between the breasts, prostheses, and complications resulting from a mastectomy, including lymphedema? Your annual notice may be the same notice provided when you enrolled in the plan if it contains the information described above.

My State Also Requires Health-Insurance Companies to Cover Minimum Hospital Stays in Connection with a Mastectomy (Which Is Not Required by WHCRA). If I Have a Mastectomy and Breast Reconstruction, Am I Also Entitled to the Minimum Hospital Stay?

If your employer's group health plan provides coverage through an insurance company, you are entitled to the minimum hospital stay required by the state law. Many state laws provide more protections than WHCRA for coverage provided by an insurance company or "insured coverage."

To find out if your group health coverage is "insured" or "self-insured," check your health plan's Summary Plan Description (SPD) or contact your plan administrator.

Table 78.1. Your Rights after a Mastectomy

If Your Employer's Group Health Plan Provides	You Are Entitled To
Coverage through an insurance company	Federal and state protections (in states that provide them)
Self-insured coverage	Federal protections only

If your coverage is "insured" and you want to know if you have additional state law protections, contact your state insurance department.

I Have Health Coverage through an Individual Policy, Not through an Employer. Am I Covered under WHCRA?

WHCRA rights apply to individual coverage as well. These requirements are generally within the jurisdiction of the state insurance department. Call your state insurance department or the U.S. Department of Health and Human Services (HHS) toll-free at 877-267-2323, extension 6-1565.

Can I Get Breast-Cancer Screening or Similar Preventive Services for Free?

Possibly. Under the Affordable Care Act (ACA), you may receive certain recommended preventive services, such as breast-cancer mammography screenings for women aged 40 and older, with no copayment, coinsurance, deductible, or other cost-sharing.

WHCRA does not require coverage for preventive services related to the detection of breast cancer.

Chapter 79

Caregiving for Someone with Breast Cancer

It's important for cancer caregivers to understand that even though treatment has ended, cancer survivors are still coping with a lot. Often they're dealing with side effects from treatment and learning how to adjust to the many other changes they have gone through. They may not be returning back to normal life as soon as they had hoped.

What Caretakers Need to Do after the End of Treatment

Once treatment ends, most people want to put the cancer experience behind them. Still, one of the most common reactions by caregivers is to ask themselves, "Now what do I do?" They were used to having many roles, such as helping with medical care, managing household tasks, and coordinating visits and calls from friends. Many have to think about how to adjust to this "new normal."

Until now, your focus has been on getting the patient through treatment. So it can be a time of mixed emotions—you may be happy treatment is over. But at the same time, the full impact of what you've gone through with your loved one may start to hit you.

This chapter includes text excerpted from "Caregiving after Treatment Ends," National Cancer Institute (NCI), November 6, 2017.

Be Aware of Your Feelings

It's normal to have many different feelings after treatment ends. Some caregivers say that their feelings are even more intense after treatment because they have more time to process it all.

You may be glad and relieved that your loved one completed treatment. But you could also feel anxious because you're no longer doing something directed at fighting cancer. You may feel a sense of sadness and loss at still seeing your friend or family member in a weakened state. This can also be a time when you feel more lonely and isolated than before.

Common feelings that you may have included:

- Missing the support you had from the patient's healthcare team

- Feeling pressure to return to your old self

- Missing being needed or being busy

- Feeling lonely. Friends and family may go back to their daily lives, leaving you with more to do. They may not be checking in with you as they did when your loved one was getting treatment.

- Avoiding going out with others for fear of something happening to your loved one while you are gone

- Finding it hard to relate to people who haven't been through what you have

- Having mixed feelings as you see your loved one struggle with moodiness, depression, or loss of self-esteem

- Worrying that any physical problem is a sign of the cancer returning. Yet at the same time, feeling thankful that this person is here and part of your life.

- Looking forward to putting more energy into the things that mean the most to you

These feelings are all normal. You can manage them by giving yourself time to reflect on your experience with cancer. People need different amounts of time to work through the challenges that they're facing.

Make Time for Yourself

If you've been putting your own needs aside, this may be a good time to think about how you can best care for yourself. Having some downtime to recharge your mind and spirit can help you cope.

You may want to think about:

- Getting back to activities that you enjoy
- Finding ways others can help you
- Finding new ways to connect with friends

For example, some caregivers feel the need to give back to others who are facing cancer. They turn their energy to helping people in their community, joining support groups, or volunteering with cancer organizations. For many, making a difference in the lives of others helps them to help themselves.

Let Others Help You

You may feel tempted to tell people that you and your loved one are doing fine and don't need help. It may be that you don't want to trouble people any longer. Chances are that both of you are tired and are still getting used to life after treatment. It may help to tell others that you're still adjusting and let them know ways they can help. Family, friends, neighbors, and coworkers who stayed away during treatment may now be willing or able to support you. Think about what types of support would be helpful. The clearer you can be about your needs, the easier it will be to get the help you need.

However, be aware that others may not be there to help. They may feel awkward about helping or assume that you're getting back to your routine and don't need help anymore. Or they may have personal reasons, such as lack of time or things going on in their own lives.

Talking with Family

Try to remember that this time after treatment is new for all. Your family members may also need time to adjust to this new chapter of life for your loved one. Some points you can make:

- Let them know that recovery may take more time than expected. Your loved one may lack energy for a while and need time to adjust to this new normal.

- Ask them to continue doing your loved one's regular duties and tasks until he or she can get back to a normal routine.

- Let them know what the follow-up care will be and how your loved one will be monitored.

501

- Be honest about what types of support are needed from them now that treatment is over.

- Thank them for all they did during treatment.

Good communication is just as important now as it was during cancer treatment. Listening to each other, patience, and support can make a big difference.

Part Eight

Clinical Trials and Breast-Cancer Research

Chapter 80

What Are Clinical Trials?

Clinical trials are research studies that involve people. They are the final step in a long process that begins with research in a lab. Most treatments we use today are the results of past clinical trials.

Cancer clinical trials are designed to test new ways to:

- Treat cancer

- Find and diagnose cancer

- Prevent cancer

- Manage symptoms of cancer or side effects from its treatment

Any time you or a loved one needs treatment for cancer, clinical trials are an option to think about. Trials are available for all stages of cancer. It is a myth that they are only for people who have advanced cancer that is not responding to treatment.

Every trial has a person in charge, usually a doctor, who is called the "principal investigator." The principal investigator prepares a plan for the trial, called a "protocol." The protocol explains what will be done during the trial. It also contains information that helps the doctor decide if this treatment is right for you. The protocol includes information about:

- The reason for doing the trial

- Who can join the trial (called "eligibility requirements")

This chapter includes text excerpted from "What Are Clinical Trials?" National Cancer Institute (NCI), June 27, 2016.

- How many people are needed for the trial

- Any drugs that will be given, how they will be given, the dose, and how often

- What medical tests will be done and how often

- What types of information will be collected about the people taking part

Why Are Clinical Trials Important?

Clinical trials are key to developing new methods to prevent, detect, and treat cancer. It is through clinical trials that researchers can determine whether new treatments are safe and effective and work better than current treatments. When you take part in a clinical trial, you add to our knowledge about cancer and help improve cancer care.

Chapter 81

Breast-Cancer Clinical Trials

Chapter Contents

Section 81.1

Breast-Cancer Risk Assessment in Women Aged 40–49

This section includes text excerpted from "Breast Cancer Risk Assessment in Women Aged 40–49," ClinicalTrials.gov, National Institutes of Health (NIH), August 20, 2018.

Brief Summary

In a randomized controlled trial, the investigators will test the effect of a novel strategy for breast-cancer risk assessment and risk-based management of women in their forties seen in primary care. The investigators anticipate that this approach will lead to more optimal use of mammography screening and breast-cancer prevention interventions in women in their forties and as a result, will improve the care of these women.

Detailed Description

There is currently no standardized practice for addressing breast-cancer risk in primary care. While there are guidelines encouraging primary-care physicians (PCPs) to assess patients' breast-cancer risk, few PCPs assess patients' risk due to time constraints in primary care, lack of familiarity with risk calculators, and knowledge on how to incorporate risk into the care of women. Around 20 percent of PCPs have reported using a risk calculator but few routinely asses patients' risk. In HealthCare Associates (HCA), Beth Israel Deaconess Medical Center's primary-care based practice, the online medical record (OMR) has recently been edited to allow for PCPs to enter patients' breast-cancer risk. However, it is not known whether PCPs are using this tab. To calculate a patient's breast-cancer risk, PCPs must go to web-based calculators, ask patients their risk factors, enter the information and then add the estimated risk to OMR.

Previous studies suggest that leaving risk assessment to PCPs results in few women having their risk assessed. Instead, PCPs tend to simply use family history when deciding whether or not patients are at high risk. However, family history is only one risk factor for breast cancer. Therefore, the investigators will send women ages 40 to 49 participating in this study a questionnaire to complete before a visit to assess their risk factors for breast cancer.

Using this information, the investigators will calculate patients' breast-cancer risk using the available breast-cancer risk assessment models and will present women with a personalized breast-cancer risk report immediately before a visit with their PCP. After the visit, patients will be asked to complete a follow-up questionnaire about their experience and through their medical records will be followed to learn whether or not they are screened with mammography. The investigators will follow high-risk women to learn whether or not they receive a screening breast MRI, *BRCA* gene testing, and/or the option to take breast-cancer prevention medications. The investigators aim to recruit 445 women ages 40 to 49 years of age and years seen at HCA into a single-arm trial that allows principal investigators to learn the effect of our personalized risk-based approach to breast-cancer screening and prevention for women in their forties who are willing to be screened and provided with knowledge of the pros and cons of screening.

Specific Aims: To determine the effect of a personalized risk-based approach for breast-cancer screening and prevention for women in their forties seen in primary care on:

1. Women's intentions to be screened with mammography (primary outcome)

2. Knowledge of the pros and cons of mammography screening

3. Decisional conflict around screening, and on

4. Patient report of PCP discussion of their breast-cancer risk and of the pros and cons of mammography screening

Eligibility Criteria

Ages Eligible for Study: 40 to 49 (Adult)
Sexes Eligible for Study: Female
Gender-Based Eligibility: Yes
Accepts Healthy Volunteers: No

Inclusion Criteria

- Women

- Aged 40 to 49 years

- Read and speak English

- Scheduled for a routine visit or physical examination with a non-resident PCP in the next 4 to 12 weeks at HealthCare Associates (HCA, BIDMC's outpatient primary-care practice).

Exclusion Criteria

- Women scheduled for acute care

- Women who had or will have a mammogram within six months of their PCP visit

- Women with a history of breast cancer or a *BRCA* mutation

- Women already receiving screening breast MRIs

- Women who have been referred to genetic counseling

- Women who have taken or are taking tamoxifen or aromatase inhibitors for breast-cancer prevention

- Women with a history of an abnormal mammogram in the past two years

- Women with a history of breast enlargement or reduction

Section 81.2

Topical Calcipotriene Treatment for Breast-Cancer Immunoprevention

This section includes text excerpted from "Topical Calcipotriene Treatment for Breast Cancer Immunoprevention," ClinicalTrials.gov, National Institutes of Health (NIH), November 14, 2018.

Brief Summary

This research study is studying a topical ointment called "calcipotriene" to see if it can stimulate the immune cells against the breast lesion in ways that would prevent its recurrence after surgical removal.

Detailed Description

The investigators are doing this research study to find out how topical calcipotriene ointment affects people who have breast cancer, and what impact that may have on those who are at risk of developing breast cancer in the future. The investigators hope that what they learn will lead to the development of a new medication for the treatment and prevention of breast cancer.

Abnormal breast lesions can be benign, premalignant, or malignant. These lesions are being targeted by the topical calcipotriene ointment. The investigators aim to determine whether this topical treatment can stimulate the immune cells against the breast lesion in ways that would prevent its recurrence after surgical removal.

Calcipotriene ointment is approved by the U.S. Food and Drug Administration (FDA) to treat psoriasis, but calcipotriene ointment is not approved by the FDA to treat breast cancer.

Eligibility Criteria

Ages Eligible for Study: 45 years and older (Adult, older adult)
Sexes Eligible for Study: All
Accepts Healthy Volunteers: No

Inclusion Criteria

- Participants must have histologically confirmed benign, premalignant or early malignant breast lesions on core biopsy that will proceed directly to surgical removal without any intervening neoadjuvant chemotherapy.

- Patients diagnosed with benign breast lesions (papilloma and sclerosing lesion), flat epithelial atypia, atypical ductal hyperplasia, lobular carcinoma *in situ* (Tis N0 M0; stage 0), ductal carcinoma *in situ* (Tis N0 M0; stage 0), primary invasive ductal and lobular carcinoma (T1or2 N0or1 M0; stage I-II), who will directly receive surgery and no neoadjuvant chemotherapy.

- Patients with hormone receptor-positive, Her2 positive, and triple-negative cancers will be eligible.

- Patients with multicentric and multifocal tumors will be eligible.

- Age 45 years. To avoid the impact of menstrual cycle-associated alterations in the immune environment of the breast, the age is limited to menopausal women.

- Ability to understand and the willingness to sign a written informed consent document.

Exclusion Criteria

- Participants scheduled to undergo neoadjuvant therapy for breast cancer.

- Participants with metastatic breast cancer.

- Participants with a history of breast cancer in the past five years.

- Participants with immunosuppression (e.g., organ transplant recipients and patients with autoimmune diseases requiring immunosuppressive medications including > 5mg daily prednisone, methotrexate, cyclosporine, azathioprine, tacrolimus and TNFα-blocking agents)

- Participants with the history of hypercalcemia or clinical evidence of vitamin D toxicity.

- Participants who have had chemotherapy or radiotherapy within four weeks (six weeks for nitrosoureas or mitomycin C) prior to entering the study or those who have not recovered from adverse events due to agents administered more than four weeks earlier.

- Participants who are receiving any other investigational agents.

- Participants with known brain metastases should be excluded from this clinical trial because of their poor prognosis and because they often develop progressive neurologic dysfunction that would confound the evaluation of neurologic and other adverse events.

- History of allergic reactions attributed to compounds of similar chemical or biologic composition to topical calcipotriene ointment.

- Pregnant women are excluded from this study because topical calcipotriol ointment is a category C agent and its impact on developing fetus is unknown. In addition, premenopausal women are excluded from this study due to the impact of menstrual cycles on the immune environment of the breast.

Section 81.3

Real-Time Assessment of Breast-Cancer Lumpectomy Specimen Margins with Nonlinear Microscopy

This section includes text excerpted from "Real-Time Assessment of Breast Cancer Lumpectomy Specimen Margins with Nonlinear Microscopy," ClinicalTrials.gov, National Institutes of Health (NIH), July 26, 2018.

Brief Summary

This research is studying a new investigative-imaging instrument called a nonlinear microscope (NLM). A nonlinear microscope can produce images similar to an ordinary pathologist's microscope, but without first processing, tissue to make slides. This study will determine if an NLM can be used to evaluate tissue during lumpectomy surgery for breast cancer in order to reduce the probability that standard pathologic examination of the specimen after the end of the operation will find close or positive margins, thus possibly requiring the patient to have additional breast surgery.

Detailed Description

The purpose of this research study is to improve the treatment of breast cancer and reduce the number of patients who require repeat surgical procedures to completely remove breast malignancy.

In standard procedures, pathologists evaluate tissue samples on a microscope after the surgery is over. The new investigative-imaging instrument is an advanced type of microscope that enables evaluation during surgery.

The microscope will not be used directly on the participant or in the operating room, but instead will be used to image tissue immediately after excision but prior to the conclusion of surgery. If pathologic examination using NLM concludes that there is invasive cancer or ductal carcinoma *in situ* (DCIS) at or close to the margin of the specimen, the surgeon will be notified and may decide to do additional surgical shavings before the patient leaves the operating room, in order to improve the likelihood of achieving clean margins and reduce the probability that the patient will be advised to have another operation to achieve clean margins. For both patients on the experimental arm (NLM) and the control arm (without NLM), standard pathologic evaluation of the specimen will be done some days after the lumpectomy is completed. That pathologic evaluation will decide whether or not to recommend that the patient has additional surgery in order to achieve clean margins. The primary outcome measure is the percentage of patients in each group who are advised to have additional surgery for this reason.

Eligibility Criteria

Ages Eligible for Study: 21 years and older (Adult, older adult)
Sexes Eligible for Study: Female
Accepts Healthy Volunteers: No

Inclusion Criteria

- Patient scheduled to undergo lumpectomy for breast cancer at Beth Israel Deaconess Medical Center (BIDMC).

- Core needle biopsy revealing invasive breast cancer or DCIS.

- Female.

- Minimum age of 21 years.

- Eligible for breast-conserving surgery, lumpectomy, and radiation.

- Estrogen-receptor positive (ER+) on core needle biopsy, or if estrogen-receptor negative (ER-), have evaluable estrogen receptor status with positive internal control on core biopsy.

- Progesterone receptor positive (PR+) on core needle biopsy if biopsy indicates invasive cancer, or if progesterone receptor negative (PR-) on biopsy indicating invasive cancer, have evaluable progesterone receptor status with positive internal control on core biopsy.

- HER2 IHC and/or FISH performed on core biopsy if biopsy indicates invasive cancer. Oncotype DX or other DNA testing performed on core biopsy or not requested.

- Ability to understand and the willingness to sign a written informed-consent document.

Exclusion Criteria

- Contraindicated for radiation therapy.

- Pregnancy. (Pregnant women will be excluded from this study because radiation therapy is contraindicated during pregnancy.)

- Previous surgery for DCIS or invasive cancer.

- Any systemic neoadjuvant (or preoperative) therapy between the core biopsy and lumpectomy.

- Involvement in another therapeutic trial for breast cancer at Dana Farber or elsewhere.

- Risk of poor cosmetic outcome after initial lumpectomy and possible additional excision.

- Recommendation for mastectomy based on radiology.

- Patients that have large areas DCIS as indicated on radiology, which would require excising a large tissue volume.

- No or equivocal ER, PR or HER2 testing performed prior to surgery if biopsy indicates invasive cancer.

- No or equivocal ER testing performed prior to surgery if the biopsy indicates ductal carcinoma *in situ*.

Section 81.4

Acupuncture for Hot Flashes in Hormone-Receptor-Positive Breast Cancer, a Randomized Controlled Trial

This section includes text excerpted from "Acupuncture for Hot Flashes in Hormone Receptor-Positive Breast Cancer, a Randomized Controlled Trial," ClinicalTrials.gov, National Institutes of Health (NIH), January 21, 2019.

Brief Summary

This research study is evaluating acupuncture, a medical therapy in which hair-thin, stainless-steel needles are shallowly inserted into specific points to help the body's natural healing process, as a possible treatment to reduce hot flashes.

Detailed Description

Hot flashes are a sensation of sudden onset of body warmth, flushing, and sweating. Hot flashes are common side effects of breast-cancer treatments and can affect mood and daily life. Medications can help ease hot flashes, but many patients continue to experience symptoms despite these treatments.

Acupuncture is a complementary therapy in which, hair-thin, sterile disposable needles are inserted into various spots on the skin, with the goal of affecting a body's natural healing system. Acupuncture has been tested in clinical trials in cancer patients and has been shown to be helpful in treating a number of side effects of cancer treatment, such as nausea and vomiting from chemotherapy.

A few early studies have suggested that acupuncture may help to lessen hot flashes, but more information is needed about the benefits of acupuncture in breast-cancer patients.

This study is being done to test whether acupuncture can help to reduce the number and intensity of hot flashes in breast-cancer patients who are being treated with medications such as tamoxifen and aromatase inhibitors, such as anastrozole (Arimidex), exemestane (Aromasin), and letrozole (Femara).

Eligibility Criteria

Ages Eligible for Study: 18 years and older (Adult, older adult)
Sexes Eligible for Study: Female
Accepts Healthy Volunteers: No

Inclusion Criteria

- History of histologically or cytologically proven Stage I-III breast cancer with estrogen receptor positive with HER-2 positive or negative tumor

- Premenopausal or postmenopausal status

- Completed all primary chemotherapy and surgery

- Currently undergoing adjuvant hormonal therapy (e.g., Tamoxifen and/or Aromatase inhibitors) with or without ovarian function suppression for at least 4 weeks at study entry; the use of Trastuzumab after adjuvant chemotherapy is allowed

- Reported persistent hot flashes for at least 4 weeks AND more than 14 episodes of hot flashes per week (2 hot flashes per day) during the week prior to the study entry

- Eighteen years of age or older

- Eastern Cooperative Oncology Group (ECOG) performance status of 0 or 1

- Signed informed consent

Exclusion Criteria

- Undergoing chemotherapy or planned surgery, chemotherapy, change doses and regimen of hormonal therapy during the study period

- Unstable cardiac disease or myocardial infarction within six months prior to study entry

- Uncontrolled seizure disorder or history of seizure

- Active clinically significant uncontrolled infection

- Use of acupuncture for hot flashes within six months prior to the study entry

- Uncontrolled major psychiatric disorders, such as major depression or psychosis

- Newly starting pharmacologic treatment of hot flashes such as selective serotonin reuptake inhibitors (SSRIs) and/or anticonvulsant for less than four weeks prior to study entry. Participants may continue with medications or therapies for the treatment of hot-flashes while participating in the study if the medication has been taking for more than four weeks prior to study entry AND the dose of the medication is going to be kept consistently during the study.

Chapter 82

Breast-Cancer Research

Chapter Contents

Section 82.1

Liquid Biopsy May Predict Risk of Breast Cancer Returning Years Later

This section includes text excerpted from "Liquid Biopsy May Predict
Risk of Breast Cancer Returning Years Later," National Cancer
Institute (NCI), August 15, 2018.

Women who had cancer cells detected in their blood five years after
a breast-cancer diagnosis were 13 times more likely to have their cancer return than women who did not, results from an ongoing study
have shown.

Most women who are diagnosed with hormone-receptor-positive
(HR+) breast cancer that has not spread will not have a recurrence.
Among those who do have a recurrence, more than half have a late
recurrence, meaning their disease will return five or more years after
diagnosis.

Doctors do not currently have a reliable method to predict who is
likely to have a late recurrence and is a candidate for therapies that
might prevent or delay it. According to the study findings, a blood
test—a type of liquid biopsy—may help classify patients according to
their recurrence risk.

"This is not something that should change practice now," said
lead investigator Kathy Miller, M.D., of Indiana University, Melvin
and Bren Simon Cancer Center (SCC). "But it gives us the potential

for future clinical trials that identify patients at higher risk (of late recurrence) and study whether having that information could change treatment and improve outcomes," she added.

Though there are limitations, "this is a really well-conducted study," said Lyndsay Harris, M.D., of National Cancer Institute's (NCI) Division of Cancer Treatment and Diagnosis (DCTD), who has conducted similar research but was not involved in the study. "It's part of a clinical trial and, therefore, was carefully controlled."

The finding that detection of tumor cells in blood is associated with late recurrence of breast cancer "is a really important observation that had not been clearly shown in the setting of a large clinical trial," she added.

Detecting Breast-Cancer Cells in Blood

Tumors are solid masses, but they aren't static. In addition to growing, spreading, and changing the environment around them, tumors also shed cells into nearby blood vessels. Studies have suggested that measuring and analyzing these so-called circulating tumor cells may reveal important information about the tumor that could benefit the patient.

Liquid biopsies are being widely studied as a way to improve early detection of cancer, monitor disease progression, and help guide treatment decisions.

Dr. Miller and her colleagues wanted to determine whether a liquid biopsy test for circulating tumor cells was associated with late recurrence in women with breast cancer.

More than 700 women who were participating in a large NCI-funded clinical trial of adjuvant therapy for breast cancer also enrolled in this new study. At the time that they enrolled—around five years after their original breast-cancer diagnosis—the women did not have any evidence of a recurrence.

The researchers used a liquid biopsy test to identify and count tumor cells in a sample of blood collected from participants at the time of enrollment. The test is cleared by the U.S. Food and Drug Administration (FDA) to assess disease progression in patients with metastatic breast, prostate, and colon cancer. However, it has not been proven that using the test to inform treatment decisions improves patient outcomes, Dr. Harris stressed.

Of the 547 women whose samples could be analyzed, 26 had at least one detectable circulating tumor cell. The researchers did not observe any major differences in characteristics such as tumor size or age at diagnosis between the women who had detectable circulating tumor

521

cells and those who didn't. The proportion of women with hormone receptor-positive (HR+) and hormone receptor–negative (HR–) breast cancer who had detectable circulating tumor cells was similar.

At a median follow-up of 2.6 years after the test was performed, cancer had returned in 24 women in the study, including 7 women who had detectable circulating tumor cells and 17 who did not. For all women in the study, the detection of circulating tumor cells was associated with a 12.7-fold higher risk of recurrence.

Late recurrences are typically more common among women with HR+ than HR– breast cancer. Dr. Miller and her colleagues observed the same pattern: cancer returned in 6.5 percent of women with HR+ breast cancer and 0.5 percent of those with HR– breast cancer.

Of the 23 women with HR+ breast cancer who had a late recurrence, 7 had detectable circulating tumor cells. For women with HR+ breast cancer, the detection of circulating tumor cells was associated with a 13.1-fold higher risk of recurrence.

Among women with HR+ breast cancer who had detectable circulating tumor cells, those who had a recurrence had higher numbers of circulating tumor cells than those who did not have a recurrence.

None of the eight women with HR– disease who had detectable circulating tumor cells had a recurrence. It's not clear why circulating tumor cells are associated with recurrence only for women with HR+ disease, Dr. Miller said.

Though there's no evidence yet, one idea is that the immune system may be better at attacking and eliminating HR– tumors before they have a chance to grow back, she added.

Predicting At-Risk Patients

The research team acknowledged that the study population is small and that they need to follow the participants for a longer time. They are continuing to follow these participants.

"More patients may have a recurrence with further follow-up," Dr. Miller said.

The researchers also plan to determine if testing patients more than once is a more accurate way to predict recurrence. Circulating tumor cells might be detected later in women who had a recurrence but did not test positive at the five-year mark, said Dr. Miller.

In addition, the team will evaluate other tumor biomarkers—such as certain proteins in the blood—that might be associated with the risk of recurrence "to see if we can do an even better job of segregating patients based on their risk," Dr. Miller explained.

Dr. Harris noted that the question of how the detection of circulating tumor cells might change patient treatment and, ultimately, outcomes, still needs to be addressed.

Women with HR+ breast cancer are sometimes treated with hormone therapy for more than five years in an effort to prevent or delay a late recurrence. But it isn't clear if all patients with HR+ breast cancer need such treatment, which comes with the risk of serious side effects, for that length of time.

Having a test that could predict which HR+ breast-cancer patients are most at risk for a late recurrence and might be good candidates for extended therapy, or another treatment approach, would be helpful, Dr. Harris added.

Dr. Miller and her colleagues are beginning to talk about just such a study, using the liquid biopsy test to determine patient treatment.

Section 82.2

Olaparib Approved for Treating Some Breast Cancers with BRCA *Gene Mutations*

This section includes text excerpted from "Olaparib Approved for Treating Some Breast Cancers with *BRCA* Gene Mutations," National Cancer Institute (NCI), January 29, 2018.

The drug olaparib (Lynparza®) has become the first treatment approved by the U.S. Food and Drug Administration (FDA) for patients with metastatic breast cancer who have inherited mutations in the *BRCA1 or BRCA2* genes.

On January 12, FDA granted regular approval to olaparib for patients with metastatic breast cancer who have a *BRCA* gene mutation and have received chemotherapy previously.

"This is an important advance for women with germline *BRCA* mutations who have breast cancer," said Elise Kohn, M.D., Head of Gynecologic Cancer Therapeutics in National Cancer Institute's (NCI) Division of Cancer Treatment and Diagnosis (DCTD).

"We are always in need of new and better, more active treatments for the women we serve," Dr. Kohn continued. "The approval allows us to move forward in a new direction for treating breast cancer associated with *BRCA* mutations."

The *BRCA1* and *BRCA2* genes produce tumor suppressor proteins that help repair damaged deoxyribonucleic acid (DNA) in cells. Mutations in these genes cause about 75 to 80 percent of hereditary breast cancer and 5 to 10 percent of all breast cancers, Dr. Kohn noted.

Patients are selected for treatment with olaparib using a companion diagnostic test (CDx) called *"BRAC*-Analysis CDx," which the FDA approved for detecting mutations in *BRCA* genes in blood samples from patients with breast cancer who may be eligible for olaparib.

Olaparib belongs to a class of drugs known as pharmacological (PARP) inhibitors. These agents block the actions of PARP proteins, which, like *BRCA* proteins, help repair DNA damage in cells. Blocking PARP proteins in breast-cancer cells that already have a defect in DNA repair—because of *BRCA* mutations—may lead to further DNA damage and cell death.

Olaparib is already approved for treatment of some patients with recurrent ovarian, fallopian tube, or primary peritoneal cancer (PPC), including those with advanced cancers who have *BRCA* mutations, and as maintenance therapy for some patients with recurrent ovarian, fallopian tube, or primary peritoneal cancer.

Study Finds Improvement in Progression-Free Survival

The FDA based its new approval on the results of the OlympiAD clinical trial, which enrolled 302 patients with human epidermal growth factor receptor 2 (HER2)-negative metastatic breast cancer who carried a germline *BRCA* mutation. The trial included some patients with triple-negative breast cancer (TNBC), which can be aggressive and for which there are few treatment options.

Patients were randomly assigned to receive olaparib or standard chemotherapy selected by the patient's physician. All patients had previously received chemotherapy.

The primary endpoint of the trial—which was funded by olaparib's manufacturer, AstraZeneca—was progression-free survival.

In the study, median progression-free survival was 7.0 months for patients in the olaparib group compared with 4.2 months for patients in the standard-therapy group. In the olaparib group, 59 percent of the patients responded, compared with 28.8 percent of the standard-therapy group.

The authors also found that the median time until a patient responded was similar for olaparib and standard therapy. "This finding is an important consideration for symptomatic or rapidly progressing patients," they added.

The rate of grade 3 or higher adverse events was 36.6 percent in patients receiving olaparib and 50.5 percent in patients receiving standard therapy.

Common side effects included low levels of red blood cells (RBCs) (anemia), low levels of certain white blood cells (WBCs) (neutropenia, leukopenia), nausea, fatigue, and vomiting. Severe side effects included the development of certain blood or bone-marrow cancers (myelodysplastic syndrome (MDS)/acute myeloid leukemia (AML)) and inflammation in the lungs (pneumonitis).

"It is striking that nearly every parameter assessed in the study—from the primary endpoint to toxicity—was better with olaparib," said Dr. Kohn, adding that longer follow-up is needed to assess overall survival. "This is progress for patients."

Additional clinical trials of olaparib for breast cancer are underway. For example, a randomized phase three trial is testing the drug in patients with TNBC, and another study, which includes some patients with TNBC, is evaluating olaparib in combination with the drug onalespib.

Section 82.3

Ribociclib Approval Expanded for Some Women with Advanced Breast Cancer

This section includes text excerpted from "Ribociclib Approval Expanded for Some Women with Advanced Breast Cancer," National Cancer Institute (NCI), August 20, 2018.

The U.S. Food and Drug Administration (FDA) has expanded the approval for ribociclib (Kisqali) for some women with advanced breast cancer.

Under the approval, ribociclib can now be used in combination with some types of hormone therapy (HT) for the treatment of advanced hormone receptor-positive (HR+), human epidermal growth factor receptor 2 (HER2)-negative (HER2–) cancer in women who haven't yet reached menopause. Most breast cancers are HR+ and HER2–.

The FDA also expanded ribociclib's approval for use in postmenopausal women (PMW) with this type of advanced breast cancer. Previously, it had been approved for use in combination with a type of hormone therapy called an "aromatase inhibitor (AI)." With the expanded approval, ribociclib can now also be used with fulvestrant (Faslodex), a different type of hormone therapy (HT).

The approval for premenopausal and perimenopausal women was based on results from a randomized clinical trial called "MONALEESA-7." The expanded approval for postmenopausal women (PMW) was based on results of a related trial, called MONALEESA-3. Both trials were sponsored by Novartis, the maker of ribociclib.

The new approvals for ribociclib were the first granted through a new FDA pilot program launched earlier this year called "Real-Time Oncology Review (RTOR)." The program allows the FDA to begin reviewing a drug after results from trials are first available but before a company has officially submitted an approval application.

Under the pilot program, the expanded approval of ribociclib was granted less than a month after Novartis filed its formal approval application, FDA Commissioner Scott Gottlieb, M.D., explained in a statement.

Slowing Disease Progression

Ribociclib works by inhibiting molecules called Cyclin-dependent kinase 4 (CDK4) and Cell division protein kinase 6 (CDK6) that help control cell division. These enzymes are commonly activated by a variety of molecular mechanisms in breast-cancer cells. Other FDA-approved CDK4/6 inhibitors include palbociclib (Ibrance) and abemaciclib (Verzenio).

MONALEESA-7 enrolled 672 pre and perimenopausal women with recurrent or metastatic breast cancer. Women who had previously received hormone therapy for early-stage breast cancer, but not for advanced disease, could enroll in MONALEESA-7. Women who had received a single course of chemotherapy for advanced disease were also eligible to participate.

The researchers randomly assigned participants to receive ribociclib plus HT or a placebo plus HT. The type of HT used was based on factors such as patient and doctor preference and previous treatments, and it could be letrozole (Femara), anastrozole (Arimidex), or tamoxifen. All participants also received a monthly injection of goserelin (Zoladex), which suppresses hormone production in PMW and allows hormone therapy to work better. Goserelin is usually given with standard hormone therapy for PMW with breast cancer.

Women who received ribociclib plus hormone therapy lived longer without their disease progressing (progression-free survival) than women who received placebo plus HT: a median of 24 months compared with 13 months. The improvement in progression-free survival in women treated with ribociclib was about the same regardless of what type of HT was used.

Earlier trials of other CDK4/6 inhibitors had included some PMW but weren't exclusively designed for them, explained Jairam Krishnamurthy, M.D., from the University of Nebraska Medical Center, who was not involved in MONALEESA-7.

Based on results from the earlier trials, many doctors were already using CDK4/6 inhibitors in premenopausal women (with ovarian suppression), said Dr. Krishnamurthy. "MONALEESA-7 is a confirmation for that (practice)," he added.

A similar relative improvement in progression-free survival was seen in the MONALEESA-3 trial, which tested the combination of ribociclib and fulvestrant in PMW with advanced or metastatic disease.

In MONALEESA-7, more cases of a potentially dangerous change in the heart's electrical conduction (called QT interval prolongation) were seen in women who received tamoxifen, even without ribociclib, than in women who received the other forms of hormone therapy, explained Debu Tripathy, M.D., of the University of Texas, MD Anderson Cancer Center, who led the trial. "As a precaution, the new approval does not include the use of ribociclib in combination with tamoxifen," he added.

Some of the most common side effect seen in women in both trials included a drop in the number of white blood cells (WBC), infection, fatigue, and nausea. Quality of life (QOL) remained higher for longer in the ribociclib group.

What Therapy for Which Patients

Follow-up for both trials is still ongoing, to see if a difference in overall survival emerges over time.

"Typically, in HR+, HER2- disease, it has been difficult to show an overall survival advantage because these patients have so many other lines of therapy available" if their disease progresses, explained Dr. Krishnamurthy. "(Improved) overall survival is something that's been kind of the holy grail" in advanced breast cancer, he added.

In both trials, patients' QOL remained high during treatment. This is important for advanced cancer said Dr. Krishnamurthy.

"A common misconception among patients (with advanced disease) and their families is they feel that we should administer chemotherapy because we have to be 'aggressive.'

"On the contrary, for HR+, HER2- disease, you have to target the estrogen receptor (ER)," for as long as possible, he added. This strategy has the potential to be both more effective and produce fewer side effects than chemotherapy, he explained.

Two trials in progress (PEARL and PASIPHAE) are testing whether giving a CDK4/6 inhibitor and HT instead of chemotherapy as an initial, or first-line, treatment for women with metastatic breast cancer improves progression-free survival.

Other questions about the best way to use CDK4/6 inhibitors remain to be answered. For instance, further studies are needed to understand which patients with advanced or metastatic breast cancer may do just as well with an HT alone and which patients have tumors that are resistant to CDK4/6 inhibition, explained Dr. Tripathy. Neither of these groups would benefit from a combination of CDK4/6 inhibitors and HT.

And for tumors that are resistant to CDK4/6 inhibitors, more research is needed to tease out "what the mechanisms of resistance are and how we can use this information—not only to make better choices for our patients but also to discover newer drugs that might reverse resistance or perform better in these patients," Dr. Tripathy said.

But "clinicians should at least discuss the possibility of adding a CDK4/6 inhibitor with everybody who's getting first-line or second-line HT (for advanced disease)," he concluded. "Because, for most patients, CDK4/6 inhibitors appear to be of benefit in terms of delaying progression and may also delay the time that they need to go on more aggressive treatment, like chemotherapy."

Section 82.4

Topical Drugs for Preventing Breast Cancer

This section includes text excerpted from "Can Topical Drugs Help Prevent Breast Cancer?" National Cancer Institute (NCI), December 4, 2018.

The drug tamoxifen can help prevent breast cancer in women at an increased risk of the disease. But many women who stand to benefit from tamoxifen do not take the drug—a pill—because of concerns about side effects, such as hot flashes and the increased risk of blood clots and stroke.

To explore alternatives to oral tamoxifen that might have fewer side effects, researchers are testing a topical form of the drug in two clinical trials. These randomized placebo-controlled studies are evaluating a gel formulation of tamoxifen called "4-hydroxytamoxifen (4-OHT)" that women apply directly to the breasts.

The goal of this research is to find out if delivering a form of tamoxifen topically results in the same level of the drug in the breast but leads to lower levels of the drug in the blood and other parts of the body compared with oral delivery, according to Brandy Heckman-Stoddard, Ph.D., of National Cancer Institute's (NCI) Division of Cancer Prevention (DCP).

"With lower levels of the drug in the body, women would potentially have fewer side effects," she added.

Testing a Topical Drug for Breast-Cancer Prevention

Four years ago, Seema Khan, M.D., of Northwestern University Feinberg School of Medicine led a small study that compared the proliferation of abnormal cells in the lining of the breast duct—a condition known as ductal carcinoma *in situ* (DCIS)—among women treated with the gel applied to the breast skin and women treated with oral tamoxifen. (In women with DCIS, the abnormal cells have not yet spread to other tissues in the breast.)

"We found a similar reduction in the growth of DCIS cells from both the gel and the pill form of the drug, and the concentrations (of tamoxifen) in the breasts of women who were treated with the gel were quite good," said Dr. Khan, who is leading one of the new clinical trials of the tamoxifen gel. 4-OHT has the feel and consistency of hand sanitizer gel, she noted.

Women in the gel group also had lower blood levels of certain bio-markers associated with side effects than women in the oral tamoxifen group, the researchers found.

Dr. Khan cautioned that those results need to be confirmed by the randomized placebo-controlled clinical trials now underway. She also noted that the 4-OHT gel is intended for use in a specific group of women.

"This approach is for healthy women who have an increased risk of breast cancer and for women with DCIS," said Dr. Khan. "When the problem is confined to the breast, this approach would be appropriate."

Using a topical drug would not be a viable approach once breast-cancer cells have broken through the duct walls, because those cancer cells can go elsewhere in the body, she explained.

"In such cases, the treatment for invasive breast cancer needs to be systemic, and the local approach does not achieve that," said Dr. Khan.

For women with DCIS, the topical application is "a local treatment for a local condition," said Dr. Heckman-Stoddard.

Using Breast Density as an Indicator in Clinical Trials

NCI is cosponsoring one of the 4-OHT gel clinical trials, and the company that manufactures the gel, BHR Pharma, is sponsoring the other.

"There's real excitement in the field for the results of the two studies," said Dr. Heckman-Stoddard. "And if the trials demonstrate the effectiveness of the gel, then this could lead to the next large phase three breast cancer prevention trial for NCI."

In both trials, researchers are assessing changes in breast density as a proxy for the anticancer effects of the drugs. Breast density has emerged as an important research area in breast cancer for two reasons: Dense breasts are a risk factor for breast cancer, and on mammograms dense breasts can mask breast cancers, making some tumors difficult to detect.

Clinical trials of oral tamoxifen have shown that people who have the greatest reduction in breast density also have the greatest reduction in breast-cancer risk, noted Banu K. Arun, M.D., of the University of Texas, MD Anderson Cancer Center, who is leading a second tamoxifen gel clinical trial.

Participants in this study will apply the 4-OHT gel or placebo gel to the breasts for a year. "We are measuring mammographic breast density and hoping to see a decrease," said Dr. Arun.

Although the evidence that a readily available drug—oral tamoxifen—can reduce breast-cancer risk and breast density is strong, Dr.

Arun continued, "new approaches are needed" to prevent breast cancer because many women who might benefit from oral tamoxifen do not take it because of side effects.

"We do not have a clear picture of whether the gel will avoid hot flashes," said Dr. Khan. "But the ongoing clinical trials will give us information about whether the side effects are reduced."

The clinical trials may also help answer questions about how well topical drugs are dispersed, or distributed, in the breast. Dr. Heckman-Stoddard noted that the distribution could be different for different topical agents.

Whether the amount of gel used to prevent breast cancer should differ based on breast size is also being explored in the clinical trials, Dr. Khan said.

Broadening the Approach to Include Other Drugs

In addition to its role in the 4-OHT gel studies, NCI is sponsoring two additional trials of topical drugs for breast-cancer prevention. One trial is testing a gel form of the drug bexarotene (Targretin), and the other is testing a gel form of the drug endoxifen.

If the current clinical trials demonstrate the potential of using topical drugs for preventing breast cancer, Dr. Khan plans to investigate additional agents, including topical forms of some drugs that are too toxic for patients to take orally.

"We are giving drugs for cancer prevention to healthy women, so there has to be a high standard for safety and tolerability," said Dr. Khan.

"Some drugs, such as certain types of retinoids, are not suitable for oral use by healthy women, but topical forms of these medicines might expand the options for cancer prevention if they get through the skin and have the desired effects," she added.

For the moment, the researchers are focused on the current 4-OHT gel studies and the recruitment of the few hundred women needed to advance the research.

"I'm optimistic about this approach," said Dr. Arun, referring to the use of the gel. "We know how tamoxifen works (to prevent breast cancer), and we have the results of trials testing oral tamoxifen."

Dr. Khan agreed. "The momentum is building for this agent," she said. "If both trials go in the right direction, then we'll be poised to test the approach in a study of thousands of women."

Section 82.5

Two Drugs Work Together to Block "Master Regulator" of Breast, Other Cancers

This section includes text excerpted from "Two Drugs Work Together to Block 'Master Regulator' of Breast, Other Cancers," National Cancer Institute (NCI), September 4, 2018.

A two-drug combination commonly used to treat a type of leukemia blocks an enzyme that has a central role in breast and many other cancers, a study has found. The drug combination, arsenic trioxide (Trisenox) and tretinoin (also known as "retinoic acid"), has essentially turned acute promyelocytic leukemia (APL) from a fatal disease into a curable one. But the mechanism by which it kills cancer cells has been a mystery.

In an earlier study, Kun Ping Lu, M.D., Ph.D., and Xiao Zhen Zhou, M.D., of Beth Israel Deaconess Medical Center, in Boston, and their colleagues found that retinoic acid inhibits the key enzyme, Pin1. Now, they've found that arsenic also blocks Pin1, and the combination of the two drugs inhibits the enzyme more effectively than either drug alone.

Pin1 is considered a cancer master regulator—a protein that regulates entire cellular networks that are critical to cancer progression. Some scientists consider master regulators ideal drug targets.

The findings are "an interesting launching pad for further investigation," said Joanna Watson, Ph.D., of National Cancer Institute's (NCI) Division of Cancer Biology (DCB), which helped fund the study.

The combination treatment slowed the growth of several different laboratory models of breast cancer, the researchers reported. Their findings, published in *Nature Communications*, provide the rationale to test the drug combination in a clinical trial of women with breast cancer, said Dr. Lu.

Pin1: An Ideal Drug Target

Pin1 switches the shape of the amino acid proline within proteins. This conformation change can activate 40 proteins that promote tumor growth and inactivate more than 20 proteins that suppress tumor growth.

Pin1 is overactive in many different types of cancer, including breast, lung, prostate, and colon cancer. It is also found at higher than normal levels in breast-cancer stem cells—specialized cancer cells that are thought to be responsible for tumor initiation, growth, metastasis, and drug resistance.

On the other hand, mice that lack Pin1 are protected from developing cancer even in the presence of cancer-causing mutations in other genes.

Because arsenic is often combined with retinoic acid to treat acute promyelocytic leukemia (APL), the researchers wanted to know if arsenic also targets Pin1. But rather than studying APL, they focused on triple-negative breast cancer (TNBC) because this aggressive disease has a poor prognosis and is not effectively treated with targeted therapies.

Arsenic and Retinoic Acid Work Together

First, the researchers found that arsenic inhibited Pin1 activity, which in turn slowed the growth of TNBC cells. They then showed that arsenic needed to bind to Pin1 to impede breast-cancer cell growth. Interacting with arsenic makes Pin1 unstable, explained Dr. Lu, and as a result, the protein is destroyed. Arsenic also lowered Pin1 levels and slowed the growth of breast-cancer xenograft tumors in mice. Next, the researchers examined the effects of combining arsenic and retinoic acid in cell and mouse models of TNBC.

Treating cells or mice with arsenic or retinoic acid alone lowered Pin1 levels and slowed cell growth. But the combination of the two drugs had an even greater effect. The combination also prevented Pin1 from altering the levels of certain proteins that control cancer growth, producing effects that are similar to those of inactivating the *Pin1* gene in breast-cancer cells.

The combination showed synergy, meaning that the resulting effect "is above and beyond what you would expect by just adding the two (drugs) together," explained Dr. Watson.

Synergy may reflect the fact that, in APL cells, retinoic acid treatment raises the level of a transporter that brings arsenic inside of cells. Levels of the transporter also increased when Dr. Lu and his colleagues treated TNBC with retinoic acid. By contrast, arsenic and retinoic acid did not act synergistically in TNBC cells engineered to lack this transporter.

These results suggest that, in addition to inhibiting *Pin1* directly, retinoic acid increases the amount of arsenic in cells by boosting the level of this transporter, Dr. Lu explained. The arsenic then further inhibits Pin1.

He added, this also implies that when used in combination with retinoic acid, a lower concentration of arsenic could achieve the desired effect—potentially reducing the side effects of arsenic, which is extremely toxic at high doses.

Targeting Breast-Cancer Stem Cells

Developing drugs that effectively target cancer stem cells has proven to be a challenge, and cancer stem cells that remain after treatment are thought to be a cause of cancer relapse and metastasis.

Dr. Lu's team found that to a greater extent than either drug alone, the combination of arsenic and retinoic acid eliminated TNBC stem cells. The effects of the combination treatment were similar to those of inactivating the *Pin1* gene in breast-cancer cells, they found.

The researchers also found that the combination of arsenic and retinoic acid eliminated cancer stem cells that were resistant to chemotherapy, and it eliminated cancer stem cells in mouse models of TNBC.

New Insights and Potential New Therapy

It had long been thought that arsenic's main target was a fusion protein that is found only in APL, and there were doubts that the drug would be effective against other types of cancer, despite some evidence of activity. In their earlier study, Drs. Lu and Zhou and their colleagues found that retinoic acid targets this fusion protein by inhibiting *Pin1*.

"Identifying *Pin1* as the major target of arsenic will hopefully stimulate clinical trials for other (types of) cancer," Dr. Lu said.

The researchers hope to develop a clinical trial to combine arsenic with the standard therapy for women with TNBC. And because their findings show that arsenic's activity depends on the expression of *Pin1* and its transporter, Dr. Lu said they want to select patients whose cancers express both proteins.

As for retinoic acid, it is normally broken down quickly inside the human body. To enhance its ability to reach solid tumors, the team is interested in developing a more stable form of retinoic acid. If such a form can be created, it could potentially be combined with arsenic in clinical trials, Dr. Lu said.

Another advantage of having learned one mechanism of arsenic's anticancer activity, said Dr. Watson, is being able to develop new drugs that potentially target *Pin1* more efficiently and with fewer side effects than arsenic itself. The research team is also working to develop a targeted drug that blocks Pin1 activity.

Dr. Lu noted that because *Pin1* controls multiple pathways that contribute to cancer development, cancer cells might be less able to develop resistance to drugs that block *Pin1*'s activity—something that often occurs with targeted therapies that attack a single pathway.

Section 82.6

Whole- and Partial-Breast Radiation Effective at Preventing Breast Cancer from Returning

This section includes text excerpted from "Whole- and Partial-Breast Radiation Effective at Preventing Breast Cancer from Returning," National Cancer Institute (NCI), December 19, 2018.

Results from two clinical trials suggest that either of two types of radiation therapy after breast-conserving surgery for women with early-stage breast cancer can reduce the risk of the cancer returning.

In the randomized clinical trials, both whole-breast irradiation (WBI) and accelerated partial-breast irradiation (APBI) were associated with low rates of cancer recurring in the breast where the disease originally developed. The median follow-up ranged from more than five years to more than ten years.

The United States and Canadian researchers presented results from both trials at the San Antonio Breast Cancer Symposium (SABCS).

WBI is typically given to the whole breast in a series of treatments five days a week for four to six weeks. By comparison, accelerated partial breast irradiation (APBI) is given only to the part of the breast that has or had cancer in it, and the treatments are completed in a week or less.

A Head-to-Head Comparison

Previous studies have shown that after a diagnosis of early-stage breast cancer, a lumpectomy followed by WBI decreases the risk of cancer recurring in the same breast. But many women do not receive the recommended radiation therapy for various reasons, including the inconvenience of traveling to a distant treatment center.

By delivering larger individual doses of radiation across fewer treatment sessions, APBI has emerged as an alternative approach to WBI. Studies have shown that by treating the area of the breast in the vicinity of the original tumor, APBI can reduce recurrences.

The new trials provide head-to-head comparisons of the two approaches with long-term follow-up. In the United States study, for instance, more than 95 percent of participants in each treatment group—those receiving either WBI or APBI—did not have a recurrence at a median follow-up of 10 years after their treatments ended.

Investigators with the Canadian RAPID trial reported similar results, although the median follow-up was shorter.

"In both studies—and in both treatment arms—the outcomes overall were extremely good," said Larissa Korde, M.D., of National Cancer Institute (NCI) Cancer Therapy Evaluation Program (CTEP). Patients with early-stage breast cancer, she continued, "can use this information to decide whether APBI is the right course for them individually."

Following Patients for More than a Decade

The NCI-supported National Surgical Adjuvant Breast and Bowel Project (NSABP), now part of NRG Oncology, led the U.S. phase 3 trial. NSABP researchers randomly assigned 4,216 patients with breast cancer who had received a lumpectomy to treatment with APBI or WBI.

Of this group, 25 percent had ductal carcinoma *in situ* (DCIS), 65 percent had stage 1 breast cancer, and 10 percent had stage 2 breast cancer. Eighty-one percent of the patients had hormone receptor-positive cancer, and 61 percent of the patients were postmenopausal.

Women assigned to APBI received either brachytherapy (an internal form of radiation therapy) or three-dimensional conformal external beam radiation therapy (3D-CRT).

After a median follow-up of 10.2 years, 161 patients had a breast-cancer recurrence: 90 patients who received APBI and 71 who received WBI. There were modest differences between the groups in terms of side effects.

"An Acceptable Choice for Many Women"

The two methods of radiation therapy produced similar, if not statistically equivalent, results, noted Frank Vicini, M.D., of 21st Century Oncology of Michigan, who presented the findings of the U.S. study in San Antonio. "The less burdensome radiation method of APBI may be an acceptable choice for many women," he added.

Dr. Vicini said that although APBI produced "good results for a large population of women and does remain a good option," the study results also suggested that there are "limits to the extent that we can cut back" on the schedule and dose of radiation for certain patients and still achieve good outcomes.

More research is needed to develop tools such as biomarkers that could help predict which patients with early-stage breast cancer might benefit most from WBI or APBI, according to Dr. Korde.

Rapid Results

In the RAPID study, 2,135 patients from Canada, Australia, and New Zealand (NZ) were randomly assigned to receive WBI or APBI. Of this group, 82 percent of patients had invasive breast cancer and 18 percent had DCIS only. The median follow-up was 8.6 years.

Both treatment groups had low rates of tumor recurrence: In the APBI group, the 5- and 8-year cumulative rates of recurrence were 2.3 percent and 3.0 percent, respectively, whereas the corresponding rates for the WBI group were 1.7 percent and 2.8 percent, respectively.

Although there were fewer side effects in patients receiving the APBI regimen compared with the WBI regimen after treatment, there was an increase in side effects associated with the APBI regimen after three months, the researchers reported.

Dr. Korde noted that both trials have collected data on the toxic side effects and the effects on physical appearance associated with each type of radiation therapy.

"It will be helpful to have more data that can be used to better understand which patients have a low risk of toxicity with any type of radiation therapy, and therefore, which patients might feel more comfortable with using the shorter course of APBI," said Dr. Korde.

In the future, she continued, "additional information on toxicity from the NSABP trial will further add to this important discussion."

Section 82.7

For Some Breast-Cancer Survivors, Drug May Reduce Treatment-Related Joint Pain

This section includes text excerpted from "New Approach to Immunotherapy Leads to Complete Response in Breast-Cancer Patient Unresponsive to Other Treatments," National Cancer Institute (NCI), June 4, 2018.

A novel approach to immunotherapy developed by researchers at the National Cancer Institute (NCI) has led to the complete regression of breast cancer in a patient who was unresponsive to all other

537

treatments. This patient received the treatment in a clinical trial led by Steven A. Rosenberg, M.D., Ph.D., chief of the Surgery Branch at NCI's Center for Cancer Research (CCR), and the findings were published June 4, 2018 in *Nature Medicine*. NCI is part of the National Institutes of Health (NIH).

"We've developed a high-throughput method to identify mutations present in cancer that are recognized by the immune system," Dr. Rosenberg said. "This research is experimental right now. But because this new approach to immunotherapy is dependent on mutations, not on cancer type, it is in a sense a blueprint we can use for the treatment of many types of cancer."

The new immunotherapy approach is a modified form of adoptive cell transfer (ACT). ACT has been effective in treating melanoma, which has high levels of somatic, or acquired, mutations. However, it has been less effective with some common epithelial cancers, or cancers that start in the lining of organs, that have lower levels of mutations, such as stomach, esophageal, ovarian, and breast cancers.

In an ongoing phase 2 clinical trial, the investigators are developing a form of ACT that uses tumor-infiltrating lymphocytes (TILs) that specifically target tumor cell mutations to see if they can shrink tumors in patients with these common epithelial cancers. As with other forms of ACT, the selected TILs are grown to large numbers in the laboratory and are then infused back into the patient (who has in the meantime undergone treatment to deplete remaining lymphocytes) to create a stronger immune response against the tumor.

A patient with metastatic breast cancer came to the trial after receiving multiple treatments, including several chemotherapy and hormonal treatments, that had not stopped her cancer from progressing. To treat her, the researchers sequenced deoxyribonucleic acid (DNA) and ribonucleic acid (RNA) from one of her tumors, as well as normal tissue to see which mutations were unique to her cancer, and identified 62 different mutations in her tumor cells.

The researchers then tested different TILs from the patient to find those that recognized one or more of these mutated proteins. TILs recognized four of the mutant proteins, and the TILs then were expanded and infused back into the patient. She was also given the checkpoint inhibitor pembrolizumab to prevent the possible inactivation of the infused T cells by factors in the tumor microenvironment. After the treatment, all of this patient's cancer disappeared and has not returned more than 22 months later.

"This is an illustrative case report that highlights, once again, the power of immunotherapy," said Tom Misteli, Ph.D., Director of CCR at NCI. "If confirmed in a larger study, it promises to further extend the reach of this T-cell therapy to a broader spectrum of cancers."

Investigators have seen similar results using mutation-targeted TIL treatment for patients in the same trial with other epithelial cancers, including liver cancer and colorectal cancer. Dr. Rosenberg explained that results like this in patients with solid epithelial tumors are important because ACT has not been as successful with these kinds of cancers as with other types that have more mutations.

He said the "big picture" here is this kind of treatment is not cancer-type specific. "All cancers have mutations, and that's what we're attacking with this immunotherapy," he said. "It is ironic that the very mutations that cause the cancer may prove to be the best targets to treat the cancer."

Section 82.8

NIH Scientists Find That Breast-Cancer Protection from Pregnancy Starts Decades Later

This section includes text excerpted from "NIH Scientists Find That Breast Cancer Protection from Pregnancy Starts Decades Later," National Cancer Institute (NCI), December 14, 2018.

In general, women who have had children have a lower risk of breast cancer compared to women who have never given birth. However, research has found that moms don't experience this breast cancer protection until many years later and may face an elevated risk for more than 20 years after their last pregnancy.

Scientists at the National Institutes of Health (NIH), along with members of the international Premenopausal Breast Cancer Collaborative Group, found breast-cancer risk increases in the years after birth, with the highest risk of developing the disease about five years later. The findings, which appeared online in the *Annals of Internal Medicine*, suggest breast-cancer protection from pregnancy may not begin until as many as 30 years after the birth of the last child.

According to senior author Dale Sandler, Ph.D., Head of the Epidemiology Branch at the National Institute of Environmental Health Sciences (NIEHS), part of NIH, a few prior studies reported an increase in breast-cancer risk after childbirth. However, most of what researchers knew about breast-cancer risk factors came from studies of women who have gone through menopause. Since breast cancer is relatively uncommon in younger women, it is more difficult to study.

Researchers combined data from approximately 890,000 women from 15 long-term studies across three continents, to understand the relationship between recent childbirth and breast-cancer risk in women age 55 and younger.

"We were surprised to find that an increase in breast-cancer risk lasted for an average of 24 years before childbirth became protective," said Sandler. "Before this study, most researchers believed that any increase in risk lasted less than 10 years."

The scientists also found that the association between recent childbirth and breast-cancer risk was stronger for women who were older at first birth, had more births, or had a family history of breast cancer. Breastfeeding did not appear to have any protective effect, even though it is generally thought to reduce breast-cancer risk. Many of these additional factors were not addressed in earlier studies, underscoring the statistical power of this larger project.

Sandler and first author Hazel Nichols, Ph.D., of the University of North Carolina Lineberger Comprehensive Cancer Center, started the study when Nichols was a research fellow at NIEHS. Nichols explained that childbirth is an example of a risk factor that is different for younger women than older women.

"This difference is important because it suggests that we may need to develop tools for predicting breast-cancer risk that is specific to young women," Nichols said. "Doing so would help women talk to their healthcare providers about when they should start mammography screening."

Nichols and Sandler both stressed the importance of keeping these findings in perspective. Breast cancer is uncommon in young women. An increase in the relative risk of breast cancer in women under age 55 translates to a very small number of additional cases of breast cancer per year.

Anthony Swerdlow, D.M., D.Sc., Ph.D., and Minouk Schoemaker, Ph.D., scientists at the Institute of Cancer Research, London, co-led the study with Sandler and Nichols.

Section 82.9

For Some Breast-Cancer Survivors, Drug May Reduce Treatment-Related Joint Pain

This section includes text excerpted from "For Some Breast Cancer Survivors, Drug May Reduce Treatment-Related Joint Pain," National Cancer Institute (NCI), January 4, 2017.

A drug most commonly used to treat depression may also reduce joint pain in some women being treated for early-stage breast cancer, according to the results of a randomized clinical trial (RCT).

After undergoing treatment for early-stage breast cancer, many postmenopausal women (PMW) take drugs known as aromatase inhibitors (AIs) to reduce the risk of the cancer returning. These drugs, however, can cause significant pain in women's joints and muscles.

The clinical trial showed that duloxetine (Cymbalta®), which is approved to treat depression and anxiety as well as fibromyalgia and nerve pain caused by diabetes, provided some relief from pain associated with AIs.

"Joint and muscle pain can lead some patients to discontinue treatment with these life-saving medications," said N. Lynn Henry, M.D., Ph.D., of the Huntsman Cancer Institute (HCI) at the University of Utah, who led the study. "Based on our results, duloxetine seems to be an effective drug for some patients who experience this pain."

Dr. Henry presented findings from the study, which was led by the National Cancer Institute (NCI)-supported clinical trials group Southwest Oncology Group (SWOG), at the San Antonio Breast Cancer Symposium (SABCS).

New Strategies Needed

The body uses an enzyme called "aromatase" to make estrogen (ER). Drugs that block the activity of this enzyme, called AIs, have been found to reduce the risk of cancer returning in postmenopausal women (PMW) whose breast tumors rely on estrogen to fuel their growth.

But many patients taking these drugs experience pain in the knees, hips, hands, and wrists, which can make everyday tasks difficult. About 20 percent of patients stop taking aromatase inhibitors due to side effects, according to Dr. Henry. She noted that patients are generally recommended to take aromatase inhibitors for 5 to 10 years, so new strategies for managing the side effects are needed.

For the duloxetine trial, the researchers enrolled 299 women at 43 NCI's Community Oncology Research Program (NCORP) sites across the United States. The women had been treated with AIs for early-stage breast cancer and were experiencing joint pain caused by treatment. The women were randomly assigned to receive a 12-week course of duloxetine or placebo.

Participants completed questionnaires about joint pain, depression, and quality of life (QOL) at the beginning of the trial, and then again after 2, 6, 12, and 24 weeks. The pain questionnaire used a 0 to 10 scale; the researchers defined a clinically significant change in average pain as a decrease of 2 or more points from the time a patient entered the study.

Duloxetine and Placebo-Reduced Pain

Over the first 12 weeks of the trial, the pain scores of women in the duloxetine group fell an average of 0.82 points more than those of the placebo group. Other measures, including worst pain, joint pain, and stiffness, underwent similar declines.

For the duloxetine group, the average pain score decreased from 5.44 at baseline to 2.91 at 12 weeks. But the average pain score also dropped in the placebo group during the same period, from 5.49 to 3.45. Both reductions were clinically significant, according to the standards of the trial.

The finding of a strong placebo effect in the control group was not entirely unexpected, noted Dr. Henry. Other studies of treatments for pain have reported similar effects, although the reasons are not clear. "This trial demonstrates the need for more research" on responsiveness to placebo, she added.

By 12 weeks, 69 percent of patients in the duloxetine group and 60 percent of patients in the placebo group had a 2-point improvement in pain compared to before starting treatment. At 24 weeks, which was 12 weeks after the patients had stopped taking duloxetine or the placebo, the average pain scores were similar for the groups (3.37 in the duloxetine group and 3.42 for the placebo group).

The most common side effects of duloxetine were nausea, fatigue, and dry mouth, which is consistent with other studies involving the drug.

Exploring Multiple Approaches

"These results of the duloxetine study are very promising," said Ann O'Mara, Ph.D., of NCI's Division of Cancer Prevention (DCP), who was

542

not involved in the study. "Duloxetine is the first drug to show a benefit for this population of patients in a large, randomized clinical trial."

Dr. O'Mara suggested that patients taking aromatase inhibitors might ultimately need to try multiple approaches to manage their pain. Exercise such as walking and acupuncture are among various strategies that are being studied as ways to reduce pain, she noted.

"Clinicians need to be clear with their patients about the potential side effects of duloxetine, but this drug may help patients decrease their pain and become functional again," she added.

Section 82.10

Survival of Women Diagnosed with Metastatic Breast Cancer Has Been Increasing

This section includes text excerpted from "Study Estimates Number of U.S. Women Living with Metastatic Breast Cancer," National Cancer Institute (NCI), May 18, 2017.

A new study shows that the number of women in the United States living with distant metastatic breast cancer (MBC), the most severe form of the disease, is growing. This is likely due to the aging of the United States population and improvements in treatment. Researchers came to this finding by estimating the number of United States women living with MBC, or breast cancer that has spread to distant sites in the body, including women who were initially diagnosed with metastatic disease, and those who developed MBC after an initial diagnosis at an earlier stage.

The researchers also found that median and five-year relative survival for women initially diagnosed with MBC is improving, especially among younger women.

The study was led by Angela Mariotto, Ph.D., chief of the Data Analytics Branch of the Division of Cancer Control and Population Sciences (DCCPS) at the National Cancer Institute (NCI), with co-authors from NCI, the Metastatic Breast Cancer Alliance, and the Fred Hutchinson Cancer Research Center. The findings appeared online on

May 18, 2017, in *Cancer Epidemiology, Biomarkers and Prevention*. NCI is part of the National Institutes of Health (NIH).

In documenting the prevalence of MBC, the findings point to the need for more research into how to address the healthcare needs of women who live with this condition. "Even though this group of patients with MBC is increasing in size, our findings are favorable," said Dr. Mariotto. "This is because, over time, these women are living longer with MBC. Longer survival with MBC means increased needs for services and research. Our study helps to document this need."

Although researchers have been able to estimate the number of women initially diagnosed with MBC, data on the number of women whose cancers spread to a distant organ site, either as a progression or a recurrence after being first diagnosed with an earlier stage of breast cancer, has been lacking because U.S. registries do not routinely collect or report data on recurrence. To develop a more accurate estimate of the total number of women living with MBC, researchers used data from NCI Surveillance, Epidemiology, and End Results (SEER) Program to include women who developed MBC after diagnosis. The researchers estimated that, as of January 1, 2017, more than 150,000 women in this country were living with MBC, and that 3 in 4 of them had initially been diagnosed with an earlier stage of breast cancer.

The study also shows that despite the poor prognosis of MBC, the survival of women initially diagnosed with MBC has been increasing, especially among women diagnosed at younger ages. The researchers estimated that between 1992 to 1994 and 2005 to 2012, five-year relative survival among women initially diagnosed with MBC at ages 15 to 49 years doubled from 18 percent to 36 percent. Median relative survival time between 1992 to 1994 and 2005 to 2012 increased from 22.3 months to 38.7 months for women diagnosed between ages 15 to 49, and from 19.1 months to 29.7 months for women diagnosed between ages 50 to 64. The researchers also reported that a small but meaningful number of women live many years after an initial diagnosis of MBC. More than 11 percent of women diagnosed between 2000 to 2004 under the age of 64 survived 10 years or more.

Based on their calculations, the researchers estimated that the number of women living with MBC increased by 4 percent from 1990 to 2000 and by 17 percent from 2000 to 2010, and they project that the number will increase by 31 percent from 2010 to 2020. Although the largest group of women with MBC consists of women who have been living with metastatic disease for two years or less (40%), one-third

(34%) of women with MBC have lived for five years or more with the disease.

To estimate the number of U.S. women living with MBC, the researchers applied a back-calculation method to breast cancer mortality and survival data from the SEER Program. SEER collects clinical, demographic, and vital status information on all cancer cases diagnosed in defined geographic areas. The method they used assumes that a breast-cancer death is preceded by MBC that was either found at diagnosis or after a recurrence with metastatic disease.

Collecting recurrence data has been challenging for cancer registries because recurrence can be diagnosed through diverse methods and in a variety of locations. To help implement the comprehensive and accurate collection of these data, NCI is funding pilot studies aimed at identifying ways to leverage existing data and informatics methods to efficiently capture information on the recurrent disease.

By including women with recurrence, this study provides a more accurate number of women in the United States currently living with MBC. This estimation can help with healthcare planning and the ultimate goal of better serving these women.

"These findings make clear that the majority of MBC patients, those who are diagnosed with nonmetastatic cancer but progress to distant disease, have never been properly documented," said Dr. Mariotto. "This study emphasizes the importance of collecting data on recurrence at the individual level in order to foster more research into the prevention of recurrence and the specific needs of this growing population."

Part Nine

Additional Help and Information

Chapter 83

Glossary of Breast-Cancer Terms

adenosis: A disease or abnormal change in a gland. Breast adenosis is a benign condition in which the lobules are larger than usual.

areola: The area of dark-colored skin on the breast that surrounds the nipple.

atrophy: Thinning or diminishing of tissue or muscle.

atypical ductal hyperplasia (ADH): A benign (not cancer) condition in which there are more cells than normal in the lining of breast ducts and the cells look abnormal under a microscope. Having ADH increases your risk of breast cancer.

biological therapy: Treatment to boost or restore the ability of the immune system to fight cancer, infections, and other diseases. Also used to lessen certain side effects that may be caused by some cancer treatments.

biopsy: The removal and examination of tissue, cells or fluid from a living body.

BRCA1: A gene on chromosome 17 that normally helps to suppress cell growth. A person who inherits certain mutations (changes) in a

---

This glossary contains terms excerpted from documents produced by several sources deemed reliable.

BRCA1 gene has a higher risk of getting breast, ovarian, prostate, and other types of cancer. *BRCA1* is short for (breast cancer 1, early onset gene).

BRCA2: A gene on chromosome 13 that normally helps to suppress cell growth. A person who inherits certain mutations (changes) in a *BRCA2* gene has a higher risk of getting breast, ovarian, prostate, and other types of cancer. *BRCA2* is short for (breast cancer 2, early onset gene).

breast-conserving surgery: An operation to remove the breast cancer but not the breast itself. Also called breast-sparing surgery.

breast density: Describes the relative amount of different tissues present in the breast. A dense breast has less fat than glandular and connective tissue.

breast implant: Any surgically implanted artificial device intended to replace missing breast tissue or to enhance a breast.

chest wall: The system of structures outside the lungs that move as a part of breathing, including bones (the rib cage) and muscles (diaphragm and abdomen).

core biopsy: The removal of a tissue sample with a wide needle for examination under a microscope.

cyst: A sac or capsule in the body. It may be filled with fluid or other material.

diagnostic mammogram: X-ray of the breasts used to check for cancer after a lump or other sign or symptom of breast cancer has been found.

ductal carcinoma *in situ***:** A noninvasive condition in which abnormal cells are found in the lining of a breast duct. The abnormal cells have not spread outside the duct to other tissues in the breast.

excisional biopsy: A surgical procedure in which an entire lump or suspicious area is removed for diagnosis. The tissue is then examined under a microscope to check for signs of disease.

fat necrosis: A benign condition in which fat tissue in the breast or other organs is damaged by injury, surgery, or radiation therapy. The fat tissue in the breast may be replaced by a cyst or by scar tissue, which may feel like a round, firm lump.

fibroadenoma: A benign (not cancer) tumor that usually forms in the breast from both fibrous and glandular tissue. Fibroadenomas are the most common benign breast tumors.

grade: A description of a tumor based on how abnormal the cancer cells look under a microscope and how quickly the tumor is likely to grow and spread.

hematoma: A collection of blood inside the body, for example in skin tissue.

hormonal therapy: Treatment that adds, blocks, or removes hormones. For certain conditions (such as diabetes or menopause), hormones are given to adjust low hormone levels.

implant displacement views: A procedure used to do a mammogram (X-ray of the breasts) in women with breast implants.

incisional biopsy: A surgical procedure in which a portion of a lump or suspicious area is removed for diagnosis. The tissue is then examined under a microscope to check for signs of disease.

inflammation/irritation: The response of the body to infection or injury characterized by swelling, redness, warmth and/or pain.

lactation: The production and secretion of milk by the breast glands.

lobe: A portion of an organ, such as the breast, liver, lung, thyroid, or brain.

lobule: A small lobe or a subdivision of a lobe.

local anesthesia: A temporary loss of feeling in one small area of the body caused by special drugs or other substances called anesthetics. The patient stays awake but has no feeling in the area of the body treated with the anesthetic.

lumpectomy: Surgery to remove abnormal tissue or cancer from the breast and a small amount of normal tissue around it. It is a type of breast-sparing surgery.

lymph node: A rounded mass of lymphatic tissue that is surrounded by a capsule of connective tissue. Lymph nodes filter lymph (lymphatic fluid), and they store lymphocytes (white blood cells). They are located along lymph vessels. Also called a lymph gland.

lymph vessel: A thin tube that carries lymph (lymphatic fluid) and white blood cells through the lymphatic system. Also called lymphatic vessel.

lymph: The clear fluid that travels through the lymphatic system and carries cells that help fight infections and other diseases. Also called lymphatic fluid.

lymphocyte: A type of immune cell that is made in the bone marrow and is found in the blood and in lymph tissue. The two main types of lymphocytes are B lymphocytes and T lymphocytes. B lymphocytes make antibodies, and T lymphocytes help kill tumor cells and help control immune responses. A lymphocyte is a type of white blood cell.

macrocalcification: A small deposit of calcium in the breast that cannot be felt but can be seen on a mammogram. It is usually caused by aging, an old injury, or inflamed tissue and is usually not related to cancer.

mammography: A type of X-ray examination of the breasts used for detection of cancer.

mastectomy: Partial or complete removal of the breast.

menopausal hormone therapy (MHT): Hormones (estrogen, progesterone, or both) given to women after menopause to replace the hormones no longer produced by the ovaries. Also called hormone replacement therapy and HRT.

menopause: The time of life when a woman's ovaries stop working and menstrual periods stop. Natural menopause usually occurs around age 50. A woman is said to be in menopause when she hasn't had a period for 12 months in a row.

metastatic disease: A stage of cancer after it has spread from its original site to other parts of the body.

microcalcification: A tiny deposit of calcium in the breast that cannot be felt but can be detected on a mammogram. A cluster of these very small specks of calcium may indicate that cancer is present.

mutation: Any change in the DNA of a cell. Mutations may be caused by mistakes during cell division, or they may be caused by exposure to DNA-damaging agents in the environment.

necrosis: Death of cells or tissues.

noninvasive: In cancer, it describes disease that has not spread outside the tissue in which it began. In medicine, it describes a procedure that does not require inserting an instrument through the skin or into a body opening.

perimenopausal: Describes the time in a woman's life when menstrual periods become irregular as she approaches menopause. This is usually three to five years before menopause and is often marked by many of the symptoms of menopause, including hot flashes, mood swings, night sweats, vaginal dryness, trouble concentrating, and infertility.

premalignant: A term used to describe a condition that may (or is likely to) become cancer. Also called precancerous.

premenopausal: Having to do with the time before menopause. Menopause ("change of life") is the time of life when a woman's menstrual periods stop permanently.

prosthesis: Any artificial device used to replace or represent a body part.

raloxifene: The active ingredient in a drug used to reduce the risk of invasive breast cancer in postmenopausal women who are at high risk of the disease or who have osteoporosis. It is also used to prevent and treat osteoporosis in postmenopausal women.

rupture: A hole or tear in the shell of the implant that allows silicone gel filler material to leak from the shell.

saline: Saltwater (A solution made of water and a small amount of salt).

sclerosing adenosis: A benign condition in which scar-like tissue is found in a gland, such as the breast lobules or the prostate. A biopsy may be needed to tell the difference between the abnormal tissue and cancer.

screening: Checking for disease when there are no symptoms. Since screening may find diseases at an early stage, there may be a better chance of curing the disease.

silicone: Silicone is a man-made material that can be found in several forms such as oil, gel, or rubber (elastomer). The exact composition of silicone will be different depending on its use.

sonogram: A computer picture of areas inside the body created by bouncing high-energy sound waves (ultrasound) off internal tissues or organs. Also called an ultrasonogram.

surgical biopsy: The removal of tissue by a surgeon for examination by a pathologist. The pathologist may study the tissue under a microscope.

tamoxifen: A drug used to treat certain types of breast cancer in women and men. It is also used to prevent breast cancer in women who have had ductal carcinoma in situ.

Chapter 84

Find a Breast-Cancer Screening Provider If You Are Uninsured or Underinsured

The Centers for Disease Control and Prevention's (CDC) National Breast and Cervical Cancer Early Detection Program (NBCCEDP) provides breast and cervical cancer screenings and diagnostic services to low-income, uninsured, and underinsured women across the United States.

Search for free and low-cost screenings in your state, tribe, or territory—use the interactive map (nccd.cdc.gov/dcpc_Programs/index.aspx#/1) to find local contacts for breast and cervical-cancer screening.

What Services Does the NBCCEDP Provide?

Local NBCCEDP programs offer the following services for eligible women:

- Clinical breast examinations
- Mammograms
- Papanicolaou (Pap) tests

This chapter includes text excerpted from "Find a Screening Provider Near You," Centers for Disease Control and Prevention (CDC), August 3, 2015. Reviewed February 2019.

- Pelvic examinations

- Human papillomavirus (HPV) tests

- Diagnostic testing if results are abnormal

- Referrals to treatment

Who Should Get Breast and Cervical Cancer Screenings?

All women are at risk for breast and cervical cancer, but regular screenings can prevent these diseases or find them early. The U.S. Preventive Services Task Force (USPSTF) has established the following guidelines for screening, but you should talk with your healthcare provider how often you should get screened.

- **Breast cancer:** Women between 50 and 74 years old should get a mammogram every two years. Those under 50 should talk with their provider about when they should be screened.

- **Cervical cancer:** Women should get their first Pap test at age 21 and continue screening until age 65.

Are You Eligible for Free or Low-Cost Screenings?

You may be eligible for free or low-cost screenings if you meet these qualifications:

- You are between 40 and 64 years of age for breast-cancer screening.

- You are between 21 and 64 years of age for cervical-cancer screening.

- You have no insurance, or your insurance does not cover screening exams.

- Your yearly income is at or below 250 percent of the federal poverty level.

Chapter 85

Financial Resources for People with Breast Cancer

Government Agencies That Provide Financial Assistance to People with Breast Cancer

Administration on Aging (AoA)
Toll-Free: 800-677-1116
Website: acl.gov/about-acl/administration-aging

Centers for Medicare & Medicaid Services (CMS)
Toll-Free: 877-267-2323
Website: www.cms.gov/About-CMS/Agency-Information/ContactCMS

National Breast and Cervical Cancer Early Detection Program (NBCCEDP)
Toll-Free: 800-CDC-INFO (800-232-4636)
Website: www.cdc.gov/cancer/nbccedp

U.S. Department of Health and Human Services
Toll-Free: 877-696-6775
Website: www.hhs.gov

Resources in this chapter were compiled from several sources deemed reliable; all contact information was verified and updated in February 2019.

U.S. Social Security Administration (SSA)
Toll-Free: 800-772-1213
Website: www.ssa.gov/agency/contact/phone.html

Private Agencies That Provide Financial Assistance to People with Breast Cancer

American Cancer Society (ACS)
Toll-Free: 800-227-2345
Website: www.cancer.org

The ACS offers programs for cancer patients to help pay the costs of transportation, treatment, lodging, and other expenses.

CancerCare Co-Payment Assistance Foundation
Toll-Free: 866-55-COPAY (866-552-6729)
Website: www.cancercarecopay.org

This organization offers help to those who cannot afford their insurance copayments for cancer care.

Fertile Hope
Toll-Free: 855-220-7777
Website: www.fertilehope.org

This organization provides financial help to people with cancer whose insurance will not cover fertility treatment.

NeedyMeds
Toll-Free: 800-503-6897 (Helpline)
Website: www.needymeds.org

This website collects information about patient assistance programs for medications and medical supplies sponsored by government agencies, nonprofit organizations, and pharmaceutical companies.

Partnership for Prescription Assistance (PPA)
Toll-Free: 888-4PPA-NOW (888-477-2669)
Website: www.pparx.org/wizard-help

This organization assists patients who do not have coverage for prescription medications to receive free or low-cost medications.

Patient Advocate Foundation (PAF)
Toll-Free: 800-532-5274
Website: www.patientadvocate.org

This organization assists patients with medical debt, access to insurance issues, and job retention.

Chapter 86

Directory of Organizations That Offer Information to People with Breast Cancer

Government Agencies That Provide Information about Breast Cancer

Agency for Healthcare Research and Quality (AHRQ)
Office of Communications and Knowledge Transfer
5600 Fishers Ln.
Seventh Fl.
Rockville, MD 20857
Phone: 301-427-1104
Website: www.ahrq.gov/contact/index.html

Centers for Disease Control and Prevention (CDC)
1600 Clifton Rd.
Atlanta, GA 30333
Toll-Free: 800-CDC-INFO (800-232-4636)
Phone: 404-639-3311
Toll-Free TTY: 888-232-6348
Toll-Free Fax: 800-232-4636
Website: www.cdc.gov/contact/index.htm
E-mail: CDC-INFO@cdc.gov

Resources in this chapter were compiled from several sources deemed reliable; all contact information was verified and updated in February 2019.

Federal Trade Commission (FTC)
600 Pennsylvania Ave. N.W.
Washington, DC 20580
Phone: 202-326-2222
Website: www.ftc.gov
E-mail: webmaster@ftc.gov

Healthfinder®
National Health Information
Center (NHIC)
P.O. Box 1133
Washington, DC 20013-1133
Fax: 301-984-4256
Website: www.healthfinder.gov/
NHO/FAQ.aspx
E-mail: healthfinder@hhs.gov

National Cancer Institute (NCI)
Office of Communications and
Education
9609 Medical Center Dr.
Bethesda, MD 20892-9760
Toll-Free: 800-4-CANCER
(800-422-6237)
Phone: 240-276-6600
Website: www.cancer.gov/contact
E-mail: nciocpl@mail.nih.gov

National Center for Complementary and Integrative Health (NCCIH)
NCCIH Clearinghouse
P.O. Box 7923
Gaithersburg, MD 20898-7923
Toll-Free: 888-644-6226
Toll-Free TTY: 866-464-3615
Toll-Free Fax: 866-464-3616
Website: nccih.nih.gov/about/
offices/ocpl
E-mail: info@nccam.nih.gov

National Center for Health Statistics (NCHS)
3311 Toledo Rd.
Rm. 2217
Hyattsville, MD 20782-2064
Toll-Free: 800-CDC-INFO
(800-232-4636)
Phone: 301-458-4901
Toll-Free Fax: 800-232-4636
Website: www.cdc.gov/nchs/nhis/
contact.htm
E-mail: CDC-INFO@cdc.gov

National Institute on Aging (NIA)
Bldg. 31, Rm. 5C27
31 Center Dr. MSC 2292
Bethesda, MD 20892
Toll-Free: 800-222-2225
Phone: 301-496-1752
Toll-Free TTY: 800-222-4225
Fax: 301-496-1072
Website: www.nia.nih.gov/
contact
E-mail: niaic@nia.nih.gov

National Institutes of Health (NIH)
9000 Rockville Pike
Bethesda, MD 20892
Phone: 301-496-4000
TTY: 301-402-9612
Website: www.nih.gov/about-nih/
contact-us
E-mail: NIHinfo@od.nih.gov

National Women's Health Information Center
Office on Women's Health (OWH)
200 Independence Ave. S.W.
Rm. 712 E.
Washington, DC 20201
Toll-Free: 800-994-9662
Phone: 202-690-7650
Toll-Free TDD: 888-220-5446
Fax: 202-205-2631
Website: www.womenshealth.
gov/contact-us

Sister Study
Toll-Free: 877-4SISTER
(877-474-7837)
Toll-Free TTY: 866-TTY-4SIS
(866-889-4747)
Toll-Free Fax: 866-889-4747
Website: sisterstudy.niehs.nih.
gov/English/contact.aspx
E-mail: postmaster@sisterstudy.
org

U.S. Department of Health and Human Services (HHS)
200 Independence Ave. S.W.
Washington, DC 20201
Toll-Free: 877-696-6775
Website: www.hhs.gov

U.S. Food and Drug Administration (FDA)
10903 New Hampshire Ave.
Silver Spring, MD 20993
Toll-Free: 888-INFO-FDA
(888-463-6332)
Website: www.fda.gov

U.S. National Library of Medicine (NLM)
8600 Rockville Pike
Bethesda, MD 20894
Toll-Free: 888-FIND-NLM
(888-346-3656)
Phone: 301-594-5983
Toll-Free TDD: 800-735-2258
Fax: 301-402-1384
Website: www.nlm.nih.gov
E-mail: custserv@nlm.nih.gov

Private Agencies That Provide Information about Breast Cancer

African American Breast Cancer Alliance (AABCA)
P.O. Box 8981
Minneapolis, MN 55408
Toll-Free: 800-422-6237
Phone: 612-462-6813
Fax: 612-827-2422
Website: www.aabcainc.org
E-mail: info@aabcainc.org

After Breast Cancer Diagnosis (ABCD)
5775 N. Glen Park Rd.
Ste. 201
Glendale, WI 53209
Toll-Free: 800-977-4121
Phone: 414-977-1780
Fax: 414-977-1781
Website: www.
abcdbreastcancersupport.org
E-mail: abcdinc@abcdmentor.org

American Association for Clinical Chemistry (AACC)
Lab Tests Online
900 Seventh St. N.W.
Ste. 400
Washington, DC 20001
Toll-Free: 800-892-1400
Phone: 1202-857-0717
Fax: 202-887-5093
Website: www.labtestsonline.org
Email: 2labtestsonline@aacc.org

American Cancer Society (ACS)
250 Williams St. N.W.
Atlanta, GA 30303
Toll-Free: 800-227-2345
Toll-Free TTY: 866-228-4327
Website: www.cancer.org

American College of Radiology (ACR)
1891 Preston White Dr.
Reston, VA 20191
Toll-Free: 800-227-5463
Phone: 703-648-8900
Website: www.acr.org
E-mail: info@acr.org

American Institute for Cancer Research (AICR)
1560 Wilson Blvd.
Ste. 1000
Arlington, VA 22209
Toll-Free: 800-843-8114
Phone: 202-328-7744
Fax: 202-328-7226
Website: www.aicr.org
E-mail: aicrweb@aicr.org

American Medical Association (AMA)
515 N. State St.
Chicago, IL 60654
Toll-Free: 800-621-8335
Phone: 312-123-4567
Fax: 312-123-7890
Website: www.ama-assn.org

American Society for Clinical Oncology (ASCO)
2318 Mill Rd. Ste. 800
Alexandria, VA 22314
Toll-Free: 888-651-3038
Phone: 571-483-1780
Fax: 571-366-9537
Website: www.cancer.net
E-mail: contactus@cancer.net

American Society for Radiation Oncology (ASTRO)
251 18th St. S.
Eighth Fl.
Arlington, VA 22202
Toll-Free: 800-962-7876
Phone: 703-502-1550
Fax: 703-502-7852
Website: www.astro.org

American Society of Plastic Surgeons (ASPS)
444 E. Algonquin Rd.
Arlington Heights, IL 60005
Phone: 847-228-9900
Website: www.plasticsurgery.org
E-mail: memserv@
plasticsurgery.org

Avon Foundation for Women
1 Avon Plaza, Suffern.
New York, NY 10901
Toll-Free: 800-FOR-AVON
(800-445-2866)
Phone: 212-282-5320
Website: www.avonfoundation.org
E-mail: info@avonfoundation.org

Breast Cancer Care
Chester House 1–3 Brixton Rd.
London, SW9 6DE, UK
Toll-Free: 808-800-6000
Phone: 345-092-0800
Website: www.breastcancercare.
org.uk
E-mail: info@breastcancercare.
org.uk

Breast Cancer Research Foundation (BCRF)
28 W. 44th St.
Ste. 609
New York, NY 10022
Toll-Free: 866-FIND-A-CURE
(866-346-3228)
Phone: 646-497-2600
Fax: 646-497-0890
Website: www.bcrfcure.org
E-mail: bcrf@bcrfcure.org

BreastCancerTrials.org
3450 California St.
San Francisco, CA 94118
Phone: 415-476-5777
Website: www.
breastcancertrials.org
E-mail: info@
BreastCancerTrials.org

Breastcancer.org
120 E Lancaster Ave.
Ste. 201
Ardmore, PA 19003
Phone: 610-642-6550
Website: www.breastcancer.org

Cancer and Careers, CEW Foundation
159 W. 25th St.
Eighth Fl.
New York, NY 10001
Phone: 646-929-8032
Fax: 212-685-3334
Website: www.cancerandcareers.
org
E-mail: cancerandcareers@cew.
org

Cancer Support Community
734 15th St. N.W.
Ste. 300
Washington, DC 20005
Toll-Free: 888-793-9355
Phone: 202-659-9709
Fax: 202-974-7999
Website: www.
cancersupportcommunity.org
E-mail: help@
cancersupportcommunity.org

CancerCare
275 Seventh Ave.
New York, NY 10001
Toll-Free: 800-813-HOPE
(800-813-4673)
Phone: 212-712-8400
Fax: 212-712-8495
Website: www.cancercare.org
E-mail: info@cancercare.org

Caring.com
2600 S. El Camino Real
Ste. 300
San Mateo, CA 94403
Toll-Free: 800-973-1540
Phone: 650-312-7100
Website: www.caring.com
E-mail: directory-operations@
caring.com

Cleveland Clinic
9500 Euclid Ave.
Cleveland, OH 44195
Toll-Free: 800-223-2273;
Phone: 216-636-5860 (Info Line)
TTY: 216-444-0261
Website: www.
my.clevelandclinic.org

College of American Pathologists
325 Waukegan Rd.
Northfield, IL 60093-2750
Toll-Free: 800-323-4040
Phone: 847-832-7000
Fax: 847-832-8000
Website: www.cap.org

Facing Our Risk of Cancer Empowered (FORCE)
16057 Tampa Palms Blvd. W.
PMB Ste. 373
Tampa, FL 33647
Toll-Free: 866-288-RISK (866-288-7475); 866-824-RISK (866-824-7475)
Fax: 954-827-2200
Website: www.facingourrisk.org/
about-us/about/contact-force.php
E-mail: info@facingourrisk.org

Family Caregiver Alliance (FCA)
101 Montgomery St.
Ste. 2150
San Francisco, CA 94104
Toll-Free: 800-445-8106
Phone: 415-434-3388
Website: www.caregiver.org
E-mail: info@caregiver.org

Imaginis
25 E. Ct. St.
Ste. 301
Greenville, SC 29601
Phone: 864-209-1139
Website: www.
imaginis.com/about/
imaginis-contact-information
E-mail: learnmore@imaginis.com

Inflammatory Breast Cancer (IBC) Research Foundation
P.O. Box 2805
W Lafayette, IN 47996
Toll-Free: 877-STOP-IBC
(877-786-7422)
Website: www.ibcresearch.org
E-mail: information@mail.
ibcresearch.org

Living Beyond Breast Cancer
40 Monument Rd.
Ste. 104
Bala Cynwyd, PA 19004
Toll-Free: 855-807-6386
Phone: 610-645-4567
Fax: 610-645-4573
Website: www.lbbc.org/
about-lbbc/contact-us
E-mail: mail@lbbc.org

Men Against Breast Cancer
P.O. Box 150
Adamstown, MD 21710-0150
Toll-Free: 866-547-MABC
(866-547-6222)
Fax: 301-874-8657
Website: www.
menagainstbreastcancer.org
E-mail: info@
menagainstbreastcancer.org

**Metastatic Breast Cancer
Network (MBCN)**
P.O. Box 1449
New York, NY 10159
Toll-Free: 888-500-0370
Website: www.mbcnetwork.org
E-mail: mbcn@mbcn.org

**Mothers Supporting
Daughters with Breast
Cancer (MSDBC)**
25235 Fox Chase Dr.
Chestertown, MD 21620
Phone: 410-778-1982
Fax: 410-778-1411
Website: www.
mothersdaughters.org
E-mail: msdbc@verizon.net

**National Breast Cancer
Coalition (NBCC)**
1010 Vermont Ave. N.W.
Ste. 900
Washington, DC 20005
Toll-Free: 800-622-2838
Phone: 202-296-7477
Fax: 202-265-6854
Website: www.
breastcancerdeadline2020.org
E-mail: info@
breastcancerdeadline2020.org

**National Breast Cancer
Foundation, Inc. (NBCF)**
2600 Network Blvd.
Ste. 300
Frisco, TX 75034
Website: www.
nationalbreastcancer.org

**National Coalition for
Cancer Survivorship (NCCS)**
8455 Colesville Rd.
Ste. 930
Silver Spring, MD 20910
Toll-Free: 877-NCCS-YES
(877-622-7937)
Phone: 301-650-9127
Website: www.canceradvocacy.
org
E-mail: info@canceradvocacy.org

**National Comprehensive
Cancer Network (NCCN)**
3025 Chemical Rd.
Ste. 100
Plymouth Meeting, PA 19462
Phone: 215-690-0300
Fax: 215-690-0280
Website: www.nccn.org

**National Hospice and
Palliative Care Organization
(NHPCO)**
1731 King St.
Ste. 100
Alexandria, VA 22314
Toll-Free: 800-658-8898
Phone: 703-837-1500
Fax: 703-837-1233
Website: www.nhpco.org
E-mail: nhpco_info@nhpco.org

National Lymphedema Network (NLN)
411 Lafayette St.
Sixth Fl.
New York, NY 10003
Toll-Free: 800-541-3259
Phone: 646-722-7410
Fax: 415-908-3813
Website: www.lymphnet.org
E-mail: nln@lymphnet.org

National Society of Genetic Counselors (NSGC)
330 N. Wabash Ave.
Ste. 2000
Chicago, IL 60611
Phone: 312-321-6834
Website: www.nsgc.org
E-mail: nsgc@nsgc.org

OncoLink The Perelman Center for Advanced Medicine
3400 Civic Center Blvd.
Ste. 2338
Philadelphia, PA 19104
Phone: 215-349-8895
Fax: 215-349-5445
Website: www.oncolink.org
E-mail: hampshire@uphs.upenn.edu

SHARE: Self Help for Women with Breast or Ovarian Cancer
165 W. 46th St.
Ste. 712
New York, NY 10036
844-ASK-SHARE (844-275-7427)
Phone: 212-719-0364
Website: www.sharecancersupport.org
E-mail: info@sharecancersupport.org

Sharsheret: Your Jewish Community Facing Breast Cancer
1086 Teaneck Rd.
Ste. 2G
Teaneck, NJ 07666
Toll-Free: 866-474-2774
Phone: 201-833-2341
Fax: 201-837-5025
Website: www.sharsheret.org
E-mail: info@sharsheret.org

Sisters Network Inc.
9668 Westheimer Rd.
Ste. 200-132
Houston, TX 77063
Toll-Free: 866-781-1808
Phone: 713-781-0255
Fax: 713-780-8998
Website: www.sistersnetworkinc.org
E-mail: infonet@sistersnetworkinc.org

Society of Interventional Radiology (SIR)
3975 Fair Ridge Dr.
Ste. 400 N.
Fairfax, VA 22033
Toll-Free: 800-488-7284
Phone: 703-691-1805
Fax: 703-691-1855
Website: www.sirweb.org

Society of Nuclear Medicine
1850 Samuel Morse Dr.
Reston, VA 20190
Phone: 703-708-9000
Fax: 703-708-9015
Website: www.snm.org
E-mail: feedback@snm.org

Susan G. Komen for the Cure
5005 LBJ Fwy
Ste. 526
Dallas, TX 75244
Toll-Free: 877-GO-KOMEN
(877-465-6636)
Fax: 972-855-4301
Website: ww5.komen.org/
AboutUs/PrivacyPolicy.html
E-mail: helpline@komen.org

Tigerlily Foundation
42020 Village Center Plaza
Ste. 120-156
Stone Ridge, VA 20105
Toll-Free: 888-580-6253
Fax: 703-663-9844
Website: www.
tigerlilyfoundation.org
E-mail: info@tigerlilyfoundation.
org

Triple Negative Breast Cancer Foundation
P.O. Box 204
Norwood, NJ 07648
Toll-Free: 877-880-8622
Phone: 646-942-0242
Website: www.tnbcfoundation.
org
E-mail: info@tnbcfoundation.org

Well Spouse Foundation
63 W. Main St.
Ste. H
Freehold, NJ 07728
Toll-Free: 800-838-0879
Phone: 732-577-8899
Fax: 732-577-8644
Website: www.wellspouse.org
E-mail: info@wellspouse.org

Young Survival Coalition (YSC)
75 Broad St.
Ste. 409
New York, NY 10004
Toll-Free: 877-972-1011
Fax: 646-257-3030
Website: www.youngsurvival.org

Index

Index

589